D1060849

Atlas of Ultrasound and Nerve Stimulation-Guided Regional Anesthesia

Ban C.H. Tsui, Dip Eng, B. Sc(Math),
B. Pharm, MD, MSc, FRCPC

Atlas of Ultrasound and Nerve Stimulation-Guided Regional Anesthesia

Consulting Editors
Vincent W.S. Chan, MD, FRCPC
Brendan T. Finucane, MB, BCh, BAO, FRCAC, FRCPC
Thomas Grau, MD, PhD
Anil H. Walji, MD, PhD

Contributing Authors
Ravi Bhargava, MD, FRCPC
Derek Dillane, MB, BCh, BAO, MMedSci, FFARCSI
Sugantha Ganapathy, MD, FRCPC
Lawrence Lou, MD
Michelle Noga, MD, FRCPC

Illustrations by Carol T.S. Chan

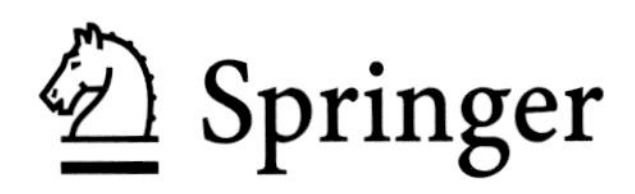

Ban C.H. Tsui, Dip Eng, B. Sc(Math), B. Pharm, MD, MSc, FRCPC
Chair, Regional Anesthesia and Acute Pain Section, Canadian Anesthesiologists' Society, Canada, *and* Pediatric and Adult Anesthesiologist, Associate Professor/Director of Clinical Research, Department of Anesthesiology and Pain Medicine, Stollery Children's Hospital/University of Alberta Hospital, Edmonton, Alberta, Canada

Consulting Editors:
Vincent W.S. Chan, MD, FRCPC (Upper and Lower Extremities)
Professor, Department of Anesthesia, University of Toronto, *and* Head of Regional Anesthesia and Pain Program, Department of Anesthesia and Pain Management, University Health Network Toronto, Ontario, Canada

Brendan T. Finucane, MB, BCh, BAO, FRCAC, FRCPC (Regional Approaches)
Professor, Department of Anesthesiology and Pain Medicine, University of Alberta Hospital, Edmonton, Alberta, Canada

Thomas Grau, MD, PhD (Central Neuraxial)
Consultant, Clinic of Anesthesiology, Intensive Care, Palliative Medicine and Pain Therapy, BG-University Hospital, Bergmannsheil, Ruhr University, Bochum, Germany

Anil H. Walji, MD, PhD (Anatomy)
Professor and Head, Division of Anatomy, Professor of Surgery, Professor of Radiology and Diagnostic Imaging, Faculty of Medicine and Dentistry, University of Alberta, Edmonton, Alberta, Canada

Library of Congress Control Number: 2006940908

ISBN: 978-0-387-68158-0 e-ISBN: 978-0-387-68159-7

Printed on acid-free paper.

9 8 7 6 5 4

springer.com

To my wife, Eliza, and my children, Jenkin and Jeremy—the real loves of my life. Without their support and understanding, I could not have completed this demanding project.

I would also like to dedicate this opus to my parents, Woon-Tak and Kau-Wan, for their love and guidance throughout my life.

Foreword

When Ban Tsui asked me to consider authoring a foreword to the *Atlas of Ultrasound Nerve Stimulation-Guided Regional Anesthesia*, I was excited because it gave me the opportunity to read the work prior to publication. The excitement stems from my knowledge of Dr. Tsui's work ethic, creativity, and knowledge of regional anesthesia.

It has been my privilege to follow Ban's career since Brendan Finucane and colleagues at the University of Alberta-Edmonton nurtured his training some years ago. Also, during my time as Editor of *Regional Anesthesia and Pain Medicine*, Dr. Tsui was a frequent contributor to our journal of soundly based research.

Upon receipt of the advance copy of this atlas I read with interest the rationale for this addition to our regional anesthesia references. The focus on nerve stimulation and ultrasound use in regional anesthesia is an area in need of wider understanding, and it is my belief that this work will help all who read it progress in both areas of regional practice. A number of us concluded some years ago that our subspecialty of regional anesthesia needed an increased focus on use of imaging in the subspecialty. It was at the turn of the Millennium that a section on imaging was added to the journal, *Regional Anesthesia and Pain Medicine*. Our idea was not unique; it was simply recognition that almost all the contemporary specialty advances across medicine as a profession made in late 1980s and 1990s were based on advances in imaging.

This atlas focuses on combining an understanding of nerve stimulation and ultrasound guidance in regional anesthesia. It is my opinion that the authors have performed their work effectively. They highlight over and over the need to keep anatomy at the center of any use of regional anesthesia. I could not agree more with that age-old, sage advice. Though not explicitly shared in this work, I continue to believe that an important element of successful use of regional anesthesia in day-to-day practice is to limit the complexity of the techniques. One caution to readers of this work is to seek to simplify rather than make complex your techniques. One way the authors have helped in this work is by placing a number of sections of *clinical pearls* at important areas of the text. Also, the authors have taken a wise course by not choosing the ideal or perfect image for their illustrations, but rather, images found in day-to-day clinical practice. This will allow an easier transition for novices in taking these techniques effectively into their own practices.

Throughout the later portions of my career I have been a vocal advocate of adding ultrasound techniques to our practices. This is primarily because of my combined interest in imaging and supraclavicular nerve block. It is my belief that with the maturation of ultrasound within the subspecialty of regional anesthesia, the technique of supraclavicular block may become the most common brachial technique for single injection blocks because of the combination of favorable anatomy and ultrasound imaging at that site. This atlas should help all of us make this a reality. This leads to the observation that most will find the use of these techniques helpful in improving peripheral nerve block techniques, in spite of the inclusion of work on neuraxial blocks guided by ultrasound. If you only have the energy to change your practice in one of those two areas, I encourage maturation of your peripheral nerve block techniques.

My only concern with this very clear advance in understanding regional anesthesia is that all of us maintain our focus first and foremost on our patients. Our gentle and yet confident hand on our patients receiving the regional technique is still the most important part of regional block. None of them should go through a regional block and be unwilling to go through the experience again. Once fully developed and used widely it is my belief that the adjunct of ultrasound should allow even more effective matching of sedation and anatomy, thus, allowing an increased willingness by patients to accept regional anesthesia for their anesthetic.

It is a privilege to author this preface and recommend the work to anyone interested in their patients and regional anesthesia.

David L. Brown, MD
Edward Rotan Distinguished Professor and Chairman
Department of Anesthesiology and Pain Medicine
UT-M. D. Anderson Cancer Center

Preface

Regional anesthesia has been long regarded as an "art" and success with these techniques appears to be confined to a small number of gifted individuals. The introduction of nerve stimulation some 30 years ago was the first step towards transforming regional anesthesia into a "science." However, nerve stimulation also has its limitations. This technique relies on physiological responses of neural structures to electrical impulses. There is considerable inter-individual variation in physiological responses to nerve stimulation. Furthermore a number of other factors influence response to nerve stimulation including injectates, physiologic solutions (e.g. blood) and disease. Despite these limitations nerve stimulation was one of the first objective methods available in regional anesthesia to place, with some reliability, a needle in close proximity to a target nerve. The introduction of nerve stimulation techniques into regional anesthesia surprisingly did not result in a renewed interest in regional anesthesia. However it was a considerable boost to those of us who were already drawn to this most interesting pursuit.

One of the most exciting advances in technology in relation to regional anesthesia in recent years has been the introduction of anatomically-based ultrasound imaging. This is the first time in close to 100 years of regional anesthesia that we can actually see an image of the nerve we would like to block. This is a quantum leap in technology for those interested in this pursuit and is sure to draw a huge number of anesthesiologists back towards regional anesthesia. However let us not forget that despite the initial excitement over this advancement, ultrasound visualization is still indirect and images are subject to individual interpretation depending on one's experiences and training and where that training and experience was obtained. Some individuals are gifted in their ability to interpret ultrasound images, however this is not the case with the majority. There is an extensive learning curve associated with ultrasound-guided regional anesthesia. To my knowledge, there is no existing textbook and/or atlas devoted entirely to ultrasound-guided regional blockade. In addition, I believe that we should not immediately abandon nerve stimulation techniques in favor of ultrasound-guided regional anesthesia. Instead I would like to suggest that we should combine the two technologies to further enhance our goal of 100% success with all of our blocks. We have already outlined some of the disadvantages of neurostimulation. Ultrasound-guided regional anesthesia is not without its flaws either. We can never be totally sure of the identity of the nerve that we are imaging, however by stimulating that nerve we can objectively determine its identity by the motor response to nerve stimulation. This atlas outlines the advantages of both technologies and I believe is the first attempt to do so.

The main objective of this book is to enable anesthesiologists who are beginning to use ultrasound-guided regional anesthesia to shorten their learning curve. For those anesthesiologists already experienced in ultrasound guidance during regional anesthesia, hopefully this atlas will further add to their knowledge in this field. Hopefully we will convince some of our readers not to hastily abandon nerve stimulation, but instead to combine it with ultrasound-guided regional anesthesia. Our ultimate goal in publishing this book is to advance knowledge in regional anesthesia and in doing so our patients will be the beneficiaries.

The central theme of this book is anatomy. Knowledge of anatomy is the backbone of regional anesthesia. Labat, the father of regional anesthesia, made the following statement about this discipline: "Anatomy is the foundation upon which the entire concept of regional anesthesia is built. Anyone who wishes to be an expert in the art of regional anesthesia must be thoroughly grounded in anatomy." It is difficult to perform ultrasound-guided regional anesthesia or nerve stimulation without some knowledge of anatomy. This atlas is generously adorned with anatomic drawings, ultrasound images, MRI images, and information about optimal use of nerve stimulation in regional anesthesia.

The book layout is consistent throughout. In the clinical chapters, there is an initial description of relevant anatomy with illustrations from cadaver dissections and corresponding MRI and ultrasound images capturing the block location. This is followed by a clinical description of how to perform ultrasound imaging during regional block. These sections describe and illustrate the positioning of the probe, the specific needling technique used, how to use nerve stimulation, and pre- and post-local anesthetic application. I believe this sequential format gives the reader a realistic simulation of the management of each clinical situation.

The images used in this book are those from our everyday practice and are achievable by any newcomer to ultrasound for regional anesthesia. We have been mindful not to concentrate on anatomically perfect ultrasound images, occasionally obtained, but on those images which are representative of what you will encounter in an average day.

Ultrasound-guided regional anesthesia is an emerging field and the literature is replete with new ideas about how to best apply this new technology. In this book, we focus on the most common approaches used and supplement these by including alternative approaches in clinical pearls and notes, as described in the literature or by the consulting editors. This way the reader can select the most suitable approach for his/her own needs.

The book starts out with brief but relevant sections providing information on both ultrasound and nerve stimulation. Equipment and setup are also discussed. Chapter 4 is perhaps the most important, including many practical ideas and approaches for performance and training of ultrasound and nerve stimulation guidance during regional blockade. For this book, all the cadaver dissections were performed under ultrasound guidance in a similar fashion to performing ultrasound-guided regional block. In other words, the structures were first localized with ultrasound and followed by "minimally invasive dissection." The dissected area was preserved with minimal distortion of the normal anatomical relationships while clearly showing the targeted nerve (i.e., direct visualization).

To further illustrate the important neuroanatomy and its relation to other anatomical structures and also to provide a realistic perspective from living persons (i.e., Dr. Finucane and myself), MRI images were captured using scanning angles similar to typical ultrasound planes for specific regional anesthesia approaches. In addition, practical schematic drawings with simplified relevant anatomy are also included to enable easy, yet comprehensive, understanding of the anatomical relationships between nerves and of the nerves relative to their surroundings.

In order to maximize recognition and identification of the structures within the ultrasonographic images, unlabelled ultrasound images (both general and during clinical procedures) are placed next to identical but well labeled images. The reader should find these figures useful learning aids, as do my residents and colleagues. They have found this layout to be most effective for familiarizing themselves with the realistic clinical images as there is no distraction from multiple labels, yet at the same time they benefit from side-by-side reference to the same image, with labeling. Furthermore, as anatomical structures are not the only relevant items to localize with ultrasound, practical ways to insert, view and control placement of the needle within the tissues are incorporated throughout the text.

In terms of nerve stimulation, a new understanding of the relevant physics of electrical stimulation is discussed. For clinical integration, readers should find the trouble-shooting tables in the nerve stimulation sections useful to help adjust needle placement in response to motor responses they may observe during needle insertion.

In preparing this book, I had the privilege of gathering close friends and colleagues as consulting editors and contributing authors. They are all highly respected experts internationally in their relevant fields. I had the opportunity to have my friend and colleague, Dr. Chan, professor at University of Toronto and current treasurer of the American Society of Regional Anesthesia, as consulting editor for the upper and lower limb sections. Dr. Chan is one of the forefront leaders in promoting ultrasound use for regional anesthesia in both Canada and the United States and indeed worldwide. Dr. Grau, a renowned colleague from Germany agreed to act as a consulting editor for the central neuraxial anesthesia portions. Dr. Grau, consultant anesthesiologist at BG-University Hospital, is one of the pioneers in introducing ultrasound use for central neuraxial blockade. It was a great honor to invite my colleague at the University of Alberta, Dr. Walji, as a consulting editor to ensure accuracy in the relevant anatomy as described in the atlas. Dr. Walji is a well known professor from the University of Alberta's Faculty of Medicine and Dentistry and was recently an editor of the latest edition of the renowned *Netter's Anatomy* atlas. I had the great pleasure to consult with Dr. Finucane, who is the past president of the American Society of Regional Anesthesia, the editor of two textbooks on regional anesthesia, the former department chair for Anesthesiology and Pain Medicine at the University of Alberta (where he still resides) and my mentor. I am forever indebted to Dr. Finucane for his continuous support and encouragement throughout my career and for introducing me to the challenges of regional anesthesia when I was his resident. Dr. Ganapathy from University of Western Ontario, a well-known Canadian regional anesthesia expert, was also kind enough to contribute an important chapter addressing ultrasound use in placing continuous catheters. My current fellow Dr. Dillane worked diligently on this project and inspired me to work together with him to create a chapter summarizing the practical tips from both the learner and trainer perspective in order to facilitate shorter learning curves in ultrasound guidance. My colleagues from the Diagnostic Imaging and Radiology department at the University of Alberta, Drs. Noga, Lou, and Bhargava, helped by facilitating me with obtaining MRI images as well as by contributing towards a basic ultrasound chapter. I also greatly appreciate Drs. Chan, Grau, and Ganapathy for sharing some of their clinical images in addition to their expert contributions, as well as Dr. Walji and the Division of Anatomy at the University of Alberta for providing assistance and facilitating me with the cadaver dissections. Last but not least, my niece, Carol Chan, a nursing student of University of Alberta, used her fine artistic talent to provide practical and meaningful medical illustrations to incorporate throughout the book.

In summary, anesthesiologists may encounter considerable difficulty identifying neural structures when learning ultrasound techniques and this may lead to frustration and failure, both of which deter anesthesiologists from adopting this technology. The concepts incorporated in this book collectively provide many reliable ways to become proficient at identifying neural structures prior to performing regional anesthesia. Throughout the book, dynamic and systematic scanning is emphasized. Instead of attempting to identify the target nerve as the initial step in performing ultrasound-assisted regional anesthesia, we strongly recommend first identifying obvious landmarks (usually blood vessels) in the vicinity of the target nerve, subsequently shifting the view to the corresponding neural structures, and tracing back along this neural structure to the specific target block location. More important, Labat's advice about the importance of anatomy is still as true today as it was some 90 odd years ago. So hold on to your anatomy books and continue to visit the dissecting rooms. Knowledge of anatomy is still the essence of regional anesthesia regardless of the advances in this field.

Ban C.H. Tsui, Dip Eng, B. Sc(Math), B. Pharm, MD, MSc, FRCPC
University of Alberta Hospital
Edmonton, Alberta, Canada
2007

Acknowledgments

I wish to acknowledge the following individuals for their support, hard work, and contributions in preparing this book. My research coordinator Jennifer Pillay, BSc, spent many extra hours and worked diligently to contribute towards and assemble the material contained in this book. Her initial drafts of many chapters and continual assistance with editing helped organize and expedite my and my colleagues' writing and editing process. Al-Karim Ramji, BSc, is a medical student who assisted with the dissections as well as organizing and labeling of the images. My department chair, Barry Finegan, provides ongoing support and encouragement. Dr. Lambert, Chair, Department of Diagnostic Imaging and Radiology, University of Alberta and Capital Health Authority, Edmonton, facilitated my access to the institution's MRI technology and operators. Staff members from the University of Alberta Hospital, the Stollery Children's Hospital and the University of Alberta always provide an excellent environment for patient care, teaching, and research that has directly facilitated the advancement of clinical practice of regional anesthesia. An investigator grant from the Alberta Heritage Foundation for Medical Research allowed me to pursue this project by helping to support my academic work. The unrestricted grant from Springer to start this project was a financial help and support, and Stacy Hague, editor, and the Springer staff are greatly appreciated for providing their expertise for this book project. The portable ultrasound machine (MicroMaxx) used for the images in this book was kindly provided by SonoSite, Inc. (Bothell, USA).

Ban C.H. Tsui, Dip Eng, B. Sc(Math), B. Pharm, MD, MSC, FRCPC
University of Alberta Hospital
Edmonton, Alberta, Canada
2007

Contents

Contributors

Ravi Bhargava, MD, FRCPC
Associate Professor, Department of Radiology and Diagnostic Imaging, University of Alberta, Edmonton, Alberta, Canada

Vincent W.S. Chan, MD, FRCPC
Professor, Department of Anesthesia, University of Toronto, *and* Head of Regional Anesthesia and Pain Program, Department of Anesthesia and Pain Management, University Health Network, Toronto, Ontario, Canada

Derek Dillane, MB, BCh, BAO, MMedSci, FFARCSI
Regional Anesthesia Clinical Fellow, Department of Anesthesiology and Pain Medicine, University of Alberta Hospital, Edmonton, Alberta, Canada

Brendan T. Finucane, MB, BCh, BAO, FRCAC, FRCPC
Professor, Department of Anesthesiology and Pain Medicine, University of Alberta Hospital, Edmonton, Alberta, Canada

Sugantha Ganapathy, MD, FRCPC
Professor, Director of Regional Anesthesia, Department of Anesthesia and Perioperative Medicine, University of Western Ontario, London, Ontario, Canada

Thomas Grau, MD, PhD
Consultant, Clinic of Anesthesiology, Intensive Care, Palliative Medicine and Pain Therapy, BG-University Hospital, Bergmannsheil, Ruhr University, Bochum, Germany

Lawrence Lou, MD
Radiology Resident, Department of Radiology and Diagnostic Imaging, University of Alberta, Edmonton, Alberta, Canada

Michelle Noga, MD, FRCPC
Assistant Professor, Department of Radiology and Diagnostic Imaging, University of Alberta, Edmonton, Alberta, Canada

Ban C.H. Tsui, Dip Eng, B. Sc(Math), B. Pharm, MD, MSc, FRCPC
Chair, Regional Anesthesia and Acute Pain Section, Canadian Anesthesiologists' Society, Canada, *and* Pediatric and Adult Anesthesiologist, Associate Professor/Director of Clinical Research, Department of Anesthesiology and Pain Medicine, Stollery Children's Hospital/ University of Alberta Hospital, Edmonton, Alberta, Canada

Anil H. Walji, MD, PhD
Professor and Head, Division of Anatomy, Professor of Surgery, Professor of Radiology and Diagnostic Imaging, Faculty of Medicine and Dentistry, University of Alberta, Edmonton, Alberta, Canada

1

Regional Block Room Setup and Equipment

Ban C.H. Tsui

1.1. Introduction

Enormous advances have been made in the discipline of anesthesiology in the last 50 years. With these advances we have seen huge changes in supportive technology. Our anesthesia machines and monitoring equipment bear no resemblance to what was available 50 years ago. This explosion in technology also involves regional anesthesia. Following is a brief overview of the equipment available for use when performing peripheral nerve blocks.

1.2. Equipment and Monitoring

Efficient, reliable, and safe regional anesthesia requires meticulous attention to equipment and patient monitoring. Although regional blocks can be performed in the operating room setting just like general anesthesia, it is preferable and desirable to perform regional anesthesia in a designated area outside the operating room environment (Figure 1.1). This requirement was recognized very early by a former master of regional anesthesia, Gaston Labat, who once wrote "regional anesthesia should be induced in a room immediately

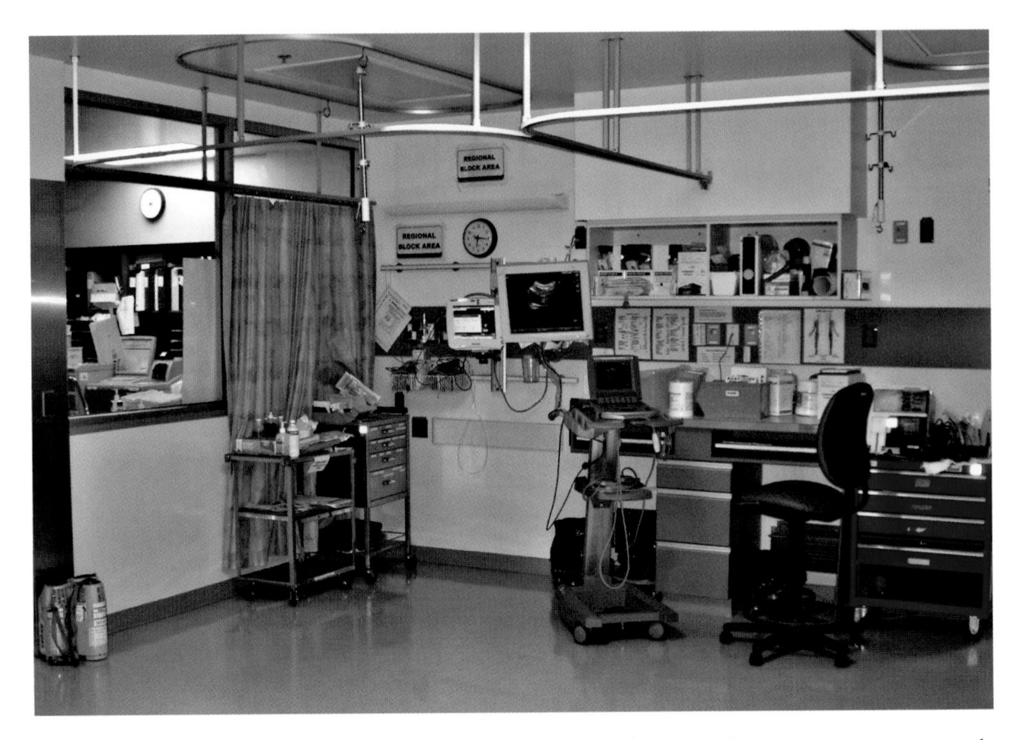

Figure 1.1. Designated regional block room adjacent to surgical suites with necessary equipment and a large ultrasound monitor.

adjoining the operating room if possible." (Adriani J, 1985, p. 14) The reason for this is that it requires a variable time for regional anesthesia to work. This is commonly referred to as *soak time*, which is the time it takes for local anesthetics to cross the cell membrane and block action potentials. This designated area must contain the necessary equipment for safe monitoring and resuscitation, but in addition the area must contain all of the supplies and equipment needed to perform common and sophisticated regional techniques. The following are the relevant requirements for block room setup and patient monitoring.

1.2.1. Block Room Setup

- A designated area for performing regional blocks, preferably adjacent to the surgical suite, is desirable.
- All supplies located in this area must be readily identifiable and accessible to the anesthesiologist.
- The area should be of ample size to allow both monitoring and resuscitation of patients.
- The block room should have the necessary equipment for oxygen delivery, emergency airway management and suction, and should have sufficient lighting.

1.2.2. Equipment Storage Cart

- The equipment storage cart (Figure 1.2) should be practically organized and include necessary equipment (including that required for emergency procedures), supplies, local anesthetics, nerve stimulators, and resuscitation drugs.
- A prepared specialty tray should include items for sterile skin preparation and draping, a marking pen and ruler for landmark identification, needles and syringes for skin infiltration, and specific block needles/catheters.
- A selection of sedatives, hypnotics, and intravenous anesthetics should be immediately available to prepare patients for regional anesthesia. These drugs should be titrated to

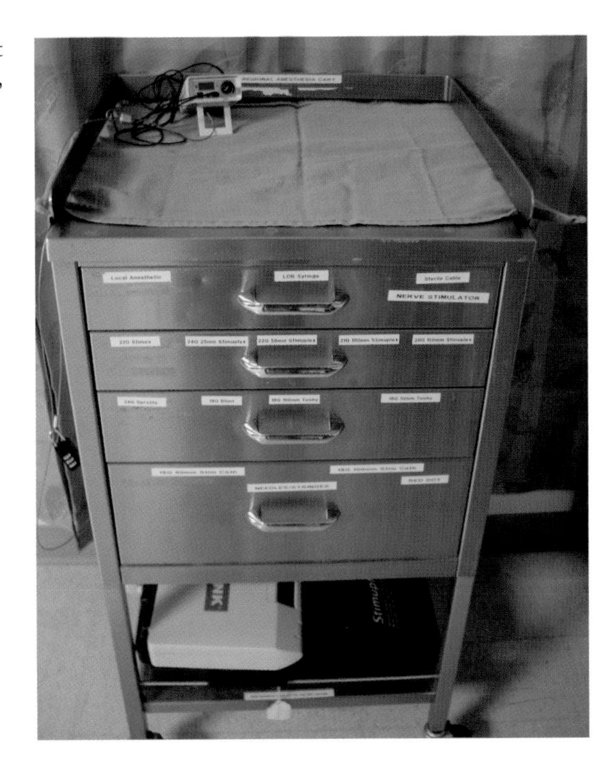

Figure 1.2. Equipment storage cart with clear identification of equipment, supplies, and medication.

maximize benefits and minimize adverse effects (High Therapeutic Index); short-acting drugs with a high safety margin are desirable.
  - Examples include propofol, midazolam, fentanyl, remifentanil, alfentanil, or a combination of the above (see Chapter 4 for specifics).

1.2.2.1. *Emergency Drugs and Equipment*

- The equipment storage cart should include emergency airway devices/equipment, for example, laryngoscopic equipment (scalpels, blades, endotracheal tubes, airways), ventilation devices, and oxygen masks.
  - Emergency drugs should include atropine, epinephrine, phenylephrine, ephedrine, propofol, thiopentone and succinylcholine, amrinone, and intralipid.

1.2.3. Monitoring

- Monitoring is essential for the diagnosis and management of complications.
  - There is the potential for systemic local anesthetic toxicity in all regional cases (e.g., intravascular injection, rapid absorption, or channeling of local anesthetics into the circulation).
  - Monitor each patient for complications for 30 min postprocedure.
- Baseline and continuous monitoring should include level of consciousness, pulse oximetry, vital signs [blood pressure (BP) and heart rate (HR)], electrocardiogram (ECG), and respiratory rate.
- Monitoring during surgery should be the same as that required for patients undergoing general anesthesia, perhaps with the exception of temperature.
- It is important to monitor injection pressures of patients undergoing regional anesthesia to minimize the risk of intraneural injection and damage from high injection pressures. The reader is referred to Chapter 4 for an example of a monitoring technique (compressed air injection technique) that may help limit and maintain pressures at a reasonable level [i.e., 25 pounds per square inch (psi) or 1293 mm Hg has been shown to be a limiting injection pressure to prevent intraneural damage].

1.2.4. Needles, Catheters, and Related Equipment

There are numerous combinations of needles and catheters used and the choice often depends on the depth of the target neural structures, whether catheters are employed (referring to needle gauge), and personal comfort with the amount of manual control offered. In addition to needle and catheter parameters, accessories can be utilized for their added benefits. Extension tubing is often pre-attached to needles for stabilization and facilitates aspiration and syringe changes. Additionally, a small pressure gauge may be used to monitor injection pressures in order to decrease risk of intraneural damage.

1.2.4.1. *Needles*

1.2.4.1.1. Needle Tip Design

- The type of needle tip used may influence the risk of neural damage; however, scientific information on this topic is still inconclusive.
- A blunt bevel (Figure 1.3) design is popular for use with a single injection.
- Blunt tip Tuohy or pencil-point (e.g., Sprotte) designs are commonly used for continuous blocks (Figure 1.4).
- Tip design also influences the subjective feel of tissue layers.
  - Designs that provide moderate resistance and a "pop" feel are generally preferred.
- With superficial blocks, sharp and smaller gauge (e.g., 25–26 ga) needles are preferable.

1.2.4.1.2. Needle Length

- Desired needle length will depend on the specific block and patient characteristics.
- Shorter needles carry a lower risk of complications and allow easier manipulation, but the target distance should be the ultimate consideration.
- The choice of needle comes down to personal preference and partly depends on experience; the examples referred to in this book are the authors' preferences.
- Clear markings throughout the entire length of the needle is also very important for measuring depth of penetration (Figure 1.5).

1.2.4.1.3. Needle Gauge

- Gauge will depend on whether the block is single shot or continuous.
- Midsized gauges (22 ga) are often used for deep blocks to compromise between small (25–26 ga) gauges (with less risk of tissue trauma and less discomfort) and larger (20–21 ga) gauges (which will not bend as easily and allow ease of injection and aspiration).

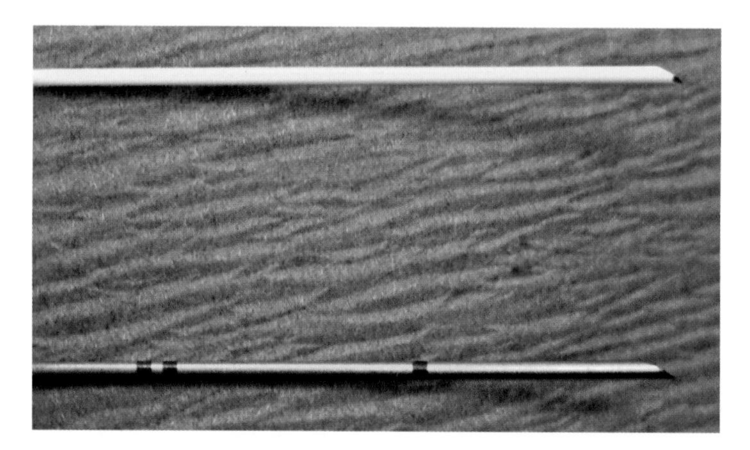

Figure 1.3. Blunt bevel needles. These are popular for single-shot blocks.

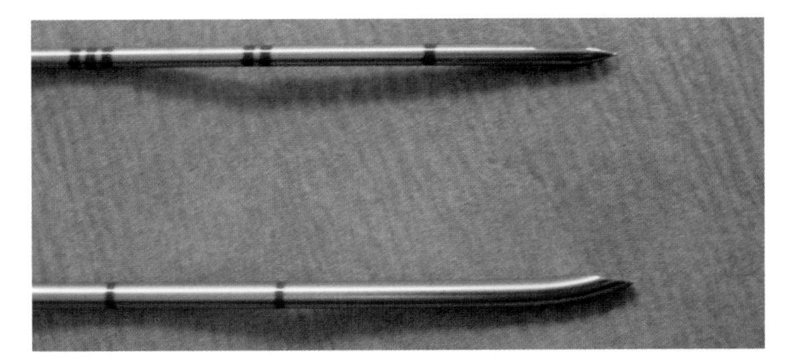

Figure 1.4. Blunted sprotte designed needles (e.g., Tuohy needle) for continuous blocks.

- The larger gauge requirement for continuous blocks allows for the passage of a catheter (e.g., often, 18-ga needles are used with a 20-ga catheter).

1.2.4.2. *Stimulating Catheters and Pumps*

Continuous peripheral nerve blocks often incorporate larger gauge needles, stylettes, and catheters designed to attach to a nerve stimulator. Accessories may include a specialized connector holding and occlusion dressings for securing catheters.

1.2.4.2.1. *Stimulating Catheters (see Chapter 16)*

- Stimulating catheters allow more predictability with catheter placement because one can follow the course of the catheter using electrical stimulation via the catheter tip (Figure 1.6).
- Normal saline is traditionally used to dilate the perineural space to facilitate catheter insertion, but nonelectrolyte solutions (e.g., nonconducting dextrose 5% in water) are now preferable for this purpose as they do not abolish the response to nerve stimulation. These nonconducting solutions allow continuous monitoring during nerve stimulation and, therefore, more precise placement of catheters.

1.2.4.2.2. *Infusion Pumps*

- A variety of pumps and systems have been introduced and the systems are either mechanical, electrical spring driven, or elastic balloon driven.
- The actual drug dosage is affected by the infusion profile, rate accuracy and consistency, temperature sensitivity of the system, and power source.
- For inpatients, most epidural pumps can be used as long as they are properly labeled.

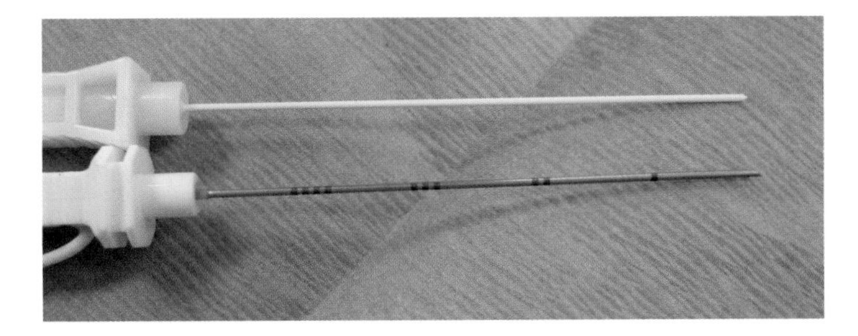

Figure 1.5. Clear markings along the entire length of needles are necessary for measuring depth of penetration.

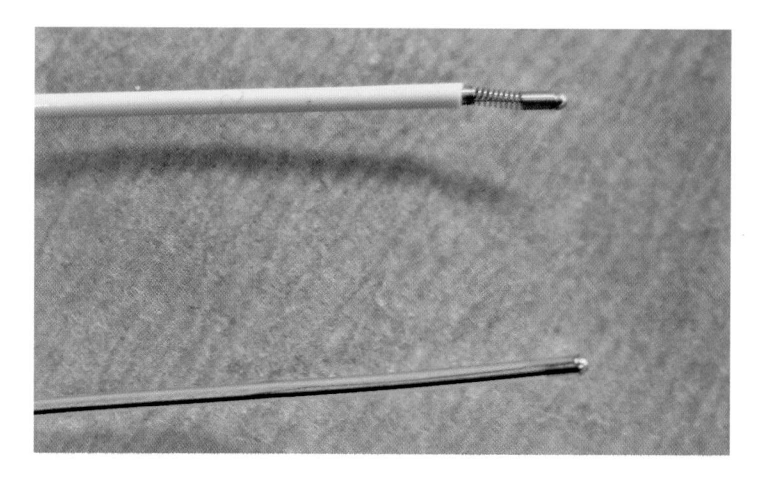

Figure 1.6. Stimulating catheters for peripheral nerve blockade.

- Infusion tubing must be clearly labeled and should be devoid of injection ports in order to prevent inadvertent injection of other medications.

1.2.5. Ultrasound Equipment

A detailed discussion about the technology of ultrasound machines and related equipment (e.g., probes) is discussed in Chapter 3 and practical aspects of ultrasound-guided anesthesia are discussed in Chapter 4. In order to facilitate performance of ultrasound-guided regional blockade and for teaching techniques of ultrasound guidance, an additional large ultrasound monitor is highly desirable (Figure 1.7).

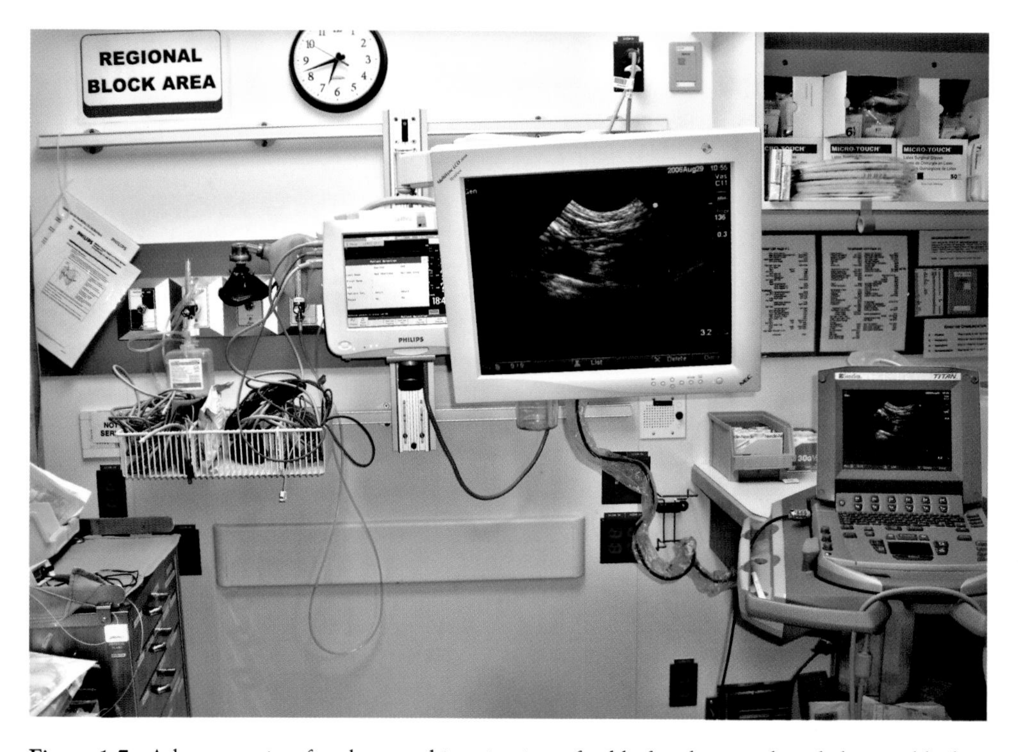

Figure 1.7. A large monitor for ultrasound imaging is preferable for ultrasound-guided nerve blocks, especially when teaching other operators.

1.2.6. Nerve Stimulator

A high-quality nerve stimulator with an appropriate current amplitude and range should be available. Lower current strength (0–5 mA) will be suitable for peripheral blocks (see Chapter 2), while epidural anesthesia will require higher limits (1–15 mA; see Chapter 18). The ability to gradually apply current (i.e., increments of 1 mA or less) is important for reliable nerve stimulation testing.

Suggested Reading and References

Adriani J. Labat's Regional Anesthesia. Techniques and Clinical Applications. 4th ed. Missouri: Warren H Green, Inc.; 1985.

Hadzic A, Vloka JD. Equipment and patient monitoring in regional anesthesia. In: Hadzic A, Vloka JD, eds. Peripheral nerve blocks: principles and practice. New York: McGraw-Hill; 2004:29–41.

Hadzic A, Dilberovic F, Shah S, et al. Combination of intraneural injection and high injection pressure leads to fascicular injury and neurologic deficits in dogs. Reg Anesth Pain Med 2004;29:417–423.

Pither CE, Raj PP, Ford DJ. The use of peripheral nerve stimulators for regional anaesthesia: a review of experimental characteristics, technique, and clinical applications. Reg Anesth 1985;10:49–58.

Raj PP, Rosenblatt R, Montgomery SJ. Use of the nerve stimulator for peripheral blocks. Reg Anesth 1980;5:14–21.

Smith BE, Allison A. Use of a low-power nerve stimulator during sciatic nerve block. Anaesthesia 1987;42:296–298.

Tsui BC, Wagner A, Finucane B. Electrophysiologic effect of injectates on peripheral nerve stimulation. Reg Anesth Pain Med 2004;29:189–193.

Tsui BCH, Kropelin B, Ganapathy S, Finucane B. Dextrose 5% in water: fluid medium for maintaining electrical stimulation of peripheral nerves during stimulating catheter placement. Acta Anaesthesiol Scand 2005;49:1562–1565.

Tsui BCH, Li LXY, Pillay JJ. Compressed air injection technique to standardize block injection pressures. Can J Anesth 2006;53:1098–1102.

Wehling MJ, Koorn R, Leddell C, Boezaart AP. Electrical nerve stimulation using a stimulating catheter: what is the lower limit? Reg Anesth Pain Med 2004;29:230–233.

2 Electrical Nerve Stimulation

Ban C.H. Tsui

2.1. Introduction

Electrical nerve stimulation is widely used for nerve localization during peripheral nerve blockade. An accurate constant current stimulator is necessary for reliable results. Electrical impulses excite nerves by inducing a flow of ions through the neuronal cell membrane, with subsequent action potential generation. The nerve membrane depolarization results in either muscle contraction or paresthesia, depending on the type of stimulated nerve fiber (motor or sensory), which is consistent with the nerve's distribution.

The general procedure for nerve stimulation with peripheral nerve blocks is as follows:

- The stimulating needle is connected to the cathode.
- After the skin is disinfected, the needle is advanced towards the nerve with the stimulator at a relatively high current intensity (1–2 mA) and with a pulse width of 100 to 200 μs.

- This higher current amplitude is necessary to stimulate the nerve at some distance from the needle (once twitches are seen, the needle is likely 1–2 cm away). Care should be exercised to avoid discomfort to the patient.
- The current intensity is then decreased as the needle approaches the nerve and the muscle twitch increases; the current at lowest twitch response (i.e., threshold current) is then recorded (usually at 0.4–0.5 mA).
- Attempting to observe a twitch at lower intensities (<0.3–0.4 mA) may result in inadvertent intraneural injection and is not necessary to increase success.
- Perineural catheters generally require more intense stimulation, especially if normal saline is used for space expansion; the ionic conductance will disperse the electrical stimulus.
- Once the acceptable threshold current is reached, aspiration for potential intravascular placement is performed. With a negative aspiration a test injection of local anesthetic or normal saline (1–2 mL) is performed. The muscle twitch should diminish following the test injection (Raj test).
- The mechanism of the Raj test was previously thought to be due to displacement of the nerve by the injectate, thereby making the minimal current insufficient to stimulate the nerve. This interpretation resulted in faulty positioning of catheters following advancement. A recent interpretation of the Raj test suggests that ionic solutions influence the response to nerve stimulation. The use of nonconducting solutions (e.g., dextrose 5% in water) for testing needle/catheter placement, which maintain the motor response, may prevent the unnecessary and faulty advancement of needles/catheters due to current leakage.
- With pure sensory nerves, the response will be a radiation of paresthesias with each pulse along the distribution of the nerve. Additionally, the pulse width used for nerve localization should be somewhat higher (300 μs–1 ms).

Recent applications of electrical stimulation include percutaneous electrode guidance, epidural catheter placement guidance, and peripheral catheter placement for continuous peripheral nerve block. Sections 2.2 and 2.3 in this chapter do not imply that the mechanisms of nerve stimulation are completely understood, and it is likely that some concepts may vary with current literature. In addition, the newly expanded application of electrical stimulation within the epidural space is addressed at length in Chapters 18 and 20.

2.2. Electrophysiology

The characteristics of the electrical impulse will determine its ability to stimulate a nerve, and the quality of stimulation will be affected by the polarity and type of electrode, the needle–nerve distance, and by potential interactions at the tissue–needle interface.

2.2.1. Characteristics of Electrical Impulses

Theoretically, a painless motor response can be produced using a low current with a short pulse width, as motor nerves are the main effectors. Conversely, the higher the current, the less preferential the stimulation is for motor nerves. Recent literature suggests other factors may also contribute to pain during peripheral nerve block, including withdrawal and repositioning of needles and strength of muscle contraction.

2.2.1.1. Current Intensity and Duration

- With applications of square current pulses, the total charge (Q) applied to a nerve equals the product of the current intensity (I) and the duration (t): $Q = I \times t$

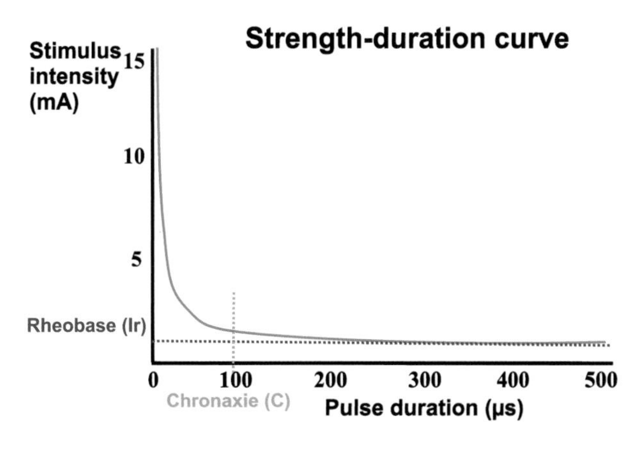

Figure 2.1. Stimulation curve plotting current intensity and pulse duration. (Reprinted from Reg Anesth; 10; Pither CE, Raj PP, Ford DJ. The use of peripheral nerve stimulators for regional anesthesia: A review of experimental characteristics, technique, and clinical implications; 49–58;10:1985. With permission from the American Society of Regional Anesthesia and Pain Medicine).

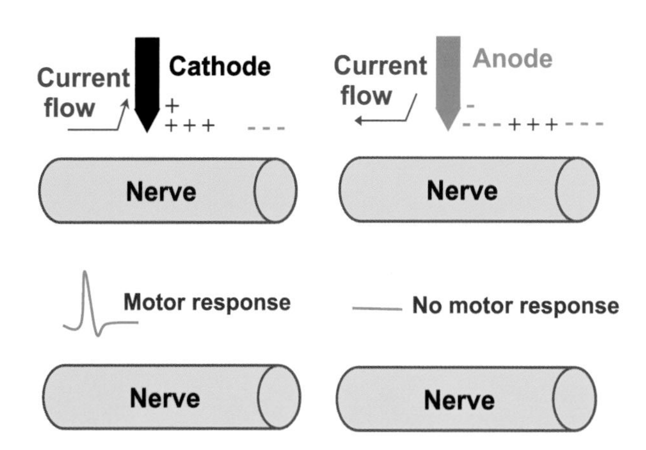

Figure 2.2. Preferential cathodal stimulation. (Reprinted from Reg Anesth; 10; Pither CE, Raj PP, Ford DJ. The use of peripheral nerve stimulators for regional anesthesia: A review of experimental characteristics, technique, and clinical implications; 49–58;10:1985. With permission from the American Society of Regional Anesthesia and Pain Medicine).

- The typical stimulation, or excitability, curve that is produced when plotting intensity versus duration results from the relationship: $I = \text{Ir}(1 + C/t)$ (Figure 2.1).
  - Ir is the rheobase: the minimum current intensity for nerve depolarization using a long pulse width.
  - C is the chronaxie: the pulse duration at an intensity twice the rheobase.
    - This variable differentiates the stimulation threshold for various nerve fibers (i.e., larger $A\alpha$ motor fibers have shorter chronaxie and are the easiest to stimulate).
- The pulse width can be varied to target different fiber types (large $A\alpha$ = 50–100 µs, smaller $A\delta$ = 150 µs, C sensory = 400 µs).

2.2.1.2. *Rate of Current Change*

- Regardless of stimulus intensity, a rate of current change that is too low will reduce nerve excitability.
- Long subthreshold intensity or slowly increasing rates will inactivate sodium conductance and prevent depolarization; this is termed *accommodation*.

2.2.2. Polarity of Stimulating and Returning Electrodes

Direct electrical current flowing through two electrodes on a given nerve will stimulate the nerve at the *cathode* (negative electrode) and resist excitation at the *anode* (positive electrode).

- Negative current from the cathode reduces voltage outside the neuronal cell membrane, causing depolarization and an action potential; the anode injects positive current outside the membrane, leading to hyperpolarization.
- Preferential cathodal stimulation (Figure 2.2) refers to the significantly reduced (one third to one quarter) current that is required to elicit a motor response when the cathode is used as the stimulating electrode.
  - The cathode is usually attached to the stimulating needle/catheter; the anode to the patient's skin as a returning electrode.
  - When using a constant current output nerve stimulator, the distance between the anode and cathode is not of particular importance, as previously thought.

2.2.3. Distance–Current Relationship

Generally, as the distance increases between the nerve and the stimulating electrode, a higher stimulus current is required. Because the current varies with the inverse of the square of the distance, a much larger stimulating current will be required as one moves away from the nerve (Figure 2.3). A shorter pulse width requires more current to stimulate the nerves at greater distances, but is a better discriminator of nerve–needle distance (Figure 2.4).

- Coulomb's law describes the relationship between distance and current intensity: $I = k(i/r^2)$.
  - I = current required; k = constant; i = minimal current; r = distance from nerve.
  - Initially, 1 to 2 mA (pulse width 100–200 μs) is used to elicit a response superficially, with the accurate placement from needle advancement indicated by an 0.2 to 0.5 mA response.
  - The potential for intraneural injection is increased as the current approaches 0.2 mA (the author now uses 0.4 mA as a limit) responses, as the electrode may be too close to the nerve.
- Percutaneous electrode guidance designates the optimal point on the skin for needle insertion in a simple, reliable, and noninvasive manner.
  - Commercially available surface electrodes with 0.5 cm diameters (Figure 2.5) connect to the negative electrode of the nerve stimulator.
  - Smaller electrodes result in greater current applied to the skin and, therefore, more tissue is affected, which may be uncomfortable for the patient.
  - The initial current used is generally 5 mA with a 200-μs pulse width, and the current is reduced to a minimal response as with the usual technique (2–8 mA currents have been used for the more superficial location of peripheral nerves).
  - With the introduction of ultrasound, the use of this method for guiding needle insertion is diminishing.

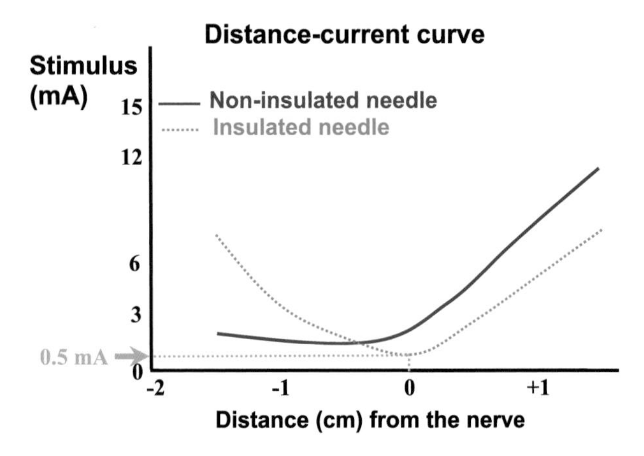

Figure 2.3. Distance–current curve. Noninsulated needles require more current than insulated needles at the same distance from the nerve and have less discrimination of distances as the needle approaches the nerve. The current threshold is minimal (0.5 mA) for insulated needles when the needle is on the nerve. (Reprinted with permission from Reg Anesth; 9; Pither CE, Ford DJ, Raj PP. Peripheral nerve stimulation with insulated and uninsulated needles: efficacy and characteristics; 42; ©1984. With permission from the American Society of Regional Anesthesia and Pain Medicine).

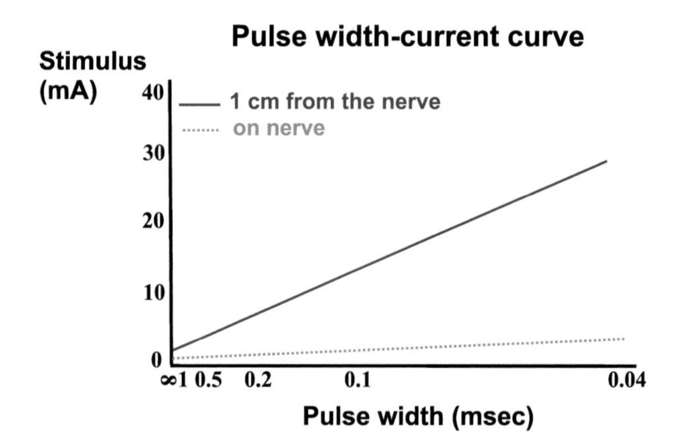

Figure 2.4. Current intensity at different pulse widths. A shorter pulse width requires more current with greater nerve–needle distances, but is a good discriminator. (Reprinted from Reg Anesth; 9; Ford DJ, Pither CE, Raj PP. Electrical characteristics of peripheral nerve stimulators: implications for nerve localization; 73–77; ©1984. With permission from the American Society of Regional Anesthesia and Pain Medicine).

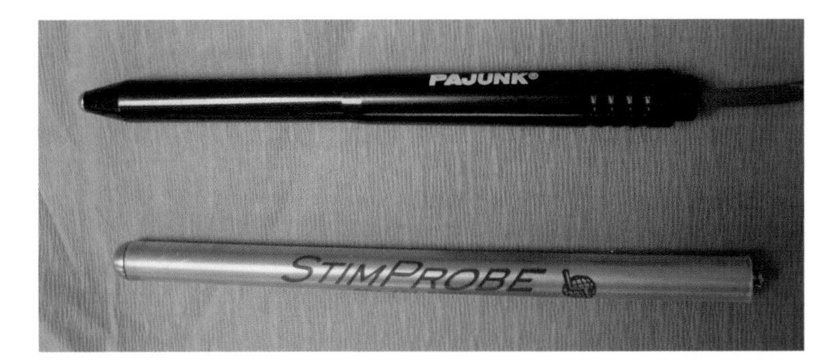

Figure 2.5. Surface electrodes for percutaneous electrode guidance. The large diameter (0.5 cm) electrodes attach to the negative electrode of the nerve stimulator.

2.2.4. Current Density of Electrodes and Injectates

At the needle tip, the conductive area for current flow will modify the current density and response threshold. Small conductive areas will condense the current and reduce the threshold current for motor responses. The needle/catheter–tissue interface can affect the density as the area of conductance can change with changing injectates (e.g., ion conductance variation) or tissue composition. The needle is an extension of the stimulating electrode. Conducting and nonconducting solutions vary significantly in their effect on the current at the needle/catheter tip.

2.2.4.1. *Electrodes*

- Types of electrodes include insulated and noninsulated needles and stimulating catheters.
- Insulated needles have nonconducting shafts (e.g., Teflon) that direct the current density to a sphere around the uncoated needle tip (i.e., small conducting area allowing low threshold current stimulation).
  - The threshold current is minimal when the needle tip contacts the nerve and is approximately 0.5 to 0.7 mA with a pulse width of 100 μs when nerves are 2 to 5 mm away.
- Stimulating catheters are similar to insulated needles, except for the requirement of a much higher threshold current with the use of saline for determining correct placement and/or dilating the perineural space.
- Noninsulated needles are bare metal and transmit current throughout their entire shaft; the current density at the tip is therefore much lower than with insulated needles.
  - Often more than 1 mA is required for nerve stimulation with noninsulated needles.

2.2.4.2. *Injectates*

- During nerve stimulation, the traditional test (Raj test) used for nerve localization includes a test injection of local anesthetic or normal saline, which abolishes the muscle twitch response.
- This effect was previously thought to result from the force of the fluid causing nerve displacement away from the needle tip. It is now known to be due to the conduction properties of these solutions (Figure 2.6).
- The use of nonelectrolyte/nonconducting injectates, for example, dextrose 5% in water (D5W), reduces the conductive area and increases the current density at the needle tip with resulting maintenance or augmentation of the motor response at a low current (<0.5 mA). Electrical resistance will also change upon injection of different injectates. The lack of such a change may serve as a warning sign of intravascular placement.
- Clearly, nerve stimulation is sensitive to changes at the tissue–needle/catheter interface. In a physiological context, the electrical field surrounding the needle tip and the

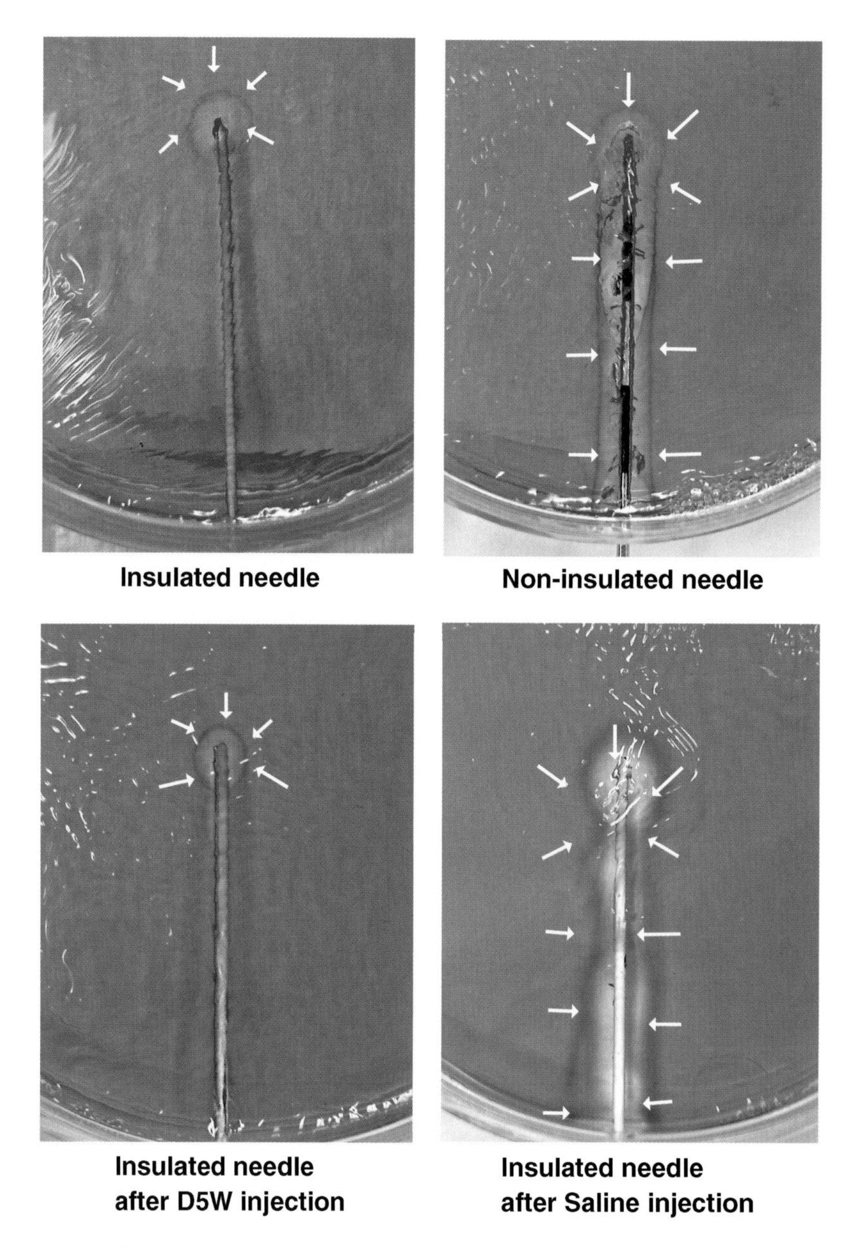

Figure 2.6. Conductive properties of electrodes and injectates. Insulated needles have a small conducting area, allowing low threshold current stimulation, while noninsulated needles transmit current through their entire length and have a lower current density at the tip. Conducting solutions (e.g., saline or local anesthetic) increase the conductive area at the needle tip and increase the threshold current requirement, whereas nonconducting (nonelectrolyte) solutions (e.g., D5W) reduce the conductive area at the tip and increase the current density. The motor response from nerve stimulation after D5W injection remains the same (or is augmented) to that during needle/catheter placement. (Reprinted from Reg Anesth Pain Med; 29; Tsui BC, Wagner A, Finucane B. Electrophysiologic effect of injectants on peripheral nerve stimulation; 189–193; ©2004. With permission from the American Society of Regional Anesthesia and Pain Medicine).

conductive area generated by the needle tip are non-uniform, which occasionally leads to unstable electrical stimulation responses.

- During advancement of the stimulating catheter, it may be beneficial to use nonconducting solutions for dilating the perineural space, as this may reduce the current leakage and promote continued motor response during advancement as long as the catheter tip stays in close proximity to the nerve.

2.3. Useful Features of Equipment Variables

There are many different makes and models of nerve stimulators on the market and anesthesiologists should familiarize themselves with the equipment available in their own institution.

2.3.1. Constant Current Output and Display

- Most modern nerve stimulators are now produced to utilize constant current (Figure 2.7), rather than the traditional voltage systems; this allows the current to remain the same regardless of resistance variation.
  - Most machines can be adjustable in frequency, pulse width, and current strength (milliamperes).
- Clear digital displays (monitors) show the current delivered to the patient and the target current setting.
  - Some stimulators have low (<6 mA) and high (<80 mA) output ranges for increased accuracy during localization of peripheral nerves and monitoring neuromuscular blockade, respectively.
- Note that the amplitude of currents required for *epidural* stimulation are much higher (1–17 mA) than the low output range of some peripheral nerve stimulators, therefore, most stimulators used solely for peripheral nerve blockade will not be suitable for this neuraxial application.

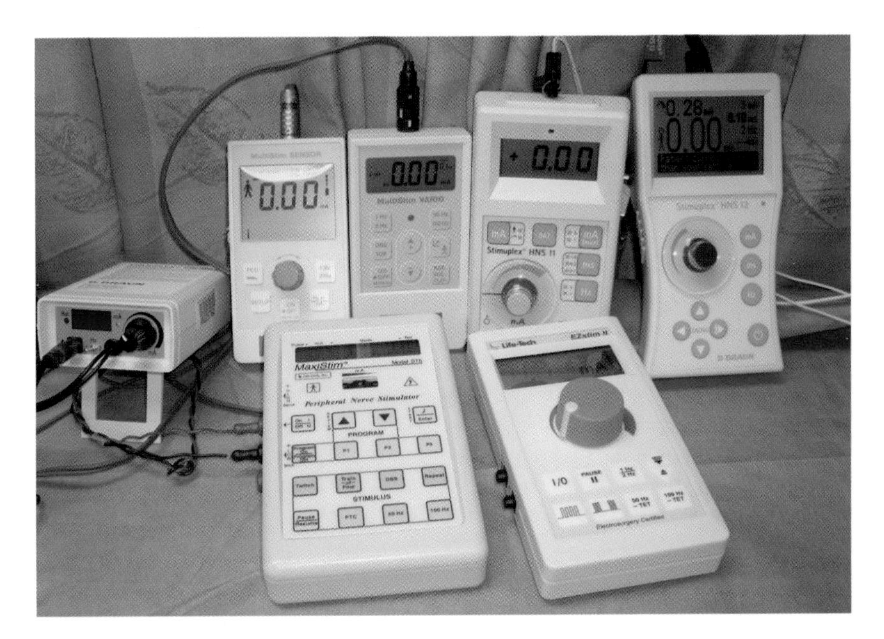

Figure 2.7. Many constant current nerve stimulators are on the market and will vary in their current output ranges.

2.3.2. Variable Pulse Width and Frequency

- Pulse width (i.e., duration of pulse) determines the amount of charge delivered and enables selective stimulation of different nerve fibers (Figure 2.1).
  - For instance, sensory fibers are more effectively stimulated with longer pulse widths (400 μs) than motor nerves (50–150 μs).
  - Some devices allow width ranges from 50 μs to 1 ms for high variation and selectivity depending on the specific nerve block location.
  - A recent study (Urmey and Grossi, 2006) suggests that utilizing pulse width variation (rather than constant width as commonly practiced) through sequential electric nerve stimuli (SENS) can increase sensitivity without compromising specificity of nerve location (see Figure 2.4, which illustrates the ratio of stimulus to pulse width at different needle–nerve distances).
    - By programming a nerve stimulator to deliver a repeating series of alternating sequential pulses of 0.1, 0.3, and 1 ms at 1/3-second period intervals between pulses, with usual current adjustments, the following results:
      - At a greater distance from the nerve, only higher durations (e.g., 0.3 and 1 ms) would stimulate the target nerve and result in 1 or 2 motor responses per second.
      - Three twitches at 0.5 mA or less indicates that three pulses were delivered successsfully for motor responses and signified the conventional endpoint for nerve location. However, this technique may increase the incidence of paresthesias due to the use of long pulse widths.
- The frequency of stimulation will affect the advancement rate of the needle, as slow stimulation frequencies may cause the target nerve to be missed due to inappropriate timing.
  - Optimal pulse frequency variation is 0.5 to 4 Hz (number of stimuli per second), with most operators using 2 Hz.

2.3.3. Specialized Polarity Electrodes

- A specialized male connector designed to fit in the female conducting portion of the stimulating needle is a newer and common feature of nerve stimulators.

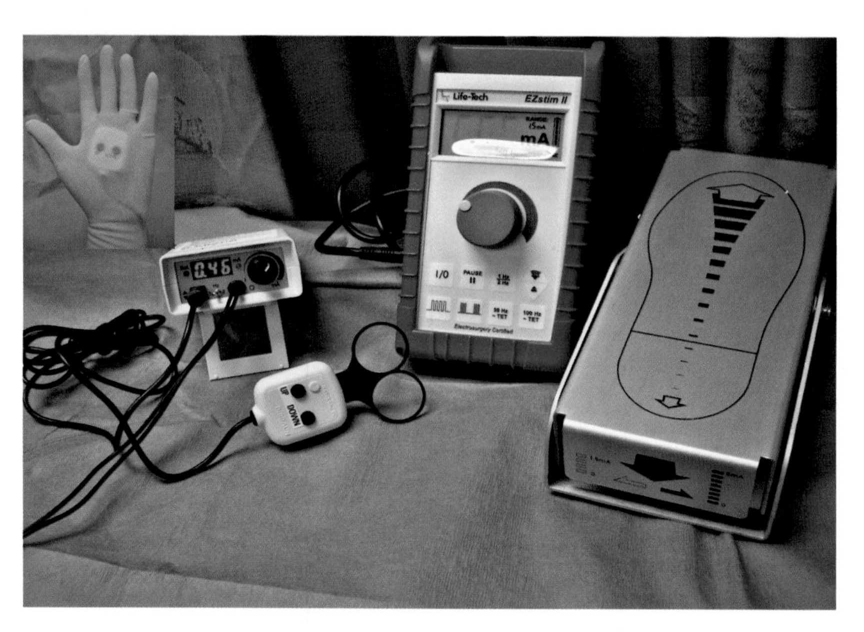

Figure 2.8. Foot pedal or hand-held remote control adjusters of current output.

2.3.4. Disconnection and Malfunction Indicators

- Indicators displaying the status of battery power as well as those warning of incomplete circuitry or pulse delivery failure are essential components of the machinery.

2.3.5. Other Accessories

- Foot pedal or small hand-held remote control adjustors of current output (Figure 2.8).
- Probes (commercially available) for the performance of surface nerve mapping during percutaneous electrode guidance procedures (Figure 2.5).

2.4. Practical Considerations

2.4.1. Documentation

- Documentation of the procedure and performance of the peripheral nerve block is very important for patient care and quality assurance, as well as for research and medicolegal purposes.
- A useful, standardized, procedure note form has recently been developed and can easily be adapted to regional anesthesia procedures.

2.4.2. Population Considerations

- Elderly, obese, and diabetic patients may have structural changes in nerves such that higher initial current thresholds may be required.

2.4.3. Does Neurostimulation Make a Difference: Can It Be Replaced by Ultrasound?

- In terms of success and safety, no clear evidence exists in the literature to support nerve stimulation as a superior approach over other traditional techniques. Some small studies have found it to be better than radiographic confirmation (obturator), and paresthesia (sciatic, axillary) and transarterial (axillary) approaches, while some have shown inferiority compared to techniques such as ultrasound (axillary, 3-in-1 femoral blocks).
- Nerve stimulation is appreciated for its objectivity and the fact that there is no need for patient reporting of paresthesias. However, it is still a variable and blind technique.
- One of the major concerns with nerve stimulation is illustrated by one study which found that up to 70% of patients had no motor response with stimulating currents of up to 1 mA despite patients experiencing paresthesias with positive verification of nerve proximity with ultrasound. This is partly due to interferences at the needle–tissue interface, as occurs with the presence of interstitial fluid or blood in the tissue. This may be resolved by using the recently introduced method utilizing nonconducting solutions (D5W; see Suggested Reading and References for this chapter).
- Studies using combined ultrasound and nerve stimulation guidance in peripheral nerve blockade have failed to demonstrate the value or added benefit of nerve stimulation to success. These studies have not been large enough to determine the safety of using ultrasound exclusively.
- Comparative studies between nerve stimulation and ultrasound have shown that ultrasound may be more beneficial during peripheral nerve blocks (e.g., 3-in-1 femoral blocks). Nevertheless, the studies have been small and variable in their power to provide best evidence.
- The main advantage of percutaneous electrode guidance to estimate the initial needle puncture site has been largely replaced by ultrasound imaging techniques.

- The inclusion of nerve stimulation during regional anesthesia procedures may be particularly helpful during training of ultrasound guidance in peripheral and neuraxial block techniques, the latter where ultrasound imaging is only able to provide indirect confirmation of needle and catheter placement (i.e., secondary to local anesthetic injection).

Suggested Reading and References

Baranoswski AP, Pither CE. A comparison of three methods of axillary brachial plexus anaesthesia. Anaesthesia 1990;45:362–365.

Bosenberg AT, Raw R, Boezaart AP. Surface mapping of peripheral nerves in children with a nerve stimulator. Paediatr Anaesth 2002;12:398–403.

Bouaziz H, Narchi P, Mercier FJ, et al. Comparison between conventional axillary block and a new approach at the midhumeral level. Anesth Analg 1997;84:1058–1062.

Capdevila X, Lopez S, Bernard N, et al. Percutaneous electrode guidance using the insulated needle for prelocation of peripheral nerves during axillary plexus blocks. Reg Anesth Pain Med 2004;29:206–211.

Chan VW, Perlas A, McCartney CJ, Brull R, Xu D, Abbas S. Ultrasound guidance improves success rate of axillary brachial plexus block. Can J Anesth 2007;54:176–182.

Ganta R, Cajee RA, Henthorn RW. Use of transcutaneous nerve stimulation to assist interscalene block. Anesth Analg 1993;76:914–915.

Goldberg ME, Gregg C, Larijani GE, et al. A comparison of three methods of axillary approach to brachial plexus blockade for upper extremity surgery. Anesthesiology 1987;66:814–816.

Guyton AC, Hall JE. Membrane potentials and action potentials. In: Textbook of medical physiology, 9th ed. Philadelphia: Saunders 1996:57–71.

Hadzic A, Vloka JD, Claudio RE, et al. Electrical nerve localization: effects of cutaneous electrode placement and duration of the stimulus on motor response. Anesthesiology 2004;100:1526–1530.

Kimura J. Facts, fallacies, and fancies of nerve stimulation techniques. In: Kimura J, ed. Electrodiagnosis in diseases of nerve and muscle: principles and practice. Philidelphia: F.A. Davis Company 1989:139–166.

Magora F, Rozin R, Ben-Menachem Y, Magora A. Obturator nerve block: an evaluation of technique. Br J Anaesth 1969;41:695–698.

Marhofer P, Schrogendorfer K, Koinig H, et al. Ultrasonographic guidance improves sensory block and onset time of three-in-one blocks. Anesth Analg 1997;85:854–857.

Pither CE, Raj PP, Ford DJ. The use of peripheral nerve stimulators for regional anaesthesia: a review of experimental characteristics, technique, and clinical applications. Reg Anesth 1985;10:49–58.

Raj PP, Rosenblatt R, Montgomery SJ. Use of the nerve stimulator for peripheral blocks. Reg Anesth 1980;5:14–21.

Shannon J, Lang SA, Yip RW, Gerard M. Lateral femoral cutaneous nerve block revisited. A nerve stimulator technique. Reg Anesth 1995;20:100–104.

Sia S, Bartoli M, Lepri A, Marchini O, Ponsecchi P. Multiple-injection axillary brachial plexus block: a comparison of two methods of nerve localization-nerve stimulation versus paresthesia. Anesth Analg 2000;91:647–651.

Tsui BC, Wagner A, Finucane B. Electrophysiologic effect of injectates on peripheral nerve stimulation. Reg Anesth Pain Med 2004;29:189–193.

Tsui BCH, Hopkins D. Electrical nerve stimulation for regional anesthesia. In: Boezaart AP, ed. Anesthesia and orthopaedic surgery. New York: McGraw-Hill; 2006, pp. 249–254.

Tsui BCH, Kropelin B, Ganapathy S, Finucane B. Dextrose 5% in water: fluid medium for maintaining electrical stimulation of peripheral nerves during stimulating catheter placement. Acta Anaesthesiol Scand 2005;49:1562–1565.

Urmey WF, Grossi P. Percutaneous electrode guidance: a noninvasive technique for prelocation of peripheral nerves to facilitate peripheral plexus or nerve block. Reg Anesth Pain Med 2002;27:261–267.

Urmey WF, Grossi P. Use of sequential electrical nerve stimulation (SENS) for location of the sciatic nerve and lumbar plexus. Reg Anesth Pain Med 2006;31:463–469.

Urmey WF, Stanton J. Inability to consistently elicit a motor response following sensory paresthesia during interscalene block. Anesthesiology 2002;96:552–554.

Williams R, Saha B. Ultrasound placement of needle in three-in-one nerve block. Emerg Med J 2006;23:401–403.

3 Ultrasound Basics

Ravi Bhargava, Michelle Noga, and Lawrence Lou

3.1. Introduction

- Numerous imaging techniques can be utilized for identifying nerve structures and block-related material, that is, needles or local anesthetic spread, but ultrasound is proving to be the most practical dynamic imaging tool available today. Real-time visualization of structures allows the operator to adjust the needle or catheter position instantaneously; thus, fewer needle attempts and improved sensory blockade occurs.
- It is particularly advantageous to have the ability to both locate the nerve structures within their musculoskeletal environment as well as determine the needle's distance from vital structures (e.g., vessels and pleura) in order to avoid complications.

- Today, technological developments have allowed ultrasound systems to deliver high-frequency (10MHz or higher) sound waves, offering the high resolution required for visualization of nerves and distinguishing them from the surrounding anatomical structures (e.g., tendons, muscles).
- The portability and relatively low expense of the equipment make the technique viable in a clinical, operating room setting.

3.2. Basic Ultrasound Physics and Technology

Ultrasound technology is based upon the detection of sound as it is reflected by various tissue interfaces in the body. Typical sound waves used in ultrasound have an acoustic fre-

Table 3.1. Practical aspects of ultrasound wave characteristics.

Frequency (Hz)
- Number of cycles per second
- High frequency provides high spatial resolution for superficial structures, but lower depth of penetration; lower frequencies are required for deeper structures

Wavelength (mm)
- Length of one cycle in one direction of propagation of the wave

Velocity (m/s)
- Displacement of the wave per unit of time
- Different acoustic impedances (densities) of tissue determine the velocity of ultrasound waves

Period(s)
- Time for one complete wave cycle

Amplitude
- Strength of the wave, calculated by the square root of the wave energy
- Amplifier gain function adjusts the strength of weak echoes to improve the signal-to-noise ratio

Attenuation
- Ultrasound wave amplitude decreases with time as it travels through tissue
- Time gain compensation (TGC) compensates for the attenuation of the wave by increasing the amplification factor of the signal as a function of time after the initial pulse; all interfaces are then uniform in signal regardless of their depth

Field (Figure 3.2)
- Characterizes the propagation of ultrasound energy within a medium
- Near field (Fresnel region) is the nondiverging portion of the beam adjacent to the transducer face; the length is a function of transducer frequency and diameter
- Far field (Fraunhofer region) is the diverging portion of the ultrasound beam with diminishing energy causing decreases in lateral resolution (or sharpness); less divergence occurs with high-frequency, large-diameter transducers
- Focused transducers can change the field interface, i.e., focal zone, being the area of greatest image resolution

Reflection
- Each interface (from various acoustic impedances) within the tissue reflects sound waves back to the emitting transducer; good contour definition thus results between different tissues
- Fluids allow perfect sound transmission, with no echoes, and result in a black image; tissues attenuate and disperse sound waves, resulting in homogeneous or heterogeneous appearances

quency of 2 to 15 MHz. Sound waves propagate through a medium and produce an echo when they encounter an interface with a different medium. Within the body, ultrasound scanners emit sound waves that produce an echo when they encounter a tissue interface. Therefore, ultrasound images reflect contours, including those of anatomical structures, based on differing acoustic impedances of human tissue or fluids. Significant reflection of sound waves occurs at interfaces between substances of different acoustic impedance, resulting in good contour definition between different tissues. Generally, fluids allow perfect sound transmission with no echoes and what results is a black image. Tissues attenuate sound and disperse sound waves, resulting in homogeneous or heterogeneous appearances. Table 3.1 describes many practical aspects related to ultrasound wave characteristics.

- A typical portable or cart-based ultrasound scanner (unit) has four main parts: a transmitter, a transducer, a receiver, and a display [Figure 3.1(A,B)]:
  - The transmitter:

    Provides the energy to the transducer using brief bursts of energy or pulses with the rate of pulses emitted by the transducer controlled by the transmitter.
  - The transducer (a.k.a. probe or scan head):

    Converts the electric energy provided by the transmitter to acoustic pulses (sound waves).

    The transducer also serves as the receiver of reflected echoes and converts the pressure changes into electric signals.
  - The receiver:

    Amplifies the signals.
  - The Display:

    Ultrasound signals can be displayed in many ways:

    A-mode displays echo information as an amplitude signal; M-mode displays motion with respect to time; and B-mode displays brightness information and produces an image of a body slice.

    The majority of imaging is done in B-mode display.
- Generally, a gray scale (a scale from black to white with several shades of gray intervening) is used with a variation in the display of brightness (or whiteness), indicating reflected signals of varying amplitude.

A

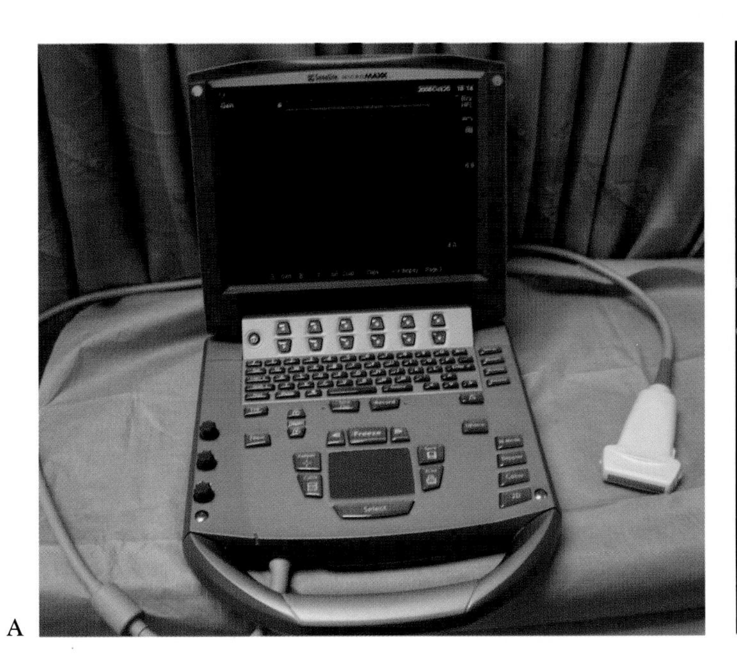

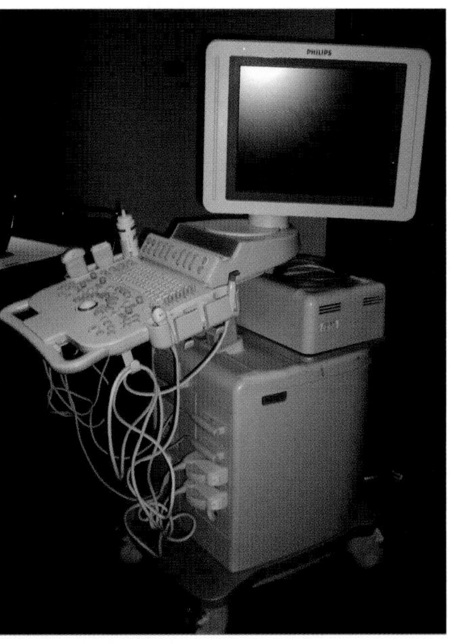

B

Figure 3.1. Portable (A) and cart-based (B) ultrasound units.

- Signals of greatest intensity appear white (hyperechoic) and signals of least intensity appear dark (hypoechoic) or black (anechoic) with intermediate intensities appearing as shades of gray.

3.2.1. Resolution and Line Density: Two Factors Influencing Image Quality

- Numerous factors can influence image quality, although resolution and line density are perhaps most relevant to regional anesthesia. The sensitivity of the system is also an important determinant of image quality; both an efficient transducer and a receiver with high signal-to-noise ratio will increase the performance of the system.

3.2.1.1. *Resolution*

- The ability to produce a clear distinction between objects is important for regional anesthesia, particularly as the nerve structures can be very small.
- The lateral resolution will be important and relates to the resolution produced at right angles to the ultrasound beam.
- With many of the locations used during ultrasound-guided regional anesthesia (e.g., supraclavicular fossa, axilla, ankle), good lateral resolution will benefit the image attained with the tangential angles of beam penetration that are often required. The artifact of anisotropy will be reduced with good lateral resolution systems.

3.2.1.2. *Line Density*

- The number of transducer elements per centimeter determines the line density and is positively related to image quality.
- The linear line density of linear transducers produces an optimal image quality.

3.2.2. Field and Gain Functions

- There are two separate regions that characterize the propagation of ultrasound energy within a medium: the *near field* (Fresnel region) and the *far field* (Fraunhofer region; Figure 3.2).

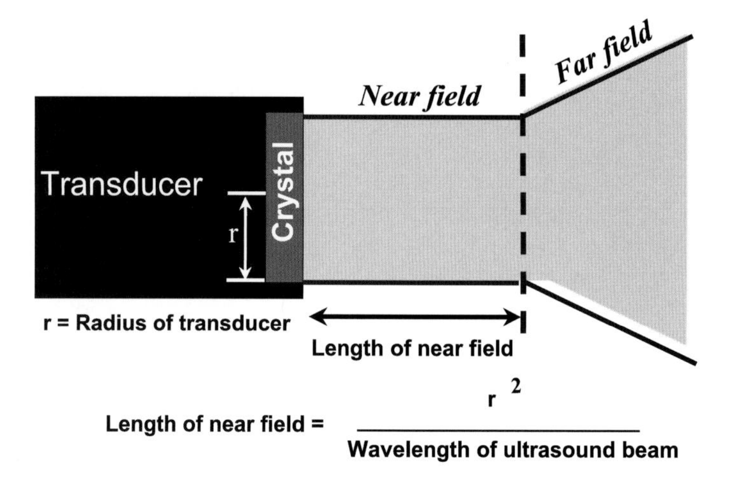

Figure 3.2. Propagation of ultrasound into near and far fields. The best lateral resolution is attained at the near field/far field interface (i.e., approximately the diameter of the transducer/probe). Focused transducers can decrease the beam diameter to a closer distance than the interface and result in a closer *focal zone* or point of best resolution.

3.2.2.1. *Near Field*

- The near field is adjacent to the transducer face and represents the nondiverging portion of the ultrasound beam.
- The diameter of the beam in the near field is no larger than the transducer diameter.
- The length of the near field is a function of transducer frequency and diameter.

3.2.2.2. *Far Field*

- The far field is the diverging portion of the ultrasound beam that possesses diminishing energy. Lateral resolution (or sharpness) decreases rapidly with depth as the beam begins to diverge in the far field.
- Less beam divergence occurs with high-frequency, large-diameter transducers.
- The near field/far field interface zone is the depth of best lateral resolution; this depth is approximately that of the transducer diameter.
- This principle is modified by the use of *focused transducers* that use an acoustic lens to decrease the beam diameter at a specified distance from the transducer. This distance is always closer than the near field/far field interface and this specified distance represents the *focal zone*, or area of greatest image resolution (Figure 3.3).

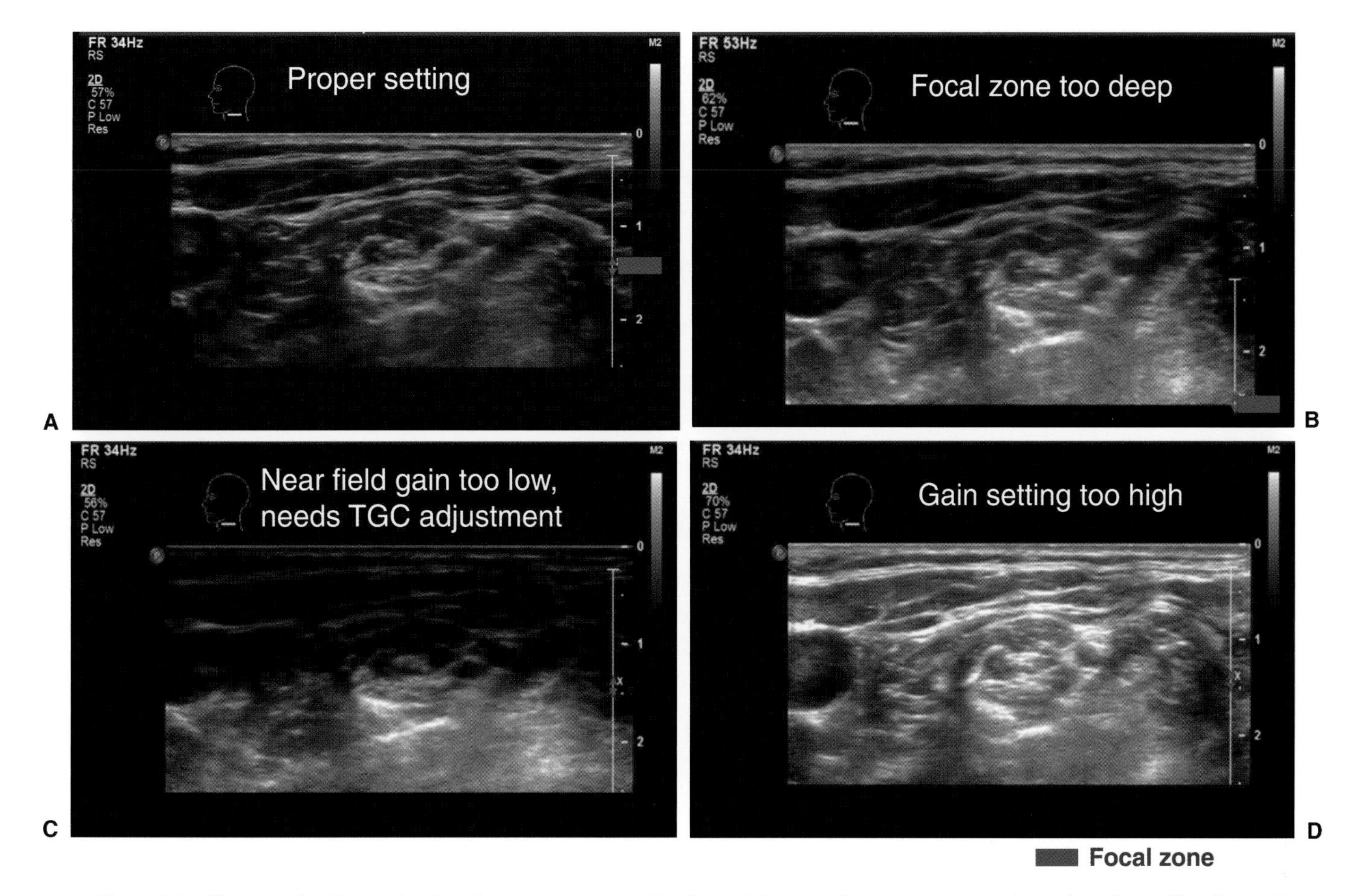

Figure 3.3. Illustrates focal zone depth and gain adjustments. Focal zone (the area of greatest image resolution) is adjusted by effectively reducing the beam diameter (B would be improved to A). Poor gain settings will result in artifactual images and poor resolution between structures (C and D). Gain adjustment will clarify the interfaces between tissues for maximum discrimination.

3.2.3. Amplifier Gain Function

- In order to detect small differences (interfaces) in tissues, the ultrasound system needs to detect weak echoes and distinguish them from other sources of noise (signal-to-noise ratio).
- The amplifier gain function of the receiver increases the amplitude of the weak echoes to improve the signal-to-noise ratio.
- The gain setting is user adjustable and can affect image quality and contrast sensitivity (the ability to detect small differences in tissues).

3.2.4. Time Gain Compensation

- There is a tendency for the amplitude of the ultrasound to decrease with time as it travels in tissue.
- Time gain compensation (TGC) compensates for the attenuation of the ultrasound wave with time as it travels through the tissues. It works by increasing the amplification factor of the signal as a function of time after the initial pulse.
- The user adjusts the amplification so that all interfaces are uniform in signal regardless of their depth. If TGC is not adjusted properly, significant artifacts may result.

3.2.5. Doppler Effect

The Doppler effect describes a phenomenon where the emitting receptor can detect the frequency of the received ultrasound waves and compare it with the emitted frequency. With the fluid flow in blood vessels, the frequency value at reception decreases with movement away from the receptor and increases as it moves towards it. The velocity of blood is measured and depicted on the screen.

- Identification of vascular structures can be very valuable for ultrasound-guided regional anesthesia. This is because many nerves are located near blood vessels at varying distances from the block location.
- Nerves to be blocked can be identified at these locations and traced back to the respective block locations quite reliably.
- This is easily achieved for the brachial plexus because the subclavian artery is clearly visualized above the midpoint of the clavicle next to the trunks and/or divisions of the plexus (Figure 3.4).
- This neurovascular relationship can be useful during numerous other nerve blocks, for example, femoral, median and radial at the elbow, ulnar in the forearm, tibial in the popliteal fossa.

3.2.6. Artifacts: The Importance of Anisotropy and Acoustic Shadowing

Artifacts are false images (i.e., echoes without an anatomical correlate) often observed due to deficiencies with ultrasound technology, equipment, or the operator. There may be incorrect attribution of the images resulting from poor anatomical knowledge of the area, for example, muscle and nerve tissue may appear similar and be difficult to differentiate due to lack of accurate knowledge of their relationship to one another. There may also be anatomical discrepancies and variations, making nerve identification difficult.

- Anisotropy is a common artifact during ultrasound-guided regional anesthesia because the tissues that require differentiation during these procedures (e.g., nerves, muscles, and tendons) are those that are subject to anisotropy the most.
  - Anisotropy results from total lack of ultrasound beam reflection (i.e., lack of any reflection back to the transducer from the tissue) that can occur with loss of a 90° incidence angle between the probe and the structure being imaged.

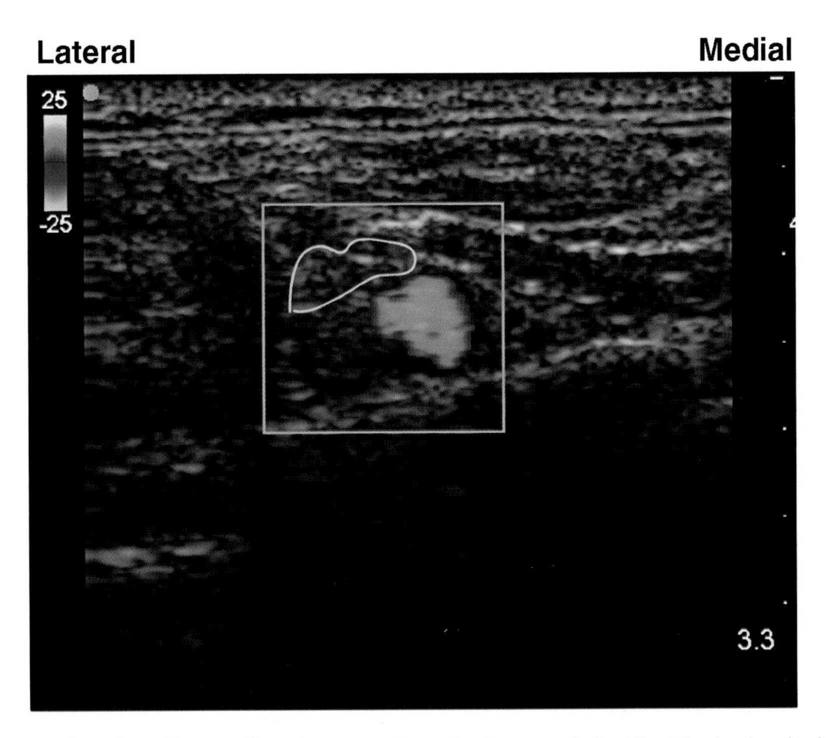

Figure 3.4. Doppler effect used at the supraclavicular fossa to help identify the brachial plexus superolateral to the illuminated subclavian artery.

- This phenomenon is common for tendons, which are linear in nature and the angle of insonation will effect the echo intensity significantly. A peculiar image (often considered as a pathological lesion during diagnostic imaging) with a hypoechoic appearance is a common finding during imaging and nerves and tendons (or muscles) tend to appear indistinguishable from each other.
- With ultrasound-guided regional anesthesia, loss of full contact between the skin and probe, that is, tangential contact with air as an interface, as, for example, in the compact supraclavicular area, may lead to peculiar images and difficulty with confirming the nerve structure's identity. Curved probes are useful in the supraclavicular region to enable the operator to have more control of the skin contact desired near the clavicle.
- Anisotropy has also occurred at the inguinal ligament location during femoral nerve blocks, making the tilt angle of the transducer important at this area. A 10° angle shift (caudad or cephalad) of the scan head has been shown to make the nerve isoechoic with the surrounding muscles (i.e., the correct angle will serve to brighten the nerve compared to the very hypoechoic iliopsoas muscle immediately deep to the nerve).

- Ultrasound waves emitted from probes are prone to attenuation by various factors, including poor skin contact, air layers, or subtle changes in interface materials (sterile covers). Beyond tangential contact of the probe to the anatomical structures being viewed, several factors may lead to artifacts and obscure imaging (e.g., air bubbles from agitated or air-producing injectates); close attention needs to be paid to this phenomenon.
- Acoustic shadowing is relevant to ultrasound guidance in regional anesthesia as many areas contain bone tissue that can greatly contribute to this artifact. Good ultrasound reflectors can obstruct the passage of the ultrasound beam and result in loss of beam penetration to the distal structures. A good example of this shadowing is the compact thoracic spine, where the calcified vertebrae greatly affect the viewing of the underlying neural structures.

3.3. Echogenic Appearance of Various Tissues

- The echogenic appearance of different tissues is often somewhat similar, although there are distinguishable characteristics depending on the location (Table 3.2).
- The axial resolution (that in the same direction as the ultrasound beam) of transducers lower than 10MHz may not be sufficient to differentiate between the fascicular (nerves) and fibrillar (tendons) appearing structures in superficial locations; thus higher resolutions are suggested to allow greater differentiation between tissues. Regardless, in locations where nerves and numerous tendons are located in close proximity (e.g., at the wrist or ankle), there may still be difficulty interpreting the image (Figures 3.5 and 3.6).
- Imaging of the tissues may be carried out in transverse or longitudinal planes. Generally, the terms short axis, transverse, or cross-sectional are interchangeable, as well as long axis and longitudinal imaging.

3.3.1. Nerves and Tendons

- Long-axis views of the nerves in the periphery make them appear as hyperechoic tubular structures (connective tissue) with parallel linear internal echoes against a background of elongated and well-defined hypoechoic spaces (neuronal fascicles).
- A short-axis view will show round to slightly elliptical hypoechoic structures (fascicles) with a gross punctate internal pattern seen within a homogeneous hyperechoic connective tissue background (often termed *honeycomb*).
- In contrast, nerve roots, particularly cervical, may appear monofascicular when compared to peripheral nerves. On examination of the brachial plexus with 7.5- to 10-MHz transducers, the fascicular pattern in the nerves can be appreciated in the plexus trunks (which are surrounded by thick epineurium) and proximal cords, but not in the roots, due to the depth of the latter.

Table 3.2. Echographic characteristics of various tissues.

Tissue/cavity	Sonographic appearance
Nerves	Fascicular appearance
Long axis	Hyperechoic tubular connective tissue with dispersed elongated hyperechoic fascicles
Short axis	Round/elliptical hypoechoic fascicles in hyperechoic homogeneous background
Plexus level	Long-axis view more hypoechoic than in the periphery
Tendons	Fibrillar appearance
Long axis	Fine, highly linear parallel hyperechoic lines separated by fine hypoechoic lines
Short axis	Alternating hyper- and hypoechoic longitudinal areas; no round fascicular appearance
Muscle	
Long axis	Pennate or featherlike
Short axis	"Starry night" with uniform hypoechoic pattern; more hypoechoic than nerves and tendons
Bone	Linear hyperechoic bone density with hypoechoic shadow
Blood vessels	Hypo- or anechoic circular structures on short-axis viewing; arteries can be distinguished from veins by their darker, more defined circular structure, as well as their lack of easy compressibility
Fat	Generally hypoechoic, may contain pathological hyperechoic connective tissue
Fascia	Hyperechoic marking well-defined boundary
Pleura and air	Pleura appears hyperechoic with either anechoic fluid-filled cavity or diffuse hyperechoic air cavity (i.e., aerated lung)

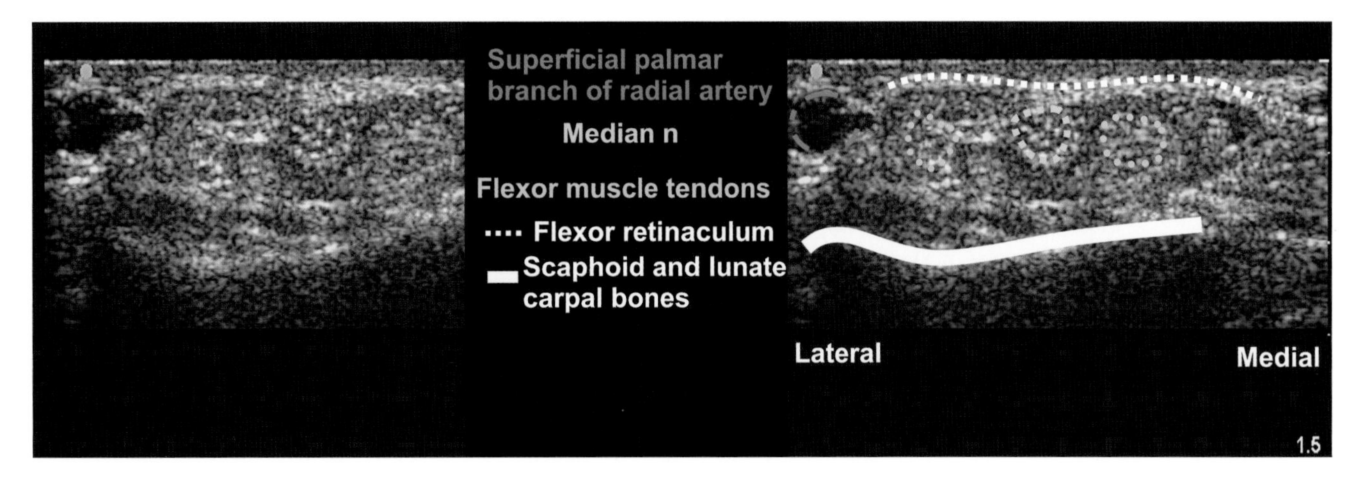

Figure 3.5. The median nerve is hard to distinguish from the numerous tendons (two illustrated here) at the wrist even when using a high-frequency linear probe.

- One observation that relates to location is the variation in the long-axis appearance of nerves that are near the neuraxis as compared with those in the periphery. For example, the long-axis view of nerve trunks of the brachial plexus appears hypoechoic as compared with the brighter, echogenic images of peripheral nerves. In a longitudinal scan such as this, the nerves may be distinguished from muscle and tendon by active or passive maneuvers as the nerves will be stationary amongst the surrounding mobile tissue (although the normal undulating course of nerve fascicles that results in a random appearance of longitudinal arrangement will appear more regular and linear when straightening the fibers). In addition, the more peripherally the nerve is scanned, the fewer the fascicles.
- When using high resolution ultrasound (15 MHz for superficial and 10–13 MHz for deeper structures), long-axis views of tendons appear with an internal texture of numerous, fine parallel hyperechoic lines (fibrillar pattern) separated by fine hypoechoic lines. This linearity in the tendons is much more pronounced than in nerves and the lines are much finer. As stated in the above section on anisotropy, this appearance will depend on an incidence angle of 90°.
- Long-axis views of nerves contain fewer echogenic lines than tendons.

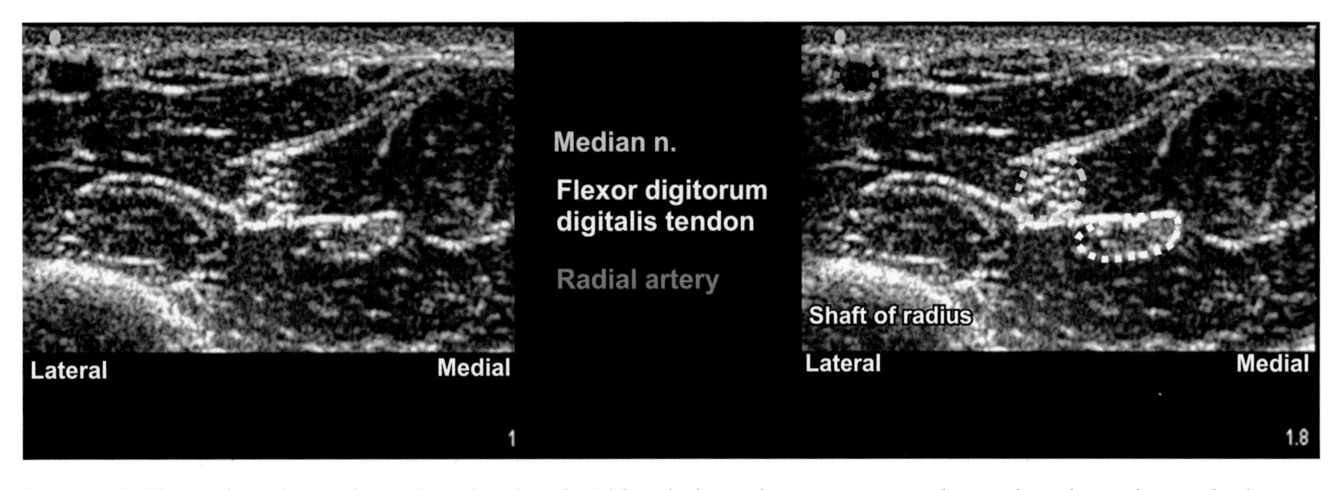

Figure 3.6. The tendons change shape along their length. Although the median nerve is more distinct from the tendons at this location (3–4 cm proximal to the wrist), accurate interpretation of the correct image of the nerve will still be difficult because the nerve and tendon appear similar. There is no reliable vascular or bony landmark at the wrist to assist accurate identification of the nerve.

- Viewed transversely, tendons still appear with alternating hyper- and hypoechoic longitudinal areas.
- One feature that distinguishes nerves from tendons is consistency in shape, with tendons often changing their profile relatively abruptly while nerves remain fairly consistent (this is shown by the differences in tendon appearance in the figures).
- Both nerves and tendons are subject to anisotropy, resulting in structures that appear largely hypoechoic, although tendons on transverse axes remain more hyperechoic than nerves.
- Generally, nerves can be considered fascicular, while tendons can be considered fibrillar.

3.3.2. Muscles

- The reflected signal from muscle tissue generates a typical pennate or featherlike appearance with long-axis scanning and what has been described as having a "starry night" appearance with a uniform hypoechoic pattern on short-axis scanning. The hyperechogenic spaces within muscle have more hypoechoic space surrounding them than do those in nerves (Figure 3.7).

3.3.3. Bone

- Bone appears as a linear, predominantly hyperechoic structure with a hypoechoic shadow underneath.
- The obvious identity of the greater trochanter of the femur makes this a good landmark for the subgluteal approach to sciatic nerve blockade (Figure 3.7).
- Additionally, the author has found the bony prominences of the humerus (i.e., radial groove/deltoid tuberosity, medial and lateral epicondyles) to be valuable landmarks for radial, median, and ulnar nerve localization, respectively.

3.3.4. Vascular Structures

- Blood vessels typically appear as hypo- or anechoic circular structures on short-axis viewing.

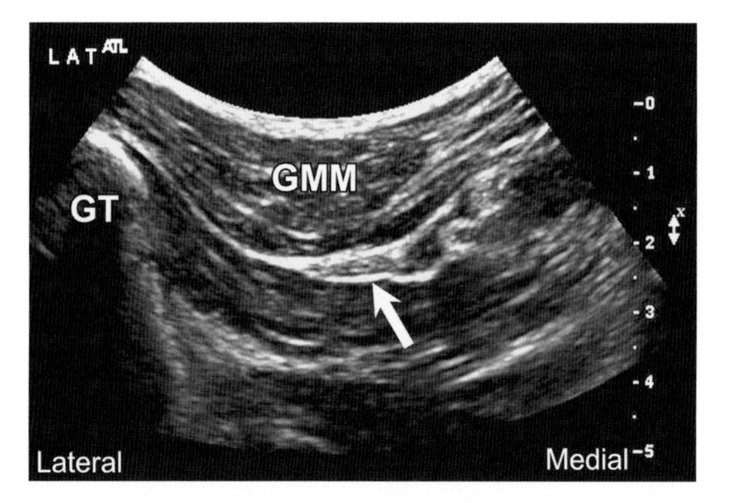

Figure 3.7. Image from a 4- to 7-MHz curved transducer and high-resolution machine (ATL HDI 5000, Philips Medical Systems, Bothell, WA, USA). The hyperechoic outline of the greater trochanter (GT) of the femur (with underlying shadowing) helps localize the sciatic nerve by using knowledge of the anatomical relationship. The "starry night" appearing gluteus maximus muscle (GMM) contains fewer hyperechoic internal areas than the nerve (*arrow*).

- Arteries can be distinguished from veins by their darker, more defined circular structure, as well as their lack of easy compressibility.

3.3.5. Fat

- Normal fatty tissue is hypoechoic, although abnormalities such as tumors may result in hyperechoic linear connective tissue encroachment.

3.3.6. Fascial Tissue

- Fascia appears hyperechoic, with a well-defined linear pattern marking tissue boundaries.

3.3.7. Pleura and Air

- Pleura often appear hyperechoic with diffuse hyperechoic air cavities (aerated lung).

3.4. Equipment Selection and Preparation

3.4.1. Equipment Selection

3.4.1.1. *Portable Ultrasound Machines* [see Figure 3.1(A)]

- Most modern ultrasound machines can be used for guidance in regional anesthesia. A compact, portable system [e.g., SonoSite MicroMaxx or TITAN, SonoSite, Inc., Bothell, WA, USA)] may be beneficial for regional block settings, while larger, cart-based systems (e.g., ATL HDI 5000, Philips Medical Systems, Bothell, WA, USA) may provide superior imaging with their added features such as compound imaging.
- Compound imaging generates higher resolution through collecting echoes from several angles and filtering artifacts.
- Cost will likely be a factor, as larger machines may be much more expensive.
- The chosen machine should have several features to enable image optimization and localization of nerves within their surroundings: color flow Doppler, contrast adjustment, gain control, freeze and save functions, as well as zoom (e.g., SonoSite MicroMaxx or TITAN).
- High-resolution systems will be equipped with software to visualize both superficial and deep musculoskeletal structures. A hard disk with high capacity stores images and short film sequences. Storing files directly in several formats with a CD burner is advantageous. The images in this book (Chapters 6–20) were captured with the SonoSite TITAN, unless stated otherwise.
- Some portable machines (e.g., SonoSite MicroMaxx or TITAN) have complex software that configures the system such that it greatly simplifies its operation. To achieve the best possible image quality, the clinician may need only to adjust the display brightness, gain, depth settings, optimization settings, and examination type.
  - Obviously, this simplification is at the expense of losing precise control over focal zones, aperture size, frequency (center and bandwidth), and waveform to optimize the best image.
  - The main advantage is that it allows the clinician to have a relative simple and quick start with reasonable image quality without the need for complex machine adjustment.
- Because the technology changes rapidly and each machine has its own features, the details related to usage of different machines will not be discussed here and the owner manuals produced by each manufacturer should be consulted.

Portable ultrasound machines are almost like a point-and-click fully automatic camera for general use that captures reasonably good pictures. In contrast, the larger cart-based systems are akin to a more complex manual camera favored by the professional photographer. In the author's experience, some of the portable machines, such as MicroMaxx or TITAN (SonoSite, Inc., Bothell, WA, USA), can capture reasonable images for successfully performing most regional blocks.

3.4.1.2. *Transducers*

Because nerves require high resolution for clear identification, the different arrays found in transducers, as well as the available frequencies, will be major factors with regional anesthesia.

3.4.1.2.1. *Array Characteristics* [Figures 3.8(A,B)]

Current technology uses a transducer composed of multiple elements, with the array formed in one of four common configurations: linear, curved, phased, or annular. Relevant for regional anesthesia are the curved (convex), linear, and, sometimes, phased array transducers. Table 3.3 includes common probe frequencies selected at each block site included in this book.

- Linear Transducer (e.g., HFL38, SLA "Hockey Stick," MicroMaxx SonoSite, Inc., Bothell, WA, USA)
  - Consists of a row of rectangular elements arranged in a linear fashion that produces a rectangular image.
  - The advantage with linear transducers is that they produce the same uniform image in both the near and far field.
  - There is a one-to-one ratio of coupling between the contact (footing) area and the image size (i.e., large coupling area) that can be a disadvantage of these transducers.
  - This array is often used for small areas or vascular applications and can be used when the nerve structures are situated superficially (generally <3–4 cm beneath the skin) in the tissue.

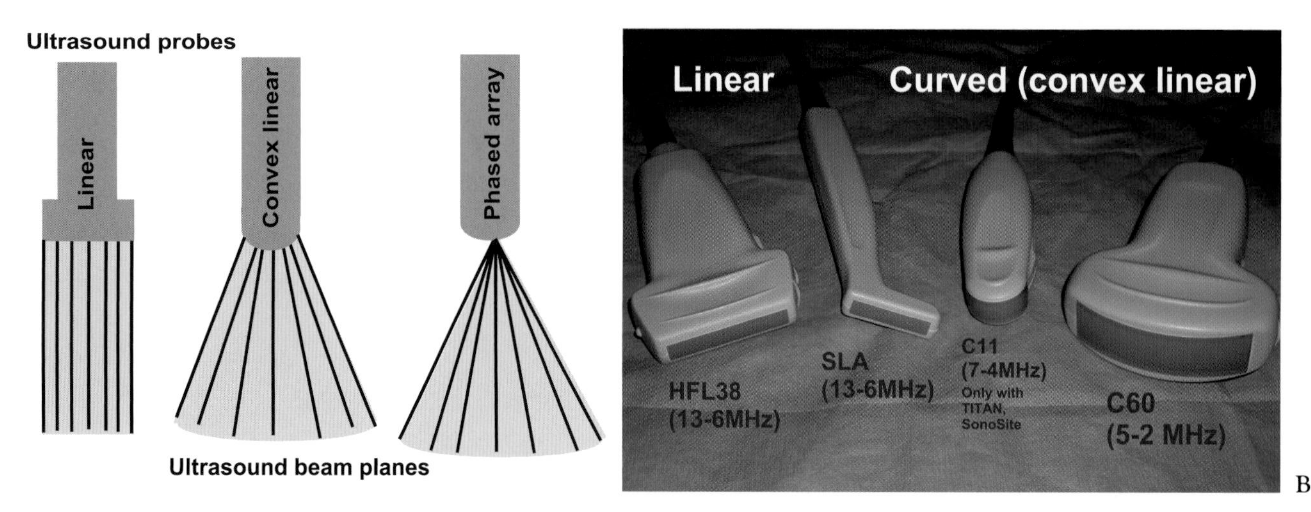

Figure 3.8. (A) Different types of ultrasound transducer arrays. The most commonly used transducers (B) (e.g., from MicroMaxx, SonoSite) used for regional anesthesia include the curved (convex linear) and linear and they all have different beam frequencies.

Table 3.3. Needle and probe selection for each peripheral block location.

Block location	Needle	Probe
Upper Extremity		
Interscalene	3.5–5 cm, 22 G	HFL38, C11
Supraclavicular	3.5–5 cm, 22 G	SLA, C11
Infraclavicular	5–8 cm, 18–22 G	HFL38, C11
Axillary	3.5–5 cm, 22 G	HFL38
Radial (anterolateral elbow)	3.5–5 cm, 22 G	HFL38
Musculocutaneous (coracobrachialis)	3.5–5 cm, 22 G	HFL38
Median (antecubital)	3.5–5 cm, 22 G	HFL38
Ulnar (mid-forearm)	2–3 cm, 22 G	SLA, HFL38
Lower Extremity		
Lumbar plexus	10 cm, 20–22 G	C60
Femoral	5–7 cm, 22–24 G	HFL38
Sciatic—anterior/posterior	5–10 cm, 22 G	C60
Popliteal—posterior	5–8 cm, 22 G	HFL38
Popliteal—lateral	5–8 cm, 20 G	HFL38
Ankle	3.5–5 cm, 22–24 G	SLA, HFL38
Trunk		
Intercostal	3.5–5 cm, 22 G	HFL38
Paravertebral	5–10 cm, 22 G	HFL38, C60

Selection based on commonnly available needle length and SonoSite probes [see Figure 3.8(B)]

- Convex Transducer (e.g., C60, SonoSite, Inc., Bothell, WA, USA)
  - The convex transducer is actually a curved linear transducer with the linear arrays shaped into convex curves, covering a large surface field of view.
  - The advantage is the larger image field produced, with less coupling to the contact (footing) area.
  - The main disadvantage is the nonlinear line density in the image, which can make it slightly more difficult for the beginner to comprehend the image.
  - A small, high-frequency, curved array scanner (e.g., C11, TITAN, SonoSite, Inc., Bothell, WA, USA) could be used for scanning superficial tissues, especially for areas where probe-skin contact can be lost (e.g., supraclavicular area) and artifacts from anisotropy are common.
- Phased Array Transducer
  - These transducers are similar to the linear by having a row of rectangular elements, but the elements in this transducer are smaller and fewer in number.
  - An advantage with these transducers is the large field of view produced despite the small coupling area.
  - The disadvantages of these transducers are the image's small near field and the non-linear line density.
  - This transducer type is used mainly in cardiology and it is not suitable for regional anesthesia performed in areas of superficial target nerve structures.

3.4.1.2.2. Wave Frequency and Tissue Penetration

- High-frequency probes allow high spatial resolution, but have limited depth of penetration; lower frequencies allow greater depth but less resolution.
- For superficial tissue visualization, optimal image frequencies are between 7.5 and 15 MHz. Lower frequencies (2–7 MHz) may be used for larger anatomical regions and deeper nerve structures (e.g., the sciatic nerve at the subgluteal location or the lumbar plexus), although the distinction between nerves and tendons will require different criteria than with higher frequencies as the fascicular (nerves) and fibrillar (tendons) echotextures

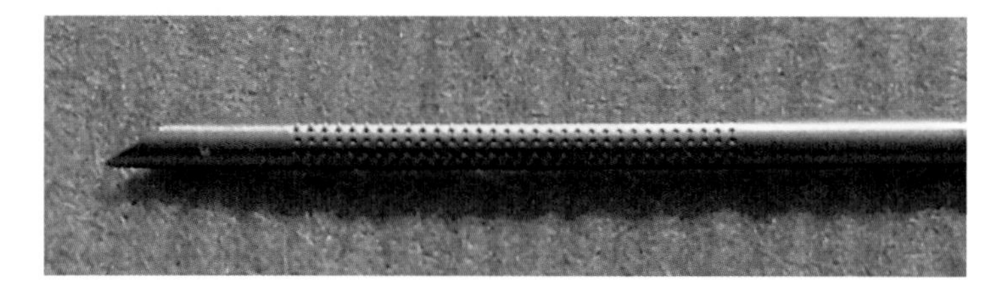

Figure 3.9. An echogenic needle with a roughened surface to maximize reflection of ultrasound beams.

may not be easily discriminated with the lower frequencies. For example, they can be distinguished by their known proximity to vascular structures, which can be illuminated with the Doppler feature.

3.4.2. Are Specific Needles Available and/or Necessary?

- Generally, smaller bored (22 ga) needles are used during ultrasound-guided nerve blocks (Table 3.3). These are particularly good for superficial nerves as they can be seen on the ultrasound screen adequately.
- Larger bored needles (e.g., 18 ga) may be beneficial for deeper locations [e.g., infraclavicular, subgluteal, or in patients with a high body mass index (BMI)] and will allow somewhat greater visibility.
- Many different maneuvers have been performed for improving needle visibility, including roughening or coating the surfaces and jiggling the needle during trajectory. These may improve visibility somewhat, but have injurious potential.
- Alternative solutions to improve needle visibility are becoming available, including the measurement of nerve depth by ultrasound and correlation of this depth to a calculated needle depth (depending on the angle of insertion). One such technique ("walk down"), described by the author, is included in Chapter 4.
- Echogenic needles are commercially available (Figure 3.9), but are not suitable for nerve block procedures as of yet, especially as they are not insulated for nerve stimulation confirmation.

3.4.3. Equipment Preparation

- Follow the manufacturer's instructions for cleaning and disinfecting the exterior surfaces of the ultrasound machine, including the monitors, cables, and transducers.
- Covering the transducer (probe) is necessary for sterility.
- It is important to apply conductivity gel above the skin to remove air–skin interfaces that are common and to allow good reflection of ultrasound waves.
- Preparation is discussed more in Chapter 4, including a discussion on practical aspects related to probe covers.

Suggested Reading and References

Bradley M, O'Donnell P. Atlas of musculoskeletal ultrasound anatomy. Cambridge: Cambridge University Press; 2002.

Chan VWS. The use of ultrasound for peripheral nerve blocks. In: Boezaart AP, ed. Anesthesia and orthopaedic surgery. New York: McGraw-Hill; 2006, pp.283–290.

Chan VWS, Nova H, Abbas S, McCartney CJL, Perlas A, Xu D. Ultrasound examination and localization of the sciatic nerve: a volunteer study. Anesthesiology 2006;104:309–314.

De Andres J, Sala-Blanch X. Ultrasound in the practice of brachial plexus anesthesia. Reg Anesth Pain Med 2002;27:77–89.

Gray AT. Ultrasound-guided regional anesthesia. Current state of the art. Anesthesiology 2006;104:368–373.

Loewy J. Sonoanatomy of the median, ulnar and radial nerves. Can Assoc Radiol J 2002;53:33–38.
Perlas A, Chan VW, Simons M. Brachial plexus examination and localization using ultrasound and electrical stimulation: a volunteer study. Anesthesiology 2003;99:429–435.
Pickuth D. Essentials of ultrasonography. A practical guide. Berlin: Springer-Verlag; 1995.
Schafhalter-Zoppoth I, McColluch CE, Gray AT. Ultrasound visibility of needles used for regional nerve block: an in vitro study. Reg Anesth Pain Med 2004;29:480–488.
Sheppard DG, Lyer RB, Fenstermacher MJ. Brachial plexus: demonstration at US. Radiology 1998;208:402–406.
Silvestri E, Martinoli C, Derchi LE, Bertolotto M, Chiaramondia M, Rosenberg I. Echotexture of peripheral nerves: correlation between US and histologic findings and criteria to differentiate tendons. Radiology 1995;197:291–296.
Soong J, Schafhalter-Zoppath I, Gray A. The importance of transducer angle to ultrasound visibility of the femoral nerve. Reg Anesth Pain Med 2005;30:505.
Yang WT, Chui PT, Metreweli C. Anatomy of the normal brachial plexus revealed by sonography and the role of sonographic guidance in anesthesia of the brachial plexus. Am J Roentgenol 1998;171:1631–1636.

For examples of images captured with the Philips HDI 5000 system, Bothell, WA, USA, see: Sites BD, Brull R. Ultrasound guidance in peripheral regional anesthesia: philosophy, evidence-based medicine, and techniques. Curr Opin Anaesthesiol 2006;19:630–639.

4

Practical and Clinical Aspects of Ultrasound and Nerve Stimulation-Guided Peripheral Nerve Blocks

Ban C.H. Tsui and Derek Dillane

4.1. Introduction

Regional anesthesia seems to work best in the hands of a small number of experts and has long been regarded as an "art" form. The introduction of nerve stimulation was the first step towards transforming regional anesthesia into a science (i.e., a predictable and reproducible technique). However, nerve stimulation is not perfect. It relies on the physiological response of neural structures to an electrical impulse. The interindividual variation of the physiological response in addition to the inconsistent physical interaction between tissues, needles, and injectates can cause nerve stimulation to appear unreliable. With the arrival of the affordable technology of anatomically based ultrasound imaging, the landscape of regional anesthesia has been propelled into a new era. However, ultrasound is still an indirect visualization technique and subject to interpretation. It therefore has a lengthy learning curve. We believe that using nerve stimulation and ultrasound in combination may compensate for the deficiencies of each individual technique.

In this chapter, we focus on some of the practical and clinical aspects of ultrasound and electrical stimulation techniques for peripheral nerve blocks, primarily based on anecdotal experience gained from training residents and fellows. A discussion of electrical stimulation and ultrasound guidance in neuraxial anesthesia is included in Chapters 18 and 20 and will not be discussed further here. Although some information may appear trivial, there are many useful tips that can improve success rates. Together, the discussed techniques and considerations will assist attainment of the three essential elements for achieving a successful surgical regional block: accurate needle placement, sufficient time to allow the local anesthetic to work, and appropriate sedation. In no way do we feel that this book will be a substitute for training in combined ultrasound–nerve stimulation techniques. Clearly, additional training is required in order to become proficient in nerve stimulation and ultrasound-assisted regional anesthesia.

4.2. Clinical Aspects of Block Accuracy and Sedation

4.2.1. Importance of Block Accuracy

If the local anesthetic is accurately placed in close proximity to the target nerve there is less need for heavy sedation. Furthermore, smaller quantities of local anesthetics are required and the risks of systemic toxicity are reduced. Ultrasound guidance enables greater precision in nerve localization, less anesthetic volume, and less time to achieve surgical anesthesia. We have recently gained considerable experience using ultrasound for supraclavicular blocks and have noted that with accurate needle placement at the brachial plexus trunks/divisions, the block onset is extremely rapid. The patient is usually ready for surgery within 10 min after the injection. The essential skills required to achieve such accuracy using ultrasound are: image acquisition, control of needle trajectory, and correct local anesthetic application. Following are some observations from performing and training others in ultrasound-guided peripheral anesthesia.

4.2.2. Image Acquisition

- The images used in this book are those from our everyday practice and are achievable by any newcomer using ultrasound for regional anesthesia. We have been mindful not to concentrate on presenting anatomically perfect ultrasound images, occasionally obtained, but on those images which are representative of what you will encounter in an average day.
- In order to maximize recognition and identification of the structures within the ultrasonographic images, unlabeled ultrasound images are placed next to identical but well-

labeled images. Our colleagues have found this layout to be most effective for familiarizing themselves with realistic clinical images as there is no distraction from multiple labels, yet at the same time they benefit from side-by-side reference to the same image, with labeling.
- More importantly, the labeling system indicates what structures are normally visualized as well as the expected locations of any relevant and important structures that may not be immediately obvious. Hopefully, this will reduce frustration and failure from unrealistic expectation when attempting to visualize all relevant structures.

4.2.2.1. *Basic Concepts*

- It is advisable to perform the block in a presurgical holding area. This is important for trainees as the block may be performed in a stress-free environment with fewer time restraints.
- The target area should be surveyed (scanned) using a generous amount of ultrasound gel prior to sterile preparation. One of the most common reasons for poor visualization is lack of sufficient gel for skin–probe contact.
- On location of a suitable puncture site the probe position is marked with a sterile marker.

4.2.2.2. *Probe Preparation*

- Both the probe and the skin of the patient should be prepared for maximum sterility and optimal imaging.
- Water-soluble conductivity gel is always used to remove the air–skin interface to allow good reflection of ultrasound waves.
- Probe sterility is paramount if performing real-time, or dynamic, ultrasound guidance during block performance. This can be maintained by standard sleeve covers but these can be expensive and cumbersome.
- When using a probe with the standard long covers, it is important to avoid air tracking between the probe and skin, which can reduce the image quality.
- For single-injection blocks, we find it quite practical to use a transparent dressing without the full cover of a sterile sleeve.
  - A sterile transparent dressing (Tegaderm; 3M Health Care, St Paul, MN, USA) can be used effectively but it must be stretched to maintain a smooth surface. The IV3000 dressing (Smith & Nephew Medical Limited, Hull, U.K.) is marketed for a similar purpose, but we have observed that, when placed over the probe surface, multiple small adhesive wells containing air form under the dressing, which lead to poor imaging and a limited ability to use the Doppler effect (Figure 4.1).
  - We also use individual sterile packs of gel.
- For continuous blocks complete sterile preparation should be performed. A complete sterile cover is used for the ultrasound probe. Both sterile gown and gloves are worn by the operator.
- After completion of the procedure, thorough cleaning of the probe and related equipment (including all surfaces and wires) is performed.

4.2.2.3. *Image Optimization*

- One of the most important factors in ultrasound-guided localization is patient position. The patient should be placed in a comfortable position to minimize motion and the target area should be well exposed. Patient position will be described for each individual block in the subsequent clinical chapters, prior to discussing the ultrasound imaging technique.
- The operator position should be optimized to enable a good view of the ultrasound screen in addition to comfortable hand positioning for needle insertion.

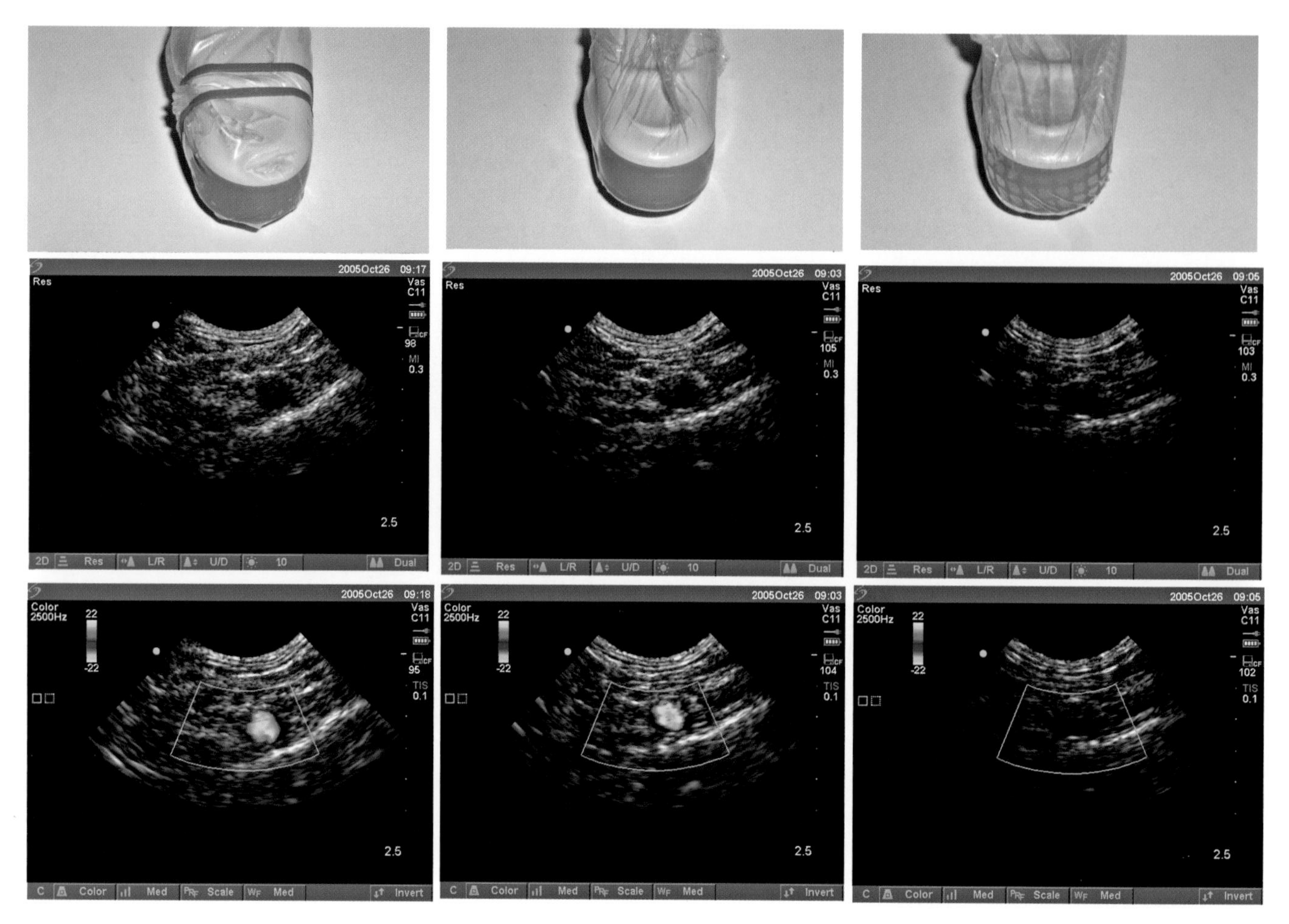

Figure 4.1. Sterile transparent dressing effects on image quality and ability to use Doppler with curved probes. The Tegaderm dressing maintains image quality and ability to use the Doppler effect as long as it is stretched (middle). The IV3000 dressing can be used (right), but multiple small adhesive wells containing air may form under the dressing, which lead to poor imaging and a limited ability to use the Doppler effect. A complete commercial sterile cover (left) would be necessary if performing catheter insertion for continuous anesthesia/analgesia. (Reprinted from Reg Anesth Pain Med; 31; Tsui BC, Twomey C, Finucane BT. Visualization of the prachial plexus in the supraclavicular region using a curved ultrasound probe with a sterile transparent dressing; 182–184; © 2006. With permission from the American Society of Regional Anesthesia and Pain Medicine).

- The reader is referred to Table 3.3 to choose the appropriate frequency of transducer at each peripheral block location; the frequency will be partly determine the type of array (linear vs. curved) that will be suitable. Often, a high-frequency linear array transducer, with approximately 10 MHz+ frequency, is most appropriate. If the area of interest is relatively deep, such as in the gluteal region, a lower frequency transducer (5–7 MHz) may be advantageous with greater penetration. Whether the probe is of curved or linear array will depend on the region and field of view required, for example, blocks in the lumbar region benefit from larger fields of view and lower frequencies which curved array probes offer.

4.2.2.4. *Probe Alignment*

- In most circumstances and particularly with transverse planes of viewing, the plane of the transducer beam should intersect the axis of the nerve structures at a perpendicular position. The lateral resolution will be optimal in this situation and artifacts such as anisotropy (see Chapter 3) will be minimized. For obtaining the best short-axis view, follow these important steps for probe handling, as discovered during ultrasound imaging for supraclavicular blockade (Figure 4.2).

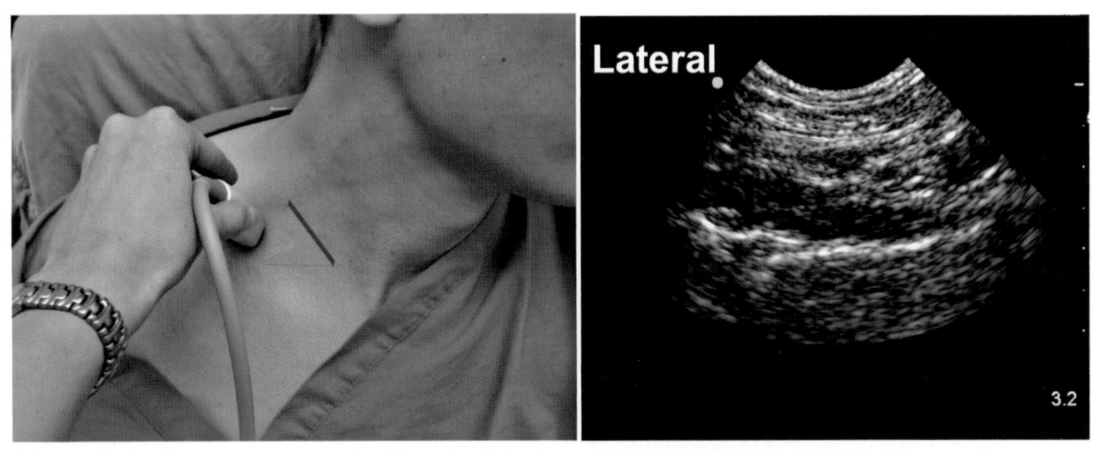

Move along the upper aspect of the clavicle to scan the short-axis of the plexus and subclavian artery

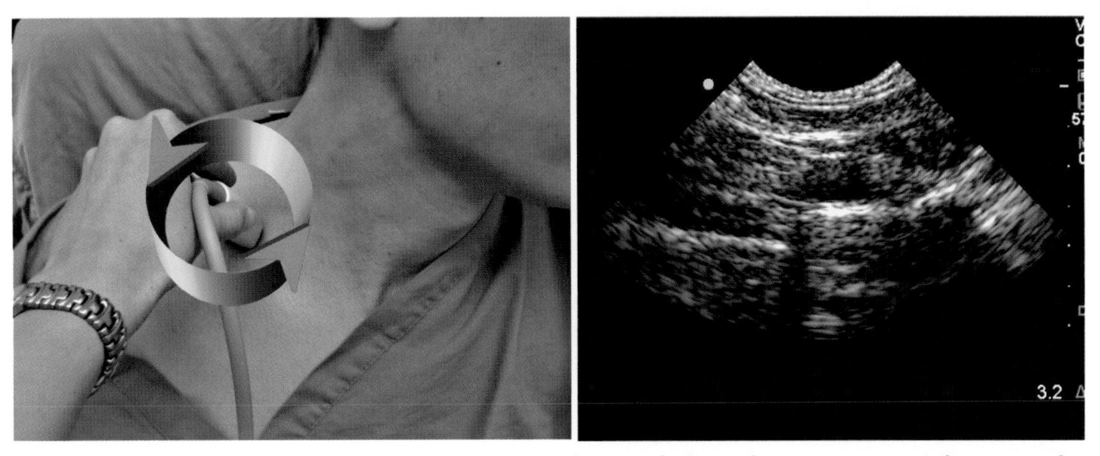

Rotate the probe to obtain the best transverse view and place the structures at the screen's center

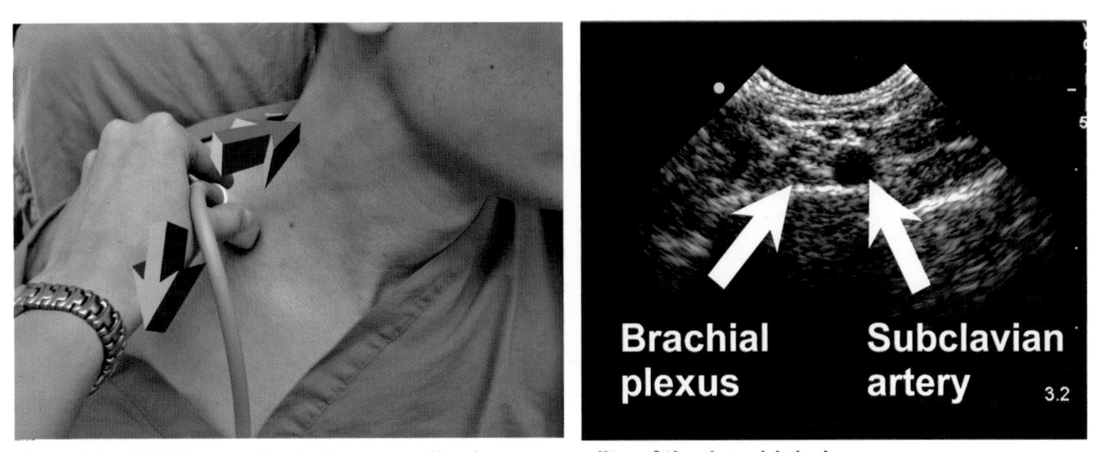

Angulate (tilt) the probe to improve the image quality of the brachial plexus

Figure 4.2. Probe handling during supraclavicular blockade with landmark identification of the subclavian artery. Move the probe in a direction perpendicular to the path of the nerve or vascular structure to capture a transverse image of the structure (in this case the subclavian artery; top). Rotate the probe axially (clockwise or counterclockwise) to obtain the best view of the transverse plane of the brachial plexus trunks/divisions and the artery at the center of the ultrasound screen (middle). Lastly, angulate the probe with anterior and posterior tilt angles to an optimal 90° angle to the neural structure to improve the image quality (bottom).

    - First, use the probe to scan across the relevant area in transverse to the vascular (e.g., subclavian artery) or nerve structure's longitudinal axis [i.e., to capture an image of the nerve structures (trunks of the brachial plexus in this location) as the probe traverses the structure]; the nerve is guaranteed to come within the beam path at one point in the scan rather than having to repeat scans if attempting to capture the nerve along its length.
    - After localizing the nerve structure, rotate the probe axially (clockwise/anticlockwise) to place the target in the desired position within the ultrasound image.
    - Angulating the probe (tilting backward or forward) to achieve a perpendicular plane of penetration will further sharpen the image.
- Adjust the time gain compensation (TGC; see Chapter 3) so that the visualized area is of uniform echotexture. Always adjust the TGC to the center when changing transducers during a study.
- Depth and focal point should be adjusted to the nerve of interest.
- Ultrasound-guided peripheral nerve blockade is not always that straightforward unless one uses a systematic approach. Most anesthesiologists attempting to learn this technique immediately try to identify the target nerve and in doing so become frustrated because images of nerves are not always easy to identify in a timely fashion. Most neural structures are accompanied by blood vessels or bony landmarks, which are far more readily identifiable using ultrasound. Thus, it is important to remind anesthesiologists about the importance of anatomy when identifying neural structures and the benefit of using a systematic, stepwise approach such as the "traceback" (see below) approach when using ultrasound in regional anesthesia.

4.2.3. Practical Approach: Traceback Method

When performing peripheral nerve blocks with the assistance of ultrasound imaging, knowledge of the relevant anatomy is of the utmost importance, as it is when using conventional approaches to regional anesthesia. The anesthesiologist must not only understand the regional anatomy and visualize neural structures spatially within their surrounding tissues, but also identify the individual nerves with ease. The issue at hand is that it is difficult to obtain reliable images based on published methodology (or lack thereof). In our experience, neural structures are not always easy to identify on the ultrasound screen and often what appears to be a neural structure is an artifact. In contrast to this, most blood vessels are readily identifiable using ultrasound and depending on the anatomical site, are often accompanied by nerves. Prior to the introduction of ultrasound for regional anesthesia, it was common practice (and still is) to use pulsatile blood vessels to identify adjacent neural structures (e.g., axillary and femoral blocks). However, there are certain block locations where the neural structures are not in close proximity to a readily identifiable artery or other highly visible structure such as bone. In these cases, it is often helpful to use a distally situated area, where such a relationship exists, to accurately identify the structures. In this section, we would like to describe a systematic traceback approach to help identify the target nerves (within various regions) of commonly used nerve blocks.

- Instead of immediately focusing on locating the target nerve at the commonly used block site, the goal of this exercise is to obtain a clear image of an obvious anatomical landmark (i.e., a blood vessel or bony landmark) not too far removed from one point along the target nerve's path.
- If suitable, it is generally preferred to perform the block at this location due to the dependable anatomical relations.
- Otherwise, the operator focuses on the nerve (often in short axis by adjusting the transducer as described above in probe alignment) and traces it towards the target area of the block by moving the ultrasound probe in a proximal or distal direction along the nerve.
- The appearance of surrounding structures (e.g., muscle and other soft tissues) change consistently with movement of the probe, whereas that of the target nerve does not change in any significant manner and is traceable.

- In this way we can more easily and reliably identify the corresponding nerve or plexus.

For illustration purposes, we present two figures (Figures 4.3 and 4.4) describing a traceback practice for facilitating identification of the sciatic nerve at the popliteal fossa (using vascular landmark identification) and the radial nerve at the anterolateral elbow (using bone landmark identification). Both approaches will allow the operator to gain confidence in their ability to recognize and locate the nerves. During the training process, we

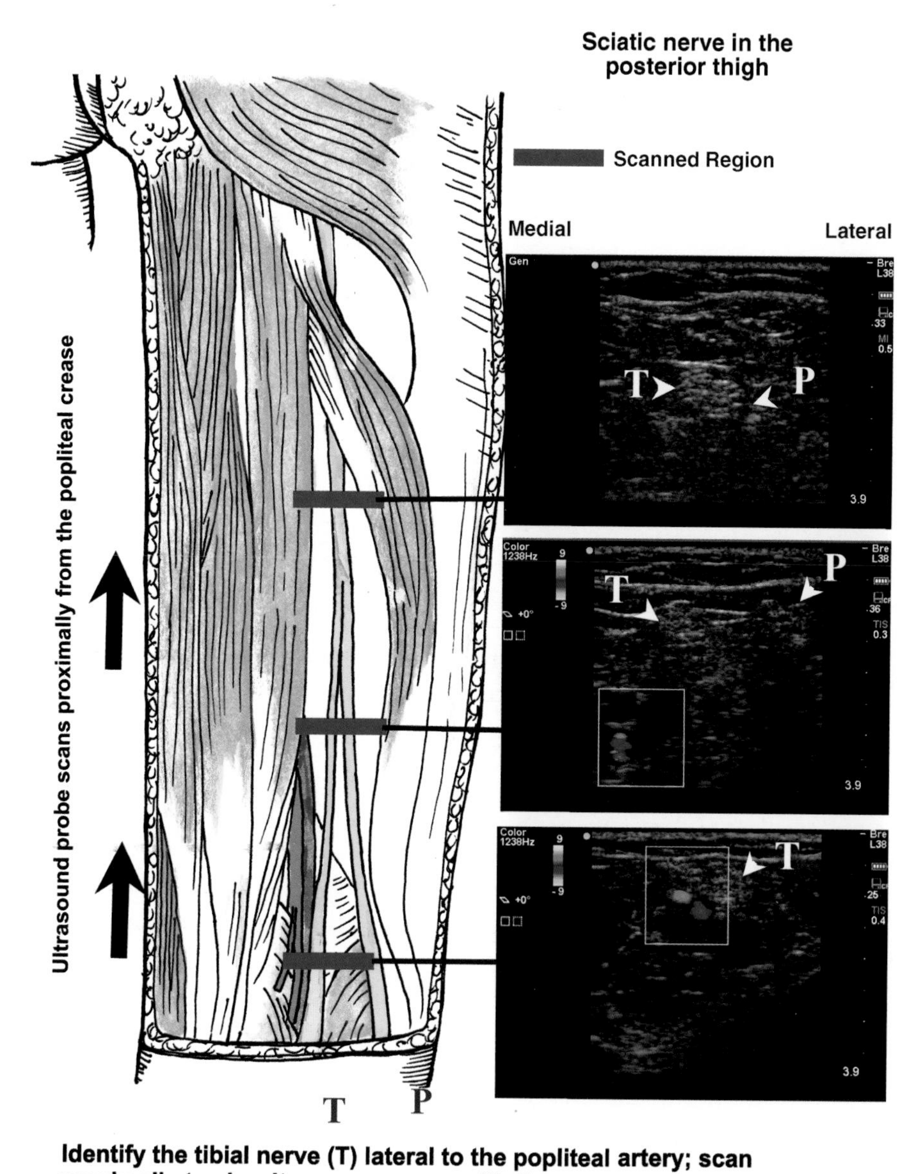

Figure 4.3. Traceback approach with a proximal scan in the posterior thigh to confidently identify the sciatic nerve. (Reprinted from Reg Anesth Pain Med; 31; Tsui BC, Twomey C, Finucane BT. Visualization of the prachial plexus in the supraclavicular region using a curved ultrasound probe with a sterile transparent dressing; 182–184; © 2006. With permission from the American Society of Regional Anesthesia and Pain Medicine).

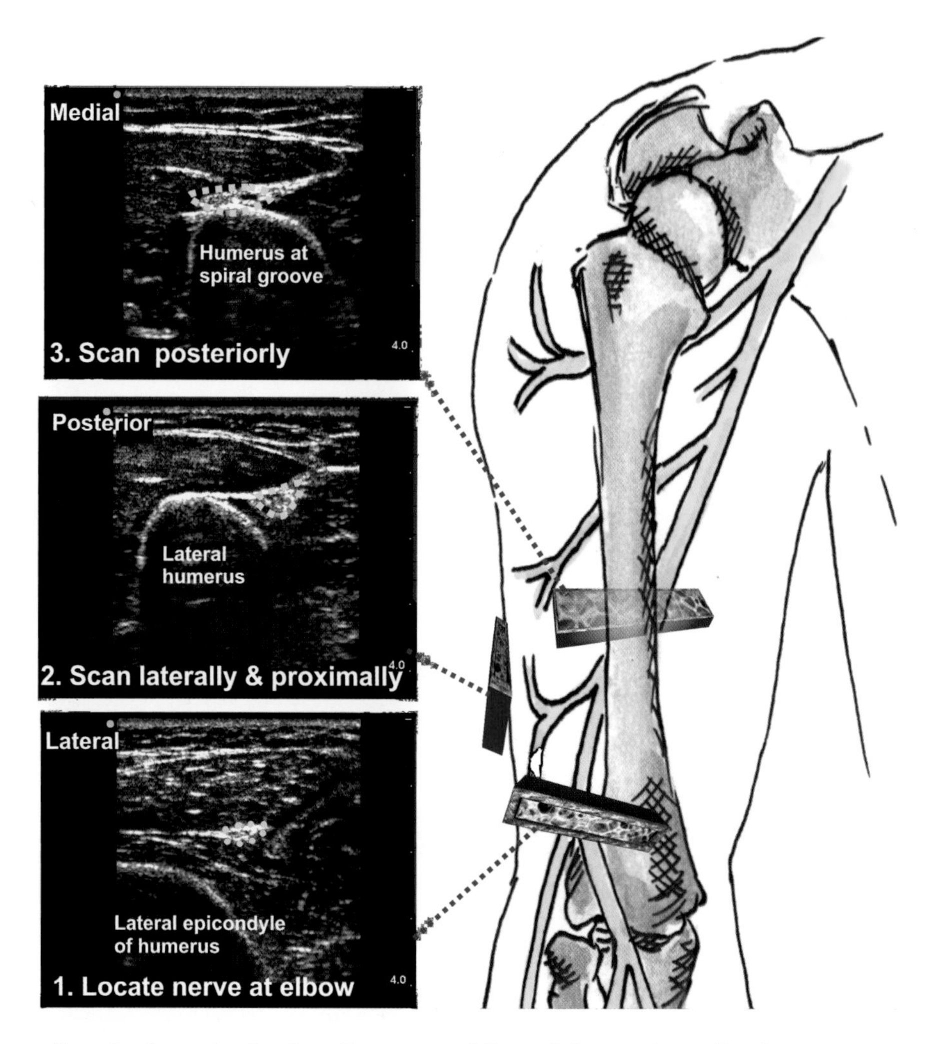

Figure 4.4. Traceback approach to confirm the radial nerve identity at the anterior elbow.

found that the traceback approach is an easy and reliable way to become proficient at identifying neural structures prior to performing regional anesthesia. Table 4.1 illustrates the numerous nerve blocks that can benefit from identification of highly visible and dependable structures [blood vessels (especially with color Doppler) and bone] for accurate nerve identification.

The examples described in this table support the importance of utilizing anatomical landmarks in regional anesthesia, regardless of recent advances in this discipline. Instead of attempting to identify the target nerve as the initial step in performing ultrasound-assisted regional anesthesia, we strongly recommend identifying obvious landmarks (usually blood vessels or bony landmarks) in the vicinity of the target nerve, then shifting the view to the corresponding neural structures and tracing back along this neural structure to the specific target location. The traceback approach may not appear to be as necessary in some locations where the larger nerves are more easily identifiable, for example, the median nerve in the axilla and the antecubital fossa and the femoral nerve in the inguinal region. However, the technique can be used for more precise location of these nerves and may be of use in special circumstances, for example, in individuals with a high body mass index (BMI) or anatomical anomalies.

4.2.4. Control of Needle Trajectory

4.2.4.1. *Needle Trajectory*

- The needle is viewed through ultrasound via movements of the shaft and tip, with the tip being highly useful for accurate nerve localization.
- Numerous techniques can be utilized to improve needle shaft and tip visibility including the use of large-bore needles (17 ga for deeper blocks); facing the bevel either directly towards or away from the ultrasound beam; roughening or coating the surface of the needle to add acoustic variation and providing maximum contrast by using a dark background from either low receiver gain or a small test dose of local anesthetic solution.
- There are, in addition, variations of the above that can be attempted depending on the plane of needling (see below).

4.2.4.2. *Hand–Eye Coordination*

One of most common errors of the beginner learning ultrasound-guided regional anesthesia is to focus their attention on the needle in their hand, instead of observing the needle position changes on the screen. This is a cardinal error, as important information relating to the needle position and the corresponding image will be missed by concentrating on the actual needle. Today's teenage population illustrates this point by focusing on the onscreen action rather than on the controller when playing a video game (Figure 4.5). Similarly, an

Table 4.1. Useful landmarks for identification of nerves using ultrasound. Many can be used in traceback approaches.

Block	Useful ultrasound landmark	Comments
Interscalene	Subclavian artery	Trace nerve proximally from the distal supraclavicular location where the artery lies medial to the nerve
Supraclavicular	Subclavian artery	Brachial plexus lies lateral and often superior to the artery
Infraclavicular	Subclavian artery and vein	Brachial plexus cords surrounding the artery
Axillary	Axillary artery	Terminal nerves surround the artery
Peripheral nerves		
Median at antecubital fossa	Brachial artery	Nerve lies immediately medial to the artery
Radial at anterior elbow	Humerus at spiral groove	Groove is found on posterolateral surface of humerus inferior to the deltoid insertion and the nerve can be located (also adjacent to the deep brachial artery) and traced to the anterior elbow
Ulnar at medial forearm	Ulnar artery	The nerve lies medial and adjacent to the artery at the midpoint of the medial forearm
Lumbar plexus	Transverse processes	Lies between and just deep to the lateral tips of the processes
Femoral	Femoral artery	Nerve lies lateral to artery (vein most medial). Insert needle above the bifurcation of the deep femoral artery
Sciatic		
Labat	Ischial bone	Nerve lies lateral to the ischial bone
Subgluteal	Greater trochanter and ischial tuberosity	Nerve lies between the two bone structures
Popliteal	Popliteal artery	Traceback from the popliteal crease where the tibial nerve is adjacent to the artery. Scanning proximally to the sciatic bifurcation, the artery becomes deeper and at a greater distance from the nerve where it is joined by the common peroneal nerve
Ankle		
Tibial (posterior tibial)	Posterior tibial artery	Nerve lies posterior to the artery
Deep peroneal	Anterior tibial artery	Nerve lies lateral to the artery

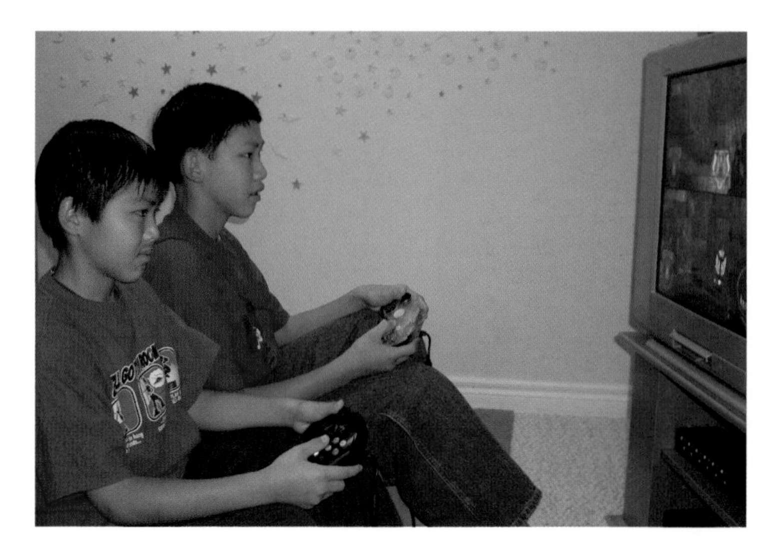

Figure 4.5. Children focusing on their video game screen rather than looking at their hand movements on the controller.

experienced laparoscopic surgeon may look directly at their instruments upon initial insertion but will transfer their focus to the screen for all subsequent instrument manipulation. Although it sounds trivial to stress good hand–eye coordination, mastering it has been extremely helpful for our trainees and ourselves.

4.2.5. Needle Insertion Technique

4.2.5.1. In-Plane Technique

- Aligning the needle to the ultrasound plane is also a very important concept to grasp and practice.
- In-plane (IP, long-axis, longitudinal, or axial) needling approaches with the needle parallel to the ultrasound scanning plane has the advantage of allowing continuous control of the needle trajectory due to clear visualization of both needle tip and shaft.
- The nerve structure is often placed at the edge of the ultrasound screen to ensure adequate viewing distance for the needle shaft.
- Good alignment of the needle shaft and scanning plane are required and can be attained by paying close attention when viewing the needle and probe from above or in an axial view.
- It has been shown that the needle for this IP alignment can be best viewed at a shallow insertion angle, while out-of-plane (OOP; short-axis, transverse) alignment benefits from steeper angles of needle insertion. However, the difference is subtle at best and can not always be relied upon. Clinically, it is best to modify the needling technique to each individual block location.
- For practical reasons, it is often advisable to use short, linear or curved probes in compact areas, such as the supraclavicular fossa. It is critical to use in-plane technique at this location (to adequately view the needle to prevent pleural puncture) and smaller probes will be beneficial.
- Most commercial needle-guiding tools involve physical fixation of the needle aligned in-plane with respect to the ultrasound beam.
  - Such an apparatus is not only expensive and cumbersome to use, but often leads to a significant limitation with fine adjustment of needle placement and requires extra long needles (Figure 4.6).
- On the other hand, the freehand technique requires excellent coordination to align and maintain the needle in plane to the ultrasound beam, in order to visually track the advancement of the needle to the target in real time.

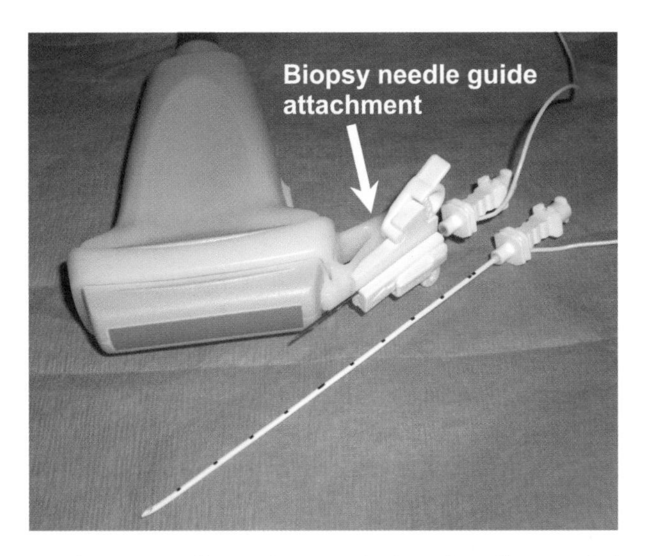

Figure 4.6. Commercial biopsy needle attachment. The fixated needle not only has a limited trajectory angle but also has to be extra long.

- Accordingly, the freehand technique often requires a steep learning curve.
- Tsui developed a method of needle-probe alignment using a laser attachment for the probe; the laser line will project onto both the needle shaft and the midline of the probe, indicating an in-plane position.

4.2.6. "Training Wheel" Laser Attachment

A practical and economical in-plane laser guide for use with ultrasound-guided needle insertion can be easily set up. Aligning the visible optical laser line with the longitudinal axis of the ultrasound probe will mimic the "invisible" beam from the ultrasound probe and allow improvements with in-plane needle alignment. With the laser-unit attachment, any misalignment of the needle to the ultrasound beam can be easily detected and adjusted in real time.

This device was based on the physical characteristics of two-dimensional (2D) ultrasound beams and laser line projections, both which produce their arrays in a single thin plane [Figure 4.7(A)]. Once the two planes are properly aligned, lining up the needle shaft to the obvious red laser line (i.e., with the corresponding line imposed on the needle shaft) will accurately align the needle in-plane to the invisible ultrasound beam [Figure 4.7(B)]. Ultimately, this alignment will enable good needle visibility under the skin surface during the needle trajectory to the target neural structure. An in vitro model was used to demonstrate how the laser line projection, and subsequently the needle, can be easily aligned with the ultrasound beam plane with a few simple steps.

A laser–ultrasound apparatus can be constructed consisting of a readily available small-line laser unit (Line Generator Laser Diode Module LML, Apinex, Montreal, Quebec, Canada) mounted onto an ultrasound transducer (HFL38 or SLA "Hockey stick", MicroMaxx, SonoSite, Inc., Bothell, WA, USA) with a commercially available plastic clamp (Aims Fasteners and Fittings, Montreal, Quebec, Canada). The procedure to align the laser attachment so as to have the laser line and ultrasound plane aligned is (Figure 4.8):

- Loosely mount the laser unit onto the ultrasound probe with the plastic clamp.
- Place the probe vertically and perpendicular to a sheet of lined paper, with the midline marking of the longitudinal axis of the probe lined up to the paper lines as accurately as possible.

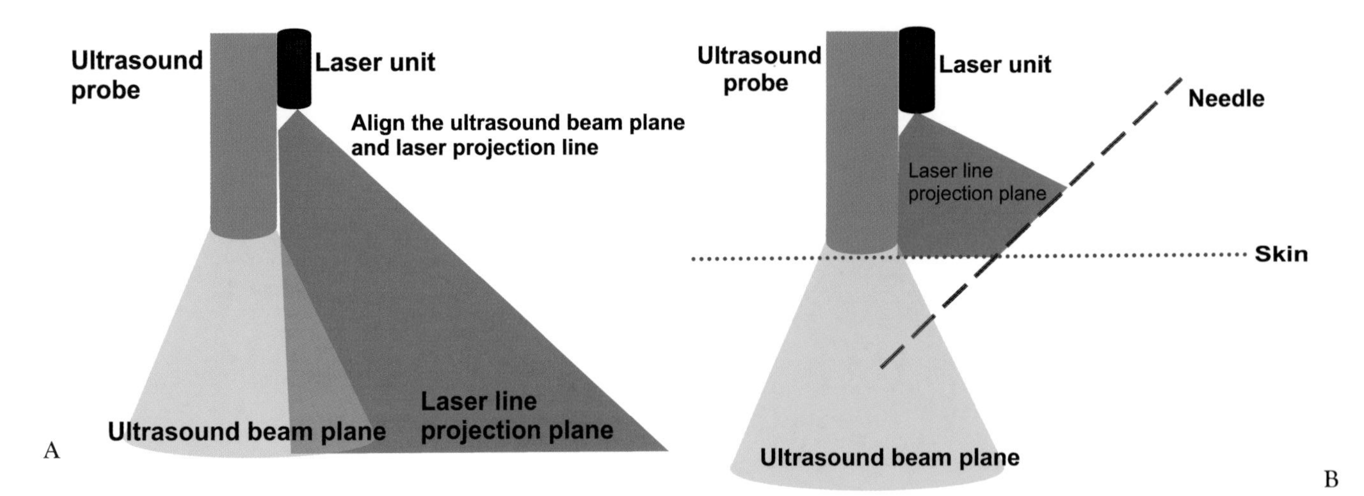

Figure 4.7. In-plane laser guide for lining block needles in plane to probes. (A) The laser line and ultrasound beam are both composed of single thin planes. (B) Once the needle is aligned with the laser line, and the laser line is projected onto the needle shaft, the needle and probe are aligned in plane. (Reprinted from Reg Anesth Pain Med; 32; Tsui BC. Facilitation needle alignment in plane to an ultrasound beam using a portable laser unit; 84–88; © 2007. With permission from the American Society of Regional Anesthesia and Pain Medicine).

- Adjust the laser unit by turning it in a clockwise or anticlockwise direction until a red laser line is projected along the midline of the probe and the lining of the paper.
- Tighten the clamp to stabilize the laser on the probe in this final position.

The limitation of this laser unit–probe apparatus is that the laser light should not be obstructed by extensive sterile covering. This device may not be suitable for cases such as those involving the insertion of catheters for continuous anesthesia because full sterile covers are required. When full sleeve covers are not necessary, as with single-injection

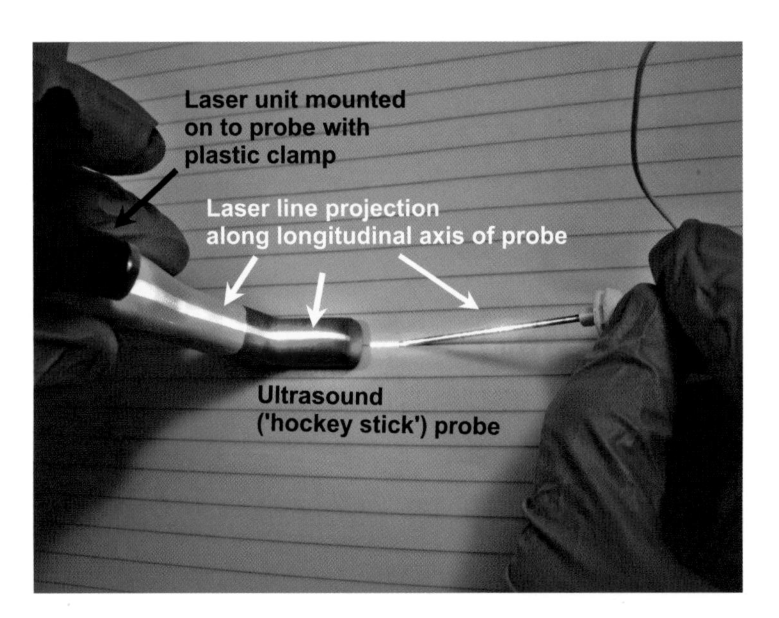

Figure 4.8. Aligning the laser line with the ultrasound beam using lined paper, a loosely clamped apparatus, and a block needle. (Reprinted from Reg Anesth Pain Med; 32; Tsui BC. Facilitation needle alignment in plane to an ultrasound beam using a portable laser unit; 84–88; © 2007. With permission from the American Society of Regional Anesthesia and Pain Medicine).

technique, the apparatus can be made sterile while maintaining the laser attachment. During a single-injection technique, the primary aim is to keep the probe surface and skin sterile.
Using this technique, the laser light can be projected to the target area without visual interference. Thus, the laser attachment can be used to effectively guide needles in a freehand fashion, while allowing maximum flexibility. The described apparatus may be extremely useful for training beginners. Both the teacher and the learner can quickly detect whether the needle is in plane (with the whole needle illuminated) or slightly off plane (i.e., at a tangential angle to the probe, with only a partial laser line projection on to the needle) from the visible laser line. It should remind the trainee that small adjustments in the needle-insertion angle can change the needle from an in-plane to off-plane position, which corresponds to poorer quality of needle trajectory visibility and control.

Regardless of their experience level, most of our residents and staff have successfully inserted needles into target areas using the in-plane laser guide. Both the laser unit and plastic clamp were obtained with minimal cost and the unit can be easily mounted on and used with any other probe. Even though the technique requires minimal specialized training, further study will be needed to demonstrate whether this apparatus can actually shorten individual learning curves.

4.2.7. Out-of-Plane Technique: Walk Down Approach

- Out-of-plane (OOP; tangential, short-axis) alignment of the needle to the scanning plane can be useful in several block locations (e.g., infraclavicular, femoral, and ankle blocks), but the separation between the needle tip and proximal shaft can be poorly defined.
- Needle tip imaging can be improved by using shallow initial puncture angles as the tip is best viewed, as a bright dot, at these angles and at the superficial location.
- An approach that can improve needle tip visibility when using OOP approaches with linear probes involves calculating the required depth of puncture (with measurement to the related neural structure recorded using ultrasound prior to the block) and using trigonometry with the needle shaft angle and length to calculate a reasonable distance to place the initial needle puncture site (Figure 4.9).
- The initial shallow puncture will be easily seen and the needle tip can be followed as it is "walked down" to the final calculated depth. For example, if the final depth of penetration for the block is 2 cm, the needle will ultimately obtain a 45° angle if the initial puncture site is 2 cm from the probe and the needle is incrementally angled to this level.
- The nerve structure is often placed in the center of the screen to guarantee that aligning the needle puncture with the center of the probe will ensure close needle tip–nerve alignment.
- The choice of probe, whether linear or curved, can be altered depending on the anatomical situation.

It is usually easier to follow the needle trajectory using linear probes rather than curved probes, particularly when using an out-of-plane alignment, as the needle tip only appears as single dot and the fanned-out nature of the image from curved probes makes it difficult to estimate the actual physical location of the dot in relation to actual footing of the probe.

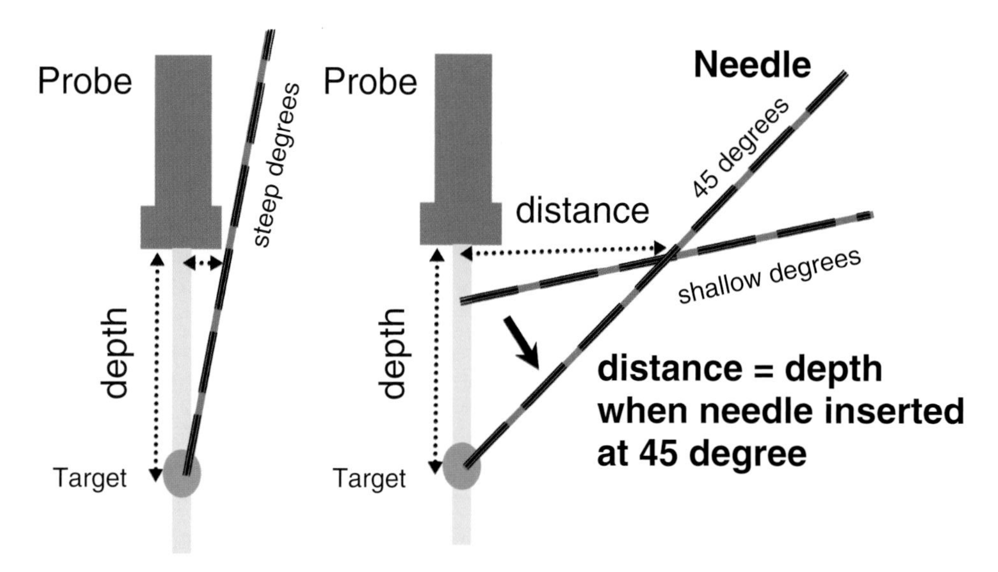

Figure 4.9. Walk down approach to optimize out-of-plane needle visibility and tracking. The steep angles (left) often used limit the visibility of needle tips, while shallower angles (right) improve visibility. The incremental needle angulation (with 2–3 insertion angles from shallow to final 45°) can improve needle tracking. The trigonometric relationship, using an ultrasound measured target depth, will allow an estimate of the target needle insertion site which will direct the needle to the target location at a final angle of 45°. (Reprinted from Reg Anesth Pain Med; 31; Tsui BC, Dillane D. Needle puncture site and a "walk down" approach for short-axis alignment during ultrasound yielded blocks; 586–587; © 2006. With permission from the American Society of Regional Anesthesia and Pain Medicine).

4.2.8. Local Anesthetic Application

- An advantage of ultrasound guidance during regional blockade is the appearance of the injectate, which is distributed (optimally circumferentially) around the target structures.
- Injection of local anesthetic or other solution around the neural structure results in a hypoechoic signal and the diffusion can be tracked.
- Unagitated solutions can be used for contrast in order to assist viewing of the nerve; alternatively, air bubbles dispersed from the needle tip can be used to improve needle tip visibility.
- After the local anesthetic application, the nerves may also be seen to float freely in the solution. The tissue surrounding the injectate is often seen to separate and expand, resulting in possible needle displacement.
- Small test injections of local anesthetic or 5% dextrose (1–2 mL) are often used to confirm proximity to the neural structure as well as ascertain whether the optimal circumferential spread of injectate will occur. If the test shows potential application near or within vessels or cavities, subsequent injection should be postponed until better localization is achieved. If suboptimal spread of injectate is viewed, the needle can be repositioned to allow another injection.
- There are many combinations of local anesthetics that can be used effectively and the dose is often reduced through accurate ultrasound-guided localization of the nerve structure. The following combinations are based on our own experiences.
  - For outpatient cases, we generally use 15 mL of 2% lidocaine and 5 mL of 0.5% bupivacaine. With a rapid onset time of 10 min and surgical time of about 3 to 4 h, this is suitable for most day case surgeries.
  - For inpatient cases, we generally use 15 mL of 2% lidocaine and 15 mL of 1% ropivacaine with a similar onset time but with an analgesic effect of up to 18 h.

- With the use of ultrasound we now very seldom rely on adjuvants for speed of onset or prolongation of blocks (e.g., epinephrine, alkalizing agent).

Test Dose with Dextrose 5% in Water Prior to Local Anesthetic Injection

- A test dose of a nonconducting solution [e.g., dextrose 5% in water (D5W)] is beneficial prior to local anesthetic injection during peripheral nerve blockade.
- The solution can be easily visualized by ultrasound, especially with color Doppler, and can indicate the approximate spread of the local anesthetic. Carefully observing the D5W spread will help confirm extravascular and extraneural needle placement, especially when threshold current during nerve stimulation is <0.4 mA.
- When used with nerve stimulation, the D5W solution will confirm needle placement near the nerve if the motor response is maintained or augmented (see Chapter 2).

4.2.9. Injection Pressure

Injection pressure can be an important factor when intraneural injection is considered. The incidence of nerve injury as a result of peripheral nerve blocks is reported, varying from <0.1% to 1%. However, manifestations of block-related neurological injuries can be severe and may be persistent. Several studies suggest that high-pressure injection into the intraneural space is a major contributing factor to neurological injury during peripheral nerve blocks. Considerable and prolonged elevation of intrafascicular pressure may cause membrane rupture or detrimentally interfere with the endoneurial microcirculation, leading to potentiation of local anesthetic toxicity.

A recent study showed that persistent motor deficits were observed in dogs injected intraneurally with pressures ≥ 25 psi [1293 mm Hg from conversion factor 1 psi = 51.71 mm Hg; 171.9 kPa (1 psi = 6894 Pa); 1.7 atm (1 psi = 0.068 atm)]. Fortunately, the intraneural injections that were not associated with high pressures did not result in persistent motor deficits, perhaps indicating that the injection pressure may be a limiting factor.

A primary issue related to high injection pressures in clinical practice is that what is perceived to be an abnormally high resistance to injection is subjective and based on experience alone. In fact, a recent study by Claudio and colleagues (2004) showed that anesthesiologists vary widely in their ability to perceive an appropriate pressure and rate of injection during peripheral nerve blocks. An additional concern is that injections are commonly performed by an assistant while the anesthesiologist maintains the correct needle position, thus making injection pressures difficult to monitor objectively.

To address both issues of limiting and reducing the variability in pressures, it is desirable to develop a method of injection monitoring which allows accurate prediction of whether injection pressures are at reasonable levels without being too complicated and at the same time conducive to contemporaneous assessment for anesthesiologists. Tsui and colleagues (Tsui, Li and Pillay, 2006) were able to demonstrate that a compressed air injection technique (CAIT), using Boyle's law (PV = constant; confirmed with an in vitro experimental system) and typical regional anesthesia equipment, could consistently maintain injection pressures below 1293 mm Hg.

4.2.9.1. *Compressed Air Injection Technique*

A compressed air injection technique involves introducing a set amount of air above a volume of injectate in a syringe, with subsequent compression and maintenance of this volume during injection to maintain the pressure at a chosen level (Figure 4.10). Depending on the percentage of air compression, the pressure can be theoretically maintained at a level

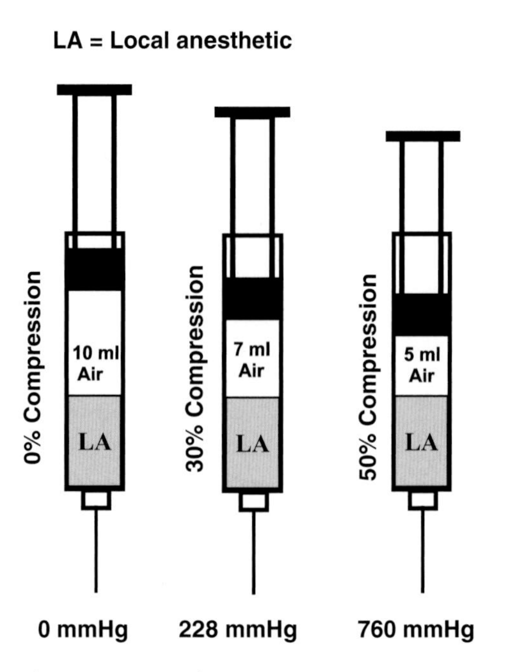

Figure 4.10. Compressed air injection technique to monitor injection pressures. An initial volume of air is withdrawn into the syringe (e.g., 10 mL) above the injectate and this air is compressed to a maximum of 50% (e.g., 5 mL remaining) prior to and during the injection. Using Boyle's law (pressure × volume = constant), the pressure will double to a net pressure of approximately 760 mm Hg (1 atm) and remain below a pressure limit of 1293 mm Hg. (Adapted with permission from Tsui BC, Li LX, Pillay JJ. Compressed air injection technique to standardize block injection pressures. Can J Anesth 2006;53:1098–102.)

determined by Boyle's law (pressure × volume = constant). Tsui and coworkers now typically use this method in the following fashion:

- A set volume of air (10 mL) is drawn into a 30-mL syringe above the 20 mL of local anesthetic and then compressed and maintained at 5 mL (50% compression).
- Theoretically, the pressure (approximated at the needle tip) should reach and be maintained at twice atmospheric pressure at 50% compression (approximately net pressure at the needle tip 760.0 mm Hg), which is well below the clinically significant figure of 1293 mm Hg.
- The key advantage is that the standardized pressure of 760 mm Hg prevents rapidly rising peak pressures and thus reduces the risk of reaching the high pressures (1293 mm Hg) associated with clinically significant neural injury.
- Two obvious limitations of this technique include potential variability of injection pressures (under manual control) and the possible risk of air injection.
    - It is important to consider the accidental injection of the withdrawn air into a blood vessel with the possibility of a venous or arterial air embolism. Embolic complications can possibly occur when performing the loss-of-resistance technique with air associated with epidural placement. Although concerns are real if enough air reaches the venous circulation (as with epidurals), the inherent air-volume monitoring aspect of this technique could carefully safeguard against any air injection.

> By using CAIT (at a maximum 50% compression), with generation of pressures well below 1293 mm Hg, the ability to monitor one's own or the assistants' injection pressures is assured. Further studies evaluating the usefulness of this technique in clinical practice are needed.

4.2.10. Appropriate Sedation

Appropriate sedation and analgesia is also an essential part of successful regional anesthesia in order to achieve the maximum benefits with minimal side effects. Effective sedation can be achieved with propofol, midazloam, fentanyl, ketamine, remifentanil, alfentanil, or a combination of these drugs. The dosages of these drugs should be titrated to reach a level of sedation appropriate for the individual patient, the specific nerve block procedure, and the length of surgery. Some examples are listed below:

- Bolus
  - Midazolam 1 to 2 mg (titrated up to 0.07 mg/kg)
  - Fentanyl 0.5 to 1 mcg/kg
  - Alfentanil 7 to 10 mcg/kg
  - Ketamine 0.1 to 0.5 mg/kg
- Infusion
  - Remifentanil 0.02 to 0.1 mcg/kg/min

4.3. Ultrasound-Guidance Training

- There are as yet no formal training recommendations for ultrasound-guided nerve localization for regional anesthesia.
- A recent World Health Organization (WHO) study group (1998) found that much work in ultrasound is carried out by essentially untrained individuals and commented that "the success of any interventional procedure is very dependant on the skill and experience of the responsible physician." (p. 3)
- A recent study published in *Regional Anesthesia and Pain Medicine* by Sites and colleagues (2004), found a "concerning novice pattern" (Sites et al, 2006; p544) of trainees advancing block needles despite failing to adequately follow the needle in the ultrasound image. This could clearly lead to dangerous outcomes, particularly at locations where inadvertent intrapleural or intravascular injection could occur (e.g., supraclavicular or femoral artery, respectively).
- As with many other techniques in regional anesthesia, ultrasound-guided regional anesthesia has a significant learning curve and there seems to be a need for a formal training curriculum, including formative and summative evaluation processes, built into the program.
- Determining the optimal technique for safe and effective block injections should be a continual process in order to maximize learning.
- As discussed above, several neural structures are best visualized using highly reliable and visually obvious landmarks. Additionally, using appropriate needling technique (i.e., in-plane vs. out-of-plane) with optimal methodology may help determine the safety of ultrasound guidance.
- Currently, the primary challenge is determining the required length of supervised training and/or the minimum number of successful ultrasound-guided blocks necessary for each practitioner to perform in order to enable reliability in practice.
- Additionally, it is unclear at this time how we should evaluate and ensure our competency with this new emerging skill. It may become evident that ultrasound use for regional anesthesia requires similar, yet less intensive, training to that required for diagnostic ultrasonography.
- Development of a suitable curriculum involving supervised training, a standard evaluation process and continuing education credits could ensure a consistent and high quality of ultrasound-guided regional anesthesia.
- Ultimately, the ability to provide competent care to our patients may occur when we can affirmatively answer the question: What are the credentials or training requirements to allow us to use ultrasound effectively?

Suggested Reading and References

Auroy Y, Narchi P, Messiah A, Litt L, Rouvier B, Samii K. Serious complications related to regional anesthesia: results of a prospective study in France. Anesthesiology 1997;87:479–486.

Borgeat A, Blumenthal S. Nerve injury and regional anaesthesia. Curr Opin Anaesthesiol 2004;17:417–421.

Chan VWS. The use of ultrasound for peripheral nerve blocks. In: Boezaart AP, ed. Anesthesia and orthopaedic surgery. New York: McGraw-Hill; 2006; pp. 283–290.

Claudio R, Hadzic A, Shih H, et al. Injection pressures by anesthesiologists during simulated peripheral nerve block. Reg Anesth Pain Med 2004;29:201–205.

Grau T. Ultrasound in the current practice of regional anesthesia. Best Pract Res Clin Anaesthesiol 2005;19:175–200.

Gray AT. Ultrasound-guided regional anesthesia. Current state of the art. Anesthesiology 2006;104:368–373.

Hadzic A, Dilberovic F, Shah S, et al. Combination of intraneural injection and high injection pressure leads to fascicular injury and neurologic deficits in dogs. Reg Anesth Pain Med 2004;29:417–423.

MacLean CA, Bachman DT. Documented arterial gas embolism after spinal epidural injection. Ann Emerg Med 2001;38:592–595.

Marhofer P, Greher M, Kapral S. Ultrasound guidance in regional anesthesia. Br J Anaesth 2005;94:7–17.

Roelants F, Veyckemans F, Van Obbergh L, et al. Loss of resistance to saline with a bubble of air to identify the epidural space in infants and children: a prospective study. Anesth Analg 2000;90:59–61.

Saberski LR, Kondamuri S, Osinubi OY. Identification of the epidural space: is loss of resistance to air a safe technique? A review of the complications related to the use of air. Reg Anesth 1997;22:3–15.

Schafhalter-Zoppoth I, McColluch CE, Gray AT. Ultrasound visibility of needles used for regional nerve block: an in vitro study. Reg Anesth Pain Med 2004;29:480–488.

Sites BD, Gallagher JD, Cravero J, Lundberg J, Blike G. The learning curve associated with a simulated ultrasound-guided interventional task by inexperienced anesthesia residents. Reg Anesth Pain Med 2004;29:544–548.

Tsui BC. "Credentials" in ultrasound-guided regional blocks. Reg Anesth Pain Med 2006;31:587–588.

Tsui BC. Facilitating needle alignment in-plane to an ultrasound beam using a portable laser unit. Reg Anesth Pain Med 2007;32:84–88.

Tsui BC, Dillane D. Needle puncture site and a "walkdown" approach for short-axis alignment during ultrasound-guided blocks. Reg Anesth Pain Med 2006;31:586–587.

Tsui BC, Finucane BT. Practical recommendations for improving needle-tip visibility under ultrasound guidance. Reg Anesth Pain Med 2005;30:596–597.

Tsui BC, Finucane BT. The importance of ultrasound landmarks: a "traceback" approach using the popliteal blood vessels for identification of the sciatic nerve. Reg Anesth Pain Med 2006;31:481–482.

Tsui BC, Twomey C, Finucane BT. Visualization of the brachial plexus in the supraclavicular region using a curved ultrasound probe with a sterile transparent dressing. Reg Anesth Pain Med 2006;31:182–184.

Tsui BCH, Li LXY, Pillay JJ. Compressed air injection technique to standardize block injection pressures. Can J Anesth 2006;53:1098–1102.

World Health Organization. Training in diagnostic ultrasound: essentials, principles and standards. Report of a WHO Study Group. Geneva: World health Organization, 1998. WHO Technical Report Series, No. 875.

5

Clinical Anatomy for Upper Limb Blocks

Ban C.H. Tsui

5.1. Origin of Spinal Nerves

A brief overview of the origin of the spinal nerves as related to peripheral nerve blockade is important to cover for a clear understanding of the formation of the different nerve plexuses and thoracic neuroanatomy.

The spinal nerves are part of the peripheral nervous system, along with the cranial and autonomic nerves and their ganglia. There are 31 pairs of spinal nerves—8 cervical (C1–C8), 12 thoracic (T1–T12), 5 lumbar (L1–L5), 5 sacral (S1–S5), and 1 coccygeal. These spinal nerves are formed by the union of the ventral (anterior) and dorsal (posterior) spinal roots. They are mixed nerves consisting of both motor and sensory fibers. In addition, all spinal nerves contain sympathetic fibers which supply blood vessels, smooth muscle, and glands in the skin. Soon after exiting the intervertebral (spinal) foramina, each spinal nerve in turn divides into a larger ventral and a smaller dorsal ramus (Figure 5.1). The ventral rami course laterally and anteriorly to supply the muscles, subcutaneous tissues (superficial fascia), and skin of the neck, trunk, and the upper and lower extremities. The dorsal rami course posteriorly and supply the paravertebral muscles, subcutaneous tissues, and skin of the back close to the midline.

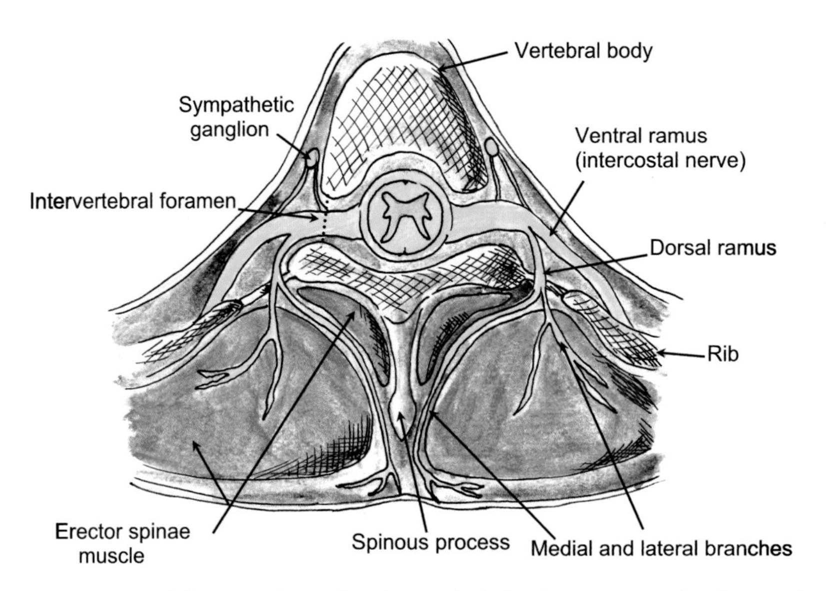

Figure 5.1. Overview of the central neural and musculoskeletal structures at the thoracic level.

It is important to realize that the first cervical (C1) nerve leaves the spinal cord and courses above the atlas (C1 vertebra), hence the cervical nerves are numbered corresponding to the vertebrae inferior to them, for example, the C8 nerve exiting below C7 and above T1 (Figure 5.2). From this point on, all the spinal nerves are named corresponding to the vertebral level above. For example, T3 and L4 spinal nerves exit below T3 and L4 vertebra, respectively.

5.2. The Brachial Plexus

The brachial plexus provides innervation to the skin, subcutaneous tissues, and muscles of the entire upper limb from the shoulder to the fingers. Surgical anesthesia and postoperative

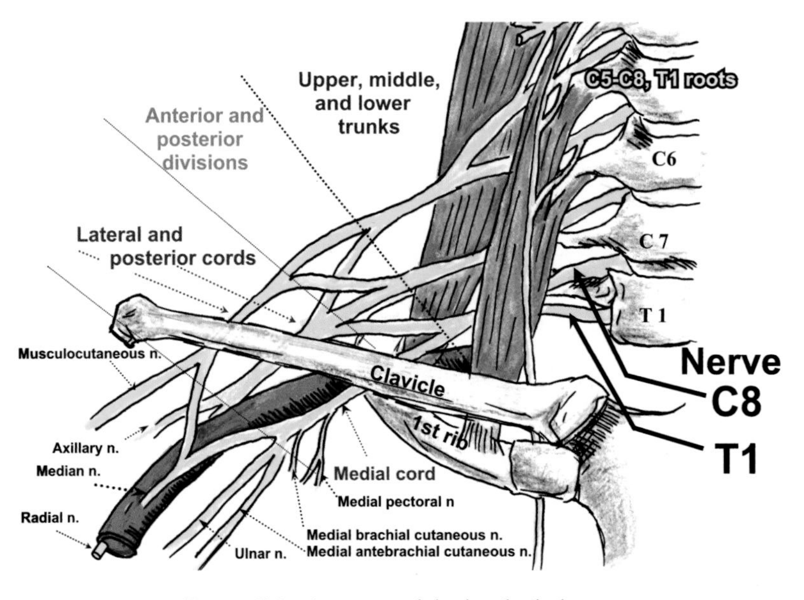

Figure 5.2. Anatomy of the brachial plexus.

analgesia can result from local anesthetic blockade of the brachial plexus at any point along its course.

The interscalene and periclavicular block approaches (e.g., supraclavicular, intersternocleidomastoid, and subclavian perivascular) target the brachial plexus at the root and trunk levels while the infraclavicular, axillary, and peripheral approaches target the cords and terminal nerves of the brachial plexus.

This chapter highlights the segmental innervation to the upper extremity, while the anatomy and distribution of the peripheral nerves are discussed at length in subsequent chapters. Figure 5.3(A,B) highlights the most clinically relevant nerves of the upper extremity.

5.2.1. The Brachial Plexus

- The brachial plexus (Figures 5.2 and 5.4) arises in the cervical region from the anterior primary rami of C5 to C8 and most of T1 spinal nerves. There are some variations. For example, the plexus may include anterior rami from C4 to C8 (prefixed), or from C5 to T2 (postfixed).
- From proximal to distal, the plexus consists of five *roots* (paravertebral), three *trunks* (interscalene), two *divisions* per trunk (subclavian), three *cords* (axillary), and five major terminal nerves (brachial; Figure 5.4).
- The C5 to T1 nerve roots emerge from their corresponding intervertebral foramina and then travel along the grooves between the anterior and posterior tubercles of the corresponding transverse processes. They finally emerge between the scalenus anterior and medius muscles (all five roots lie above the second part of subclavian artery and posterior the vertebral artery).
- C5 and C6 nerve roots unite to form the *upper (superior) trunk*, C7 continues as the *middle trunk*, and C8 and T1 converge into the *lower (inferior) trunk*.
- Two fibrous sheaths (as part of the prevertebral fascia) surround the anterior and posterior parts of the plexus and continue to envelop the plexus between the scalene muscles more distally (called the *interscalene fascial sheath* proximally and the *axillary sheath* distally). This fibrous sheath extends to surround the brachial plexus all the way to the axilla.
- The three trunks travel inferolaterally and cross the base of the posterior triangle of the neck (superficial) and the first rib (upper and middle trunks above subclavian artery and lower trunk below the artery); these are the locations of the supraclavicular, intersternocleidomastoid, and subclavian perivascular blocks.
- At the lateral border of first rib, each trunk bifurcates into *anterior* and *posterior* divisions.
- At the apex of the axilla, under the lateral border of the pectoralis minor, the divisions converge to form three *cords*: *lateral cord* [anterior divisions of upper and middle trunks (C5–7)]; *medial cord* [anterior division of lower trunk (C8, T1)]; and *posterior cord* [posterior divisions of all three trunks (C5–T1)].
  - The cords are grouped around the second part of the axillary artery [there are three parts of the axillary artery named for their positions above (medial to), behind, and below (lateral to) the pectoralis minor muscle] beginning with the *medial* cord behind and the *posterior* and *lateral cords* lateral to the first part of the axillary artery.
  - Immediately after the pectoralis minor muscle, the three cords diverge into the terminal branches; these include the median, ulnar, radial, axillary, and musculocutaneous nerves.

5.2.2. Branches of the Brachial Plexus

Branches from the roots and trunks of the plexus are given off above the clavicle (supraclavicular), while branches from the cords are given off from below the clavicle (infraclavicular). Some of these branches are illustrated in Figures 5.2 and 5.4.

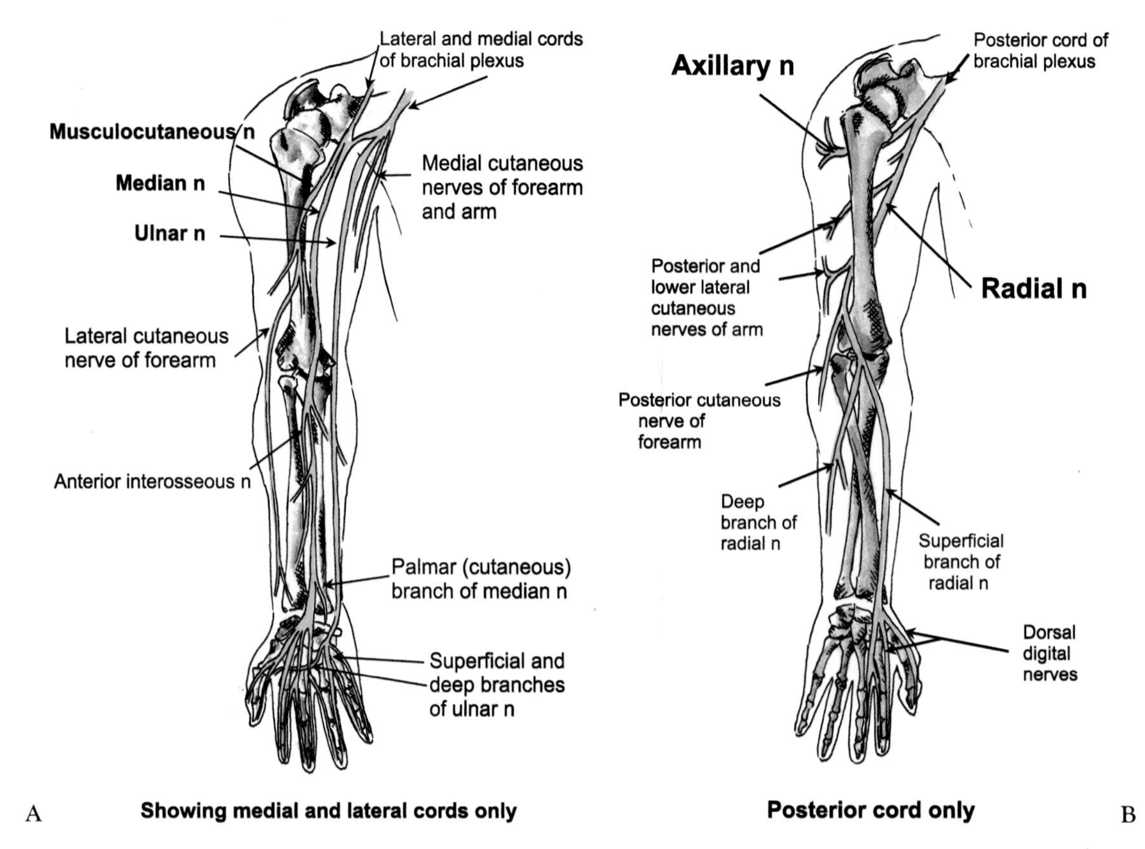

Figure 5.3. Peripheral nerves of the upper extremity. For ease of illustration, (A) the lateral and medial cords are shown in one drawing and (B) the posterior cord is shown on another.

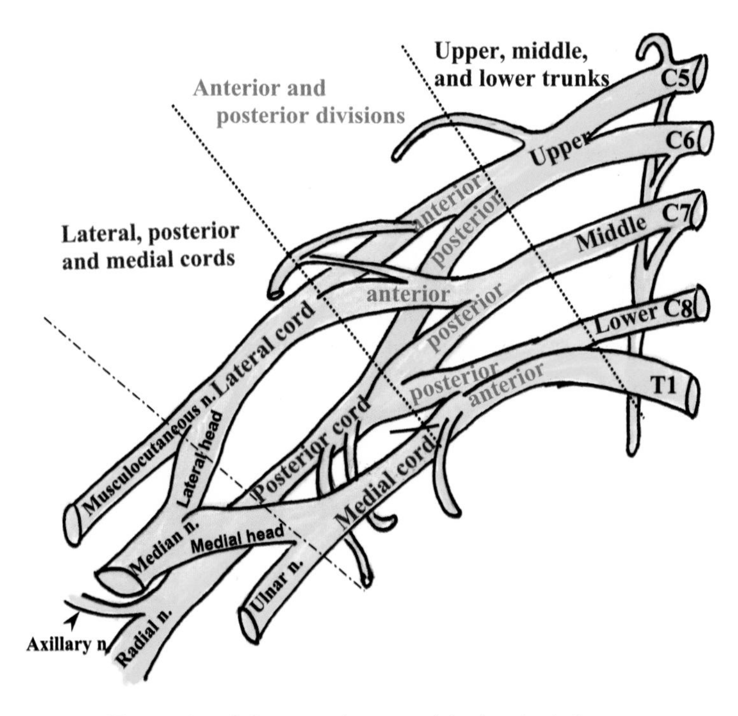

Figure 5.4. Schematic diagram of the brachial plexus.

- Root branches
  - Nerve to longus cervicis muscle (C5–C8)
  - Nerve to longus colli and scalene muscles (C5–C8)
  - Nerve to rhomboids (C5)
  - Nerve to serratus anterior (C5–C7)
  - Contribution to phrenic nerve (C5)
- Trunk branches
  - Nerve to subclavius (superior trunk, C5, C6)
  - Suprascapular nerve (superior trunk, C5, C6)
- Cord branches
  - Lateral cord
    - Lateral pectoral nerve (C5–C7); musculocutaneous nerve (C5–C7); lateral head (root) of median nerve (C6, C7)
  - Medial cord
    - Medial pectoral nerve (C8, T1); medial cutaneous nerve of arm (medial brachial cutaneous nerve; C8, T1); medial cutaneous nerve of forearm (medial antebrachial cutaneous nerve; C8, T1); medial head (root) of median nerve (C8, T1); ulnar nerve (C8, T1)
  - Posterior cord
    - Upper subscapular nerve (C5, C6); thoracodorsal nerve (C6–C8); lower subscapular nerve (C5, C6); axillary nerve (C5, C6); radial nerve (C5–C8, T1)

Terminal nerves of the brachial plexus, which provide motor innervation to the upper extremity, are summarized in Table 5.1. These nerves will be described in more detail in subsequent chapters with respect to their origins, course, and function as related to clinical practice.

Table 5.1. Target nerves of the upper extremity blocks: origin and motor responses associated with nerve stimulation.

Movement	Nerve	Cord	Division	Trunk	Root
Arm abduction	Suprascapular			Upper	C5, C6
Arm abduction	Axillary	Posterior	Posterior	Upper	C5, C6
Elbow flexion	Musculocutaneous	Lateral	Posterior and anterior	Upper	C5, C6
Extension (dorsiflexion) of elbow, wrist, hand, and fingers	Radial	Posterior	Posterior Posterior	Upper Middle	C5, C6 C7
Latissimus dorsi twitch (shoulder shrug)	Thoracodorsal	Posterior	Posterior	Middle	C7
Forearm pronation and wrist flexion	Median (lateral head)	Lateral Medial	Anterior Anterior and posterior Anterior	Upper Middle Lower	C5, C6 C7 C8, T1
Thumb flexion and opposition (flexion middle and ring finger)	Median	Medial	Anterior	Lower	C8, T1
Thumb flexion and opposition	Anterior interosseous	Medial	Anterior	Lower	C8, T1
Fifth finger flexion and opposition, ulnar deviation of wrist	Ulnar	Medial	Anterior	Lower	C8, T1

5.3. Distribution of Spinal Nerves in the Upper Extremity

Detailed knowledge and understanding of the dermatomes, myotomes, and osteotomes of the upper extremity is extremely important for providing successful surgical anesthesia and effective analgesia for any upper limb procedure. Below is a detailed examination of the dermatomes, myotomes, and osteotomes of the upper extremity. Although it is generally more useful to consider musculoskeletal regions (i.e., shoulder, elbow, etc.) for anesthesia procedures, a sound knowledge of the complex arrangement of spinal nerves and their segmentation patterns in the extremities will be beneficial for a true appreciation of the applications of regional blocks in the extremities.

5.3.1. Dermatomes

With the exception of C1 (which does not have a sensory component), sensory fibers from the dorsal roots of the spinal nerves supply a specific segment or band of skin. This skin segment is termed a *dermatome*. C5 to T1 spinal nerves provide cutaneous innervation to the upper extremity. There is considerable overlap between contiguous dermatomes and adjacent dermatomes are generally arranged as consecutive horizontal bands on the surface of the axial skeleton, and more or less vertical projections on the extremities (Figures 5.5 and 5.6). Anatomical knowledge of respective dermatomes will help to block the appropriate skin segment during peripheral nerve blockade. Dermatomes are important particularly for peripheral nerve blockade, and clinically, fairly specific areas of regional anesthesia can be achieved based on the cutaneous innervation produced by the terminal nerves in that part of the body (Figures 5.7 and 5.8).

5.3.1.1. *Segmental Cutaneous Innervation (Dermatomes) of the Upper Extremity*

- C3 and C4, upper shoulder region (supraclavicular nerves)
- C5, deltoid and lateral aspect of arm
- C6, lateral forearm and thumb
- C7, hand and middle three fingers
- C8, fifth finger and medial side of both hand and lower forearm
- T1, medial side of lower arm and upper forearm
- T2, medial side of upper arm (intercostobrachial nerve)

5.3.2. Myotomes

The ventral (motor) roots of the spinal cord provide motor innervation to the skeletal muscles by providing motor nerve fibers to the spinal nerves. A myotome is a block of skeletal muscle that is supplied segmentally by the ventral roots of a spinal nerve; movements of the extremities and trunk that are created by these myotomes can thus be classified segmentally (see segmental motor responses associated with nerve stimulation). In general, segmental innervation of the muscles can be fairly well differentiated. In addition to segmental (myotomal) distribution of innervation, there is also specific muscular distribution that is derived from the terminal nerves (Figures 5.9 and 5.10). Knowledge of this terminal nerve innervation will be extremely important when blocking the brachial plexus branches at sites beyond the root level (e.g., during axillary block it will be useful to use radial nerve motor responses to confirm posterior cord localization). Table 5.1 summarizes the origin of each terminal nerve and its objective movement upon electrical stimulation. This table is

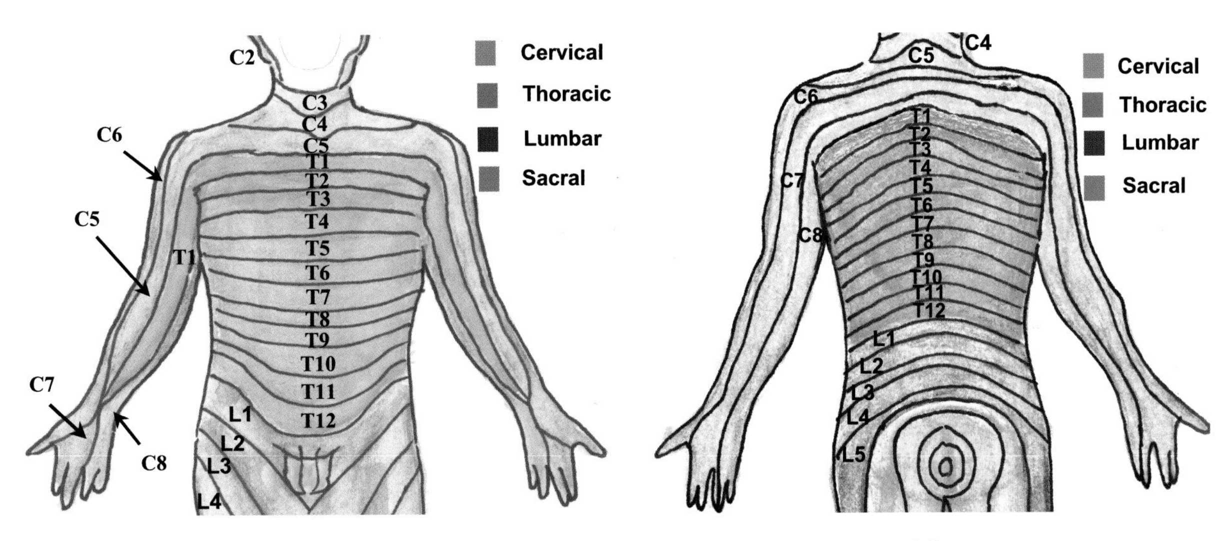

Figure 5.5. Dermatomes of the upper extremity; anterior view.

Figure 5.6. Dermatomes of the upper extremity; posterior view.

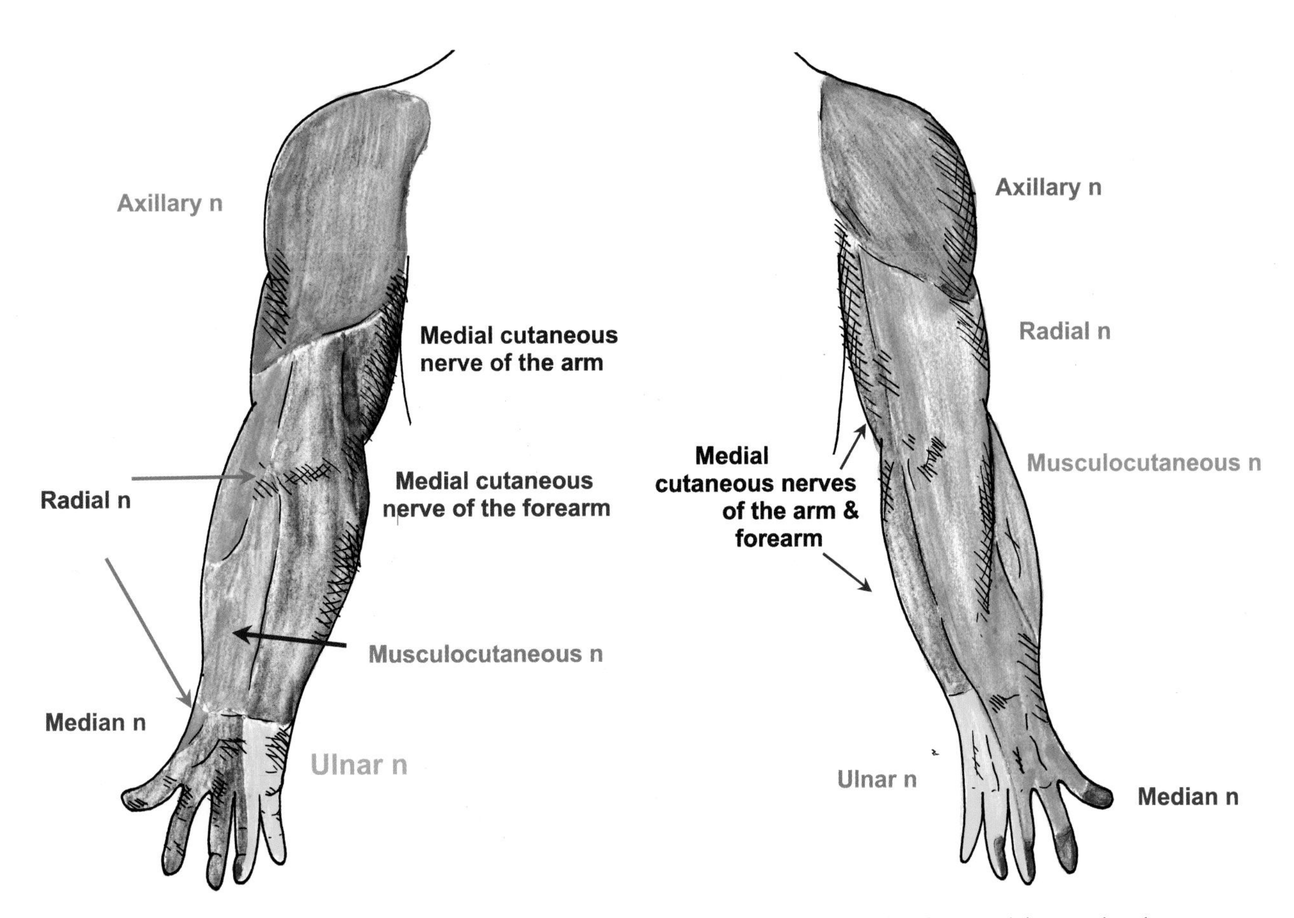

Figure 5.7. Cutaneous distribution of the peripheral nerves; anterior view.

Figure 5.8. Cutaneous distribution of the peripheral nerves; posterior view.

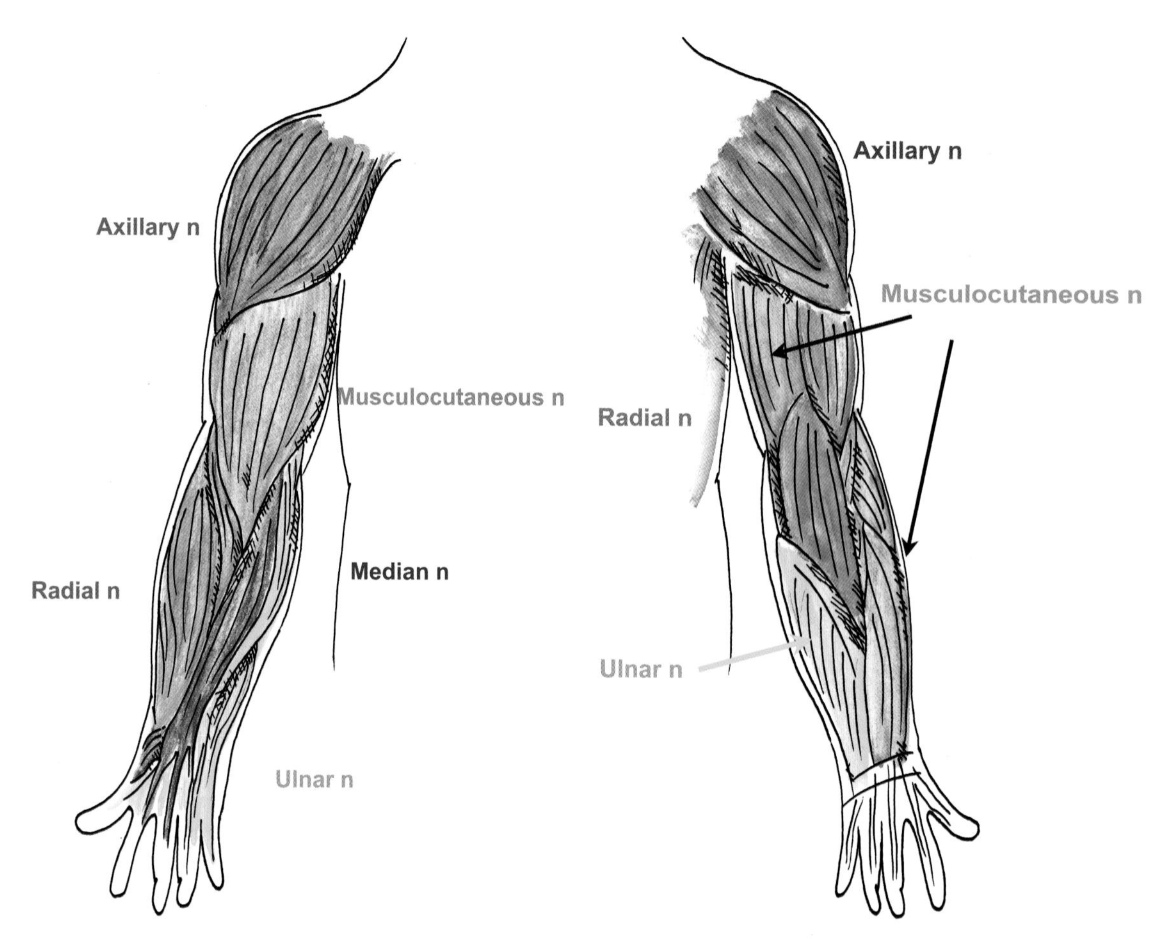

Figure 5.9. Distribution of muscular innervation by the terminal nerves of the upper extremity; anterior view.

Figure 5.10. Distribution of muscular innervation by the terminal nerves of the lower extremity; anterior view.

important for using with nerve stimulation and will also appear in the nerve stimulation sections within relevant chapters.

5.3.2.1. *Segmental Motor Responses Associated with Nerve Stimulation*

- C5, lateral rotation and abduction of the shoulder
- C6, pronation and supination of the forearm
- C5 and C6, elbow flexion
- C6 to C8, medial rotation and adduction of the shoulder
- C6 and C7, elbow extension
- C6 and C7, wrist flexion and extension (long flexor and extensor muscles of wrist)
- C7 and C8, digit flexion and extension (long flexors and extensors of fingers), opposition of thumb
- T1, intrinsic movements of the hand

5.3.2.2. *Muscular Distribution of Spinal Segments*

- C5, rhomboids, supraspinatus, infraspinatus, anterior portion of deltoid, long head of biceps

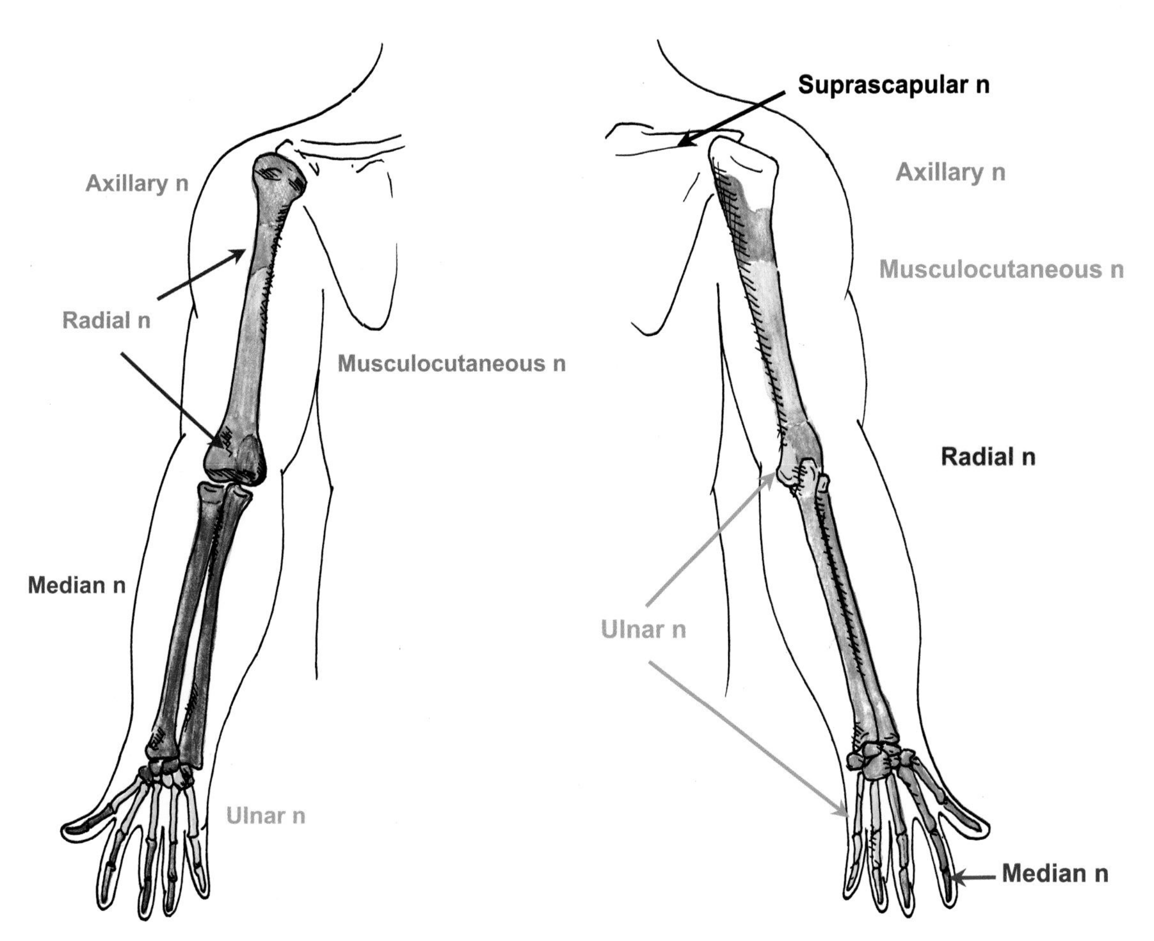

Figure 5.11. Osteomes of the upper extremity; anterior view.

Figure 5.12. Osteomes of the upper extremity; posterior view.

- C6, teres major and minor, middle and posterior deltoid, short head of biceps, coracobrachialis, brachialis, brachioradialis, extensor carpi radialis longus and brevis, supinator, pronator teres
- C7, triceps, anconeus, extensor digitorum, extensor digiti minimi, extensor carpi ulnaris, abductor pollicis longus, extensor pollicis longus and brevis, extensor indicis, flexor carpi radialis
- C8, flexor digitorum superficialis and profundus, flexor carpi ulnaris, flexor pollicis longus, pronator quadratus, abductor and flexor pollicis brevis, opponens pollicis
- T1, flexor digitorum superficialis, abductor digiti minimi, adductor pollicis, flexor digiti minimi brevis, opponens digiti minimi, palmar and dorsal interossei, lumbricals

5.3.3. Osteotomes

Terminal nerves, rather than spinal cord segments, distribute sensory innervation to specific regions of bones throughout the extremities. These regions of the bones, each supplied by a specific branch of a terminal nerve, are defined as *osteotomes* (Figures 5.11 and 5.12). In addition, these terminal nerves also send articular branches to specific joints in the extremity. The innervation of bones can be significantly different from that of the muscles and skin. A good knowledge of joint innervation is important for orthopedic surgery as well as other surgical specialties and neurology. Table 5.2 outlines the innervation of the upper extremity joints and associated motor responses for use when nerve stimulation is used during anesthesia procedures of the joints.

Table 5.2. Upper extremity joint innervation and motor responses associated with nerve stimulation.

Joint	Nerve	Root	Movement
Shoulder			
Anterior and posterior	Suprascapular	C5, C6	Arm abduction
	Axillary	C5, C6	Arm abduction
Elbow			
Anterior	Musculocutaneous	C5, C6	Elbow flexion
	Radial	C5–C7	Extension of elbow, wrist, and fingers
	Median	C5–T1	Thumb flexion and forearm pronation
Posterior	Radial	C5–C7	Extension of elbow, wrist, and fingers
	Ulnar	C8, T1	Fifth finger flexion and opposition
Wrist			
	Radial (superficial)	C5–C7	Extension of elbow, wrist, and fingers
	Median	C5–T1	Thumb flexion and forearm pronation
	Ulnar	C8, T1	Fifth finger flexion and opposition

Suggested Reading and References

Bo WJ, Meschan I, Krueger WA. Basic atlas of cross-sectional anatomy: a clinical approach. Philadelphia: Saunders; 1980.

Ellis H, Feldman S, Harrop-Griffiths W, eds. Anatomy for anaesthesiologists, 8th ed. Boston: Blackwell; 2004.

Lee B. Atlas of surgical and sectional anatomy. Stamford, CT: Appleton-Century-Crofts; 1983.

Netter FH. Atlas of human anatomy. Summit, NJ: CIBA-GEIGY Corporation; 1989.

6 Interscalene Block

Ban C.H. Tsui

Ultrasound-guided interscalene block targets the roots and proximal trunks of the brachial plexus where they are sandwiched between scalenus anterior and medius muscles (SAM and SMM) at the level of the sixth cervical vertebra (C6). The trunks are contained within a fascial sheath (interscalene sheath) at this level. Some anesthesiologists insert the needle below C6, although both approaches are successful. This block is indicated mostly for surgical anesthesia to the shoulder, upper arm, and forearm, but is often insufficient for the hand. Figure 6.1 illustrates the target level of the interscalene block (roots or trunks) with respect to the brachial plexus.

6.1. Clinical Anatomy

- From the intervertebral foramina, the five roots of the brachial plexus exit above the transverse processes of the corresponding cervical vertebrae and traverse through the interscalene groove before entering the floor of the posterior triangle of the neck (supraclavicular fossa).
- The scalenus anterior and medius muscles lie immediately anterior and posterior to the plexus in the interscalene region and then insert onto the first rib (Figure 6.2).
- The upper, middle, and lower trunks are enclosed within the interscalene fascial sheath as they emerge between the scalene muscles.
- The trunks may be crossed by the external jugular vein and transverse cervical and suprascapular arteries (both branches of the thyrocervical trunk, which can function as external collaterals of the subclavian artery) as well as supraclavicular nerves as they course inferolaterally.
- Above and at the level of the interscalene groove (C6), the plexus lies posterolateral and deep to the internal jugular vein and common carotid artery.

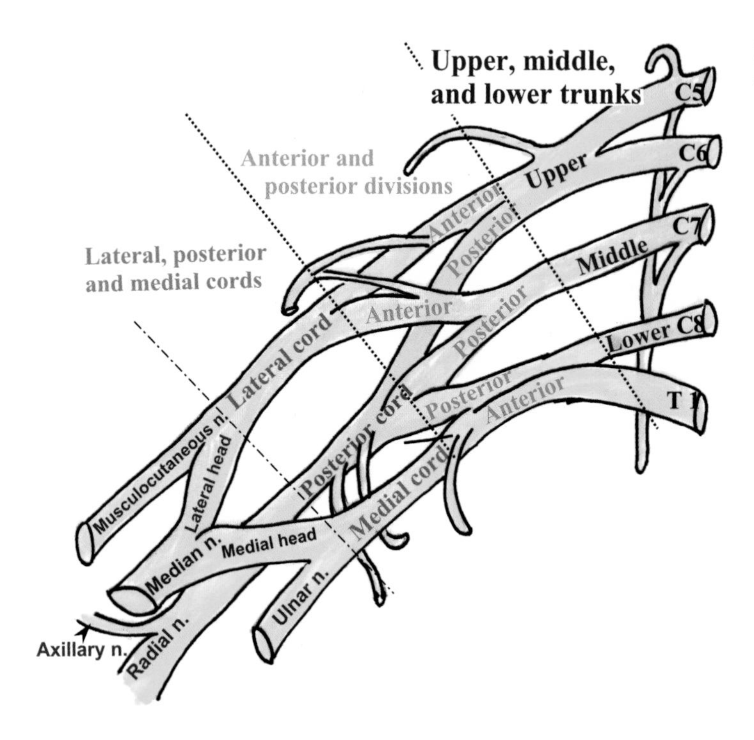

Figure 6.1. Interscalene block targets the roots and trunks within the brachial plexus.

- At the level of the interscalene groove and until it reaches the midpiont of the clavicle, the plexus lies cephaloposterior to the subclavian artery. Importantly, the subclavian vein is separated from the groove by the insertion of the scalenus anterior muscle..
- The phrenic nerve normally descends anterior to the scalenus anterior muscle; it crosses the muscle from lateral to medial as it descends and passes under the clavicle and through the superior thoracic aperture into the superior mediastinum just medial to the external jugular vein (Figure 6.3). However, there is anatomical variation in the course of the phrenic nerve and it is not always anterior to the scalenus anterior muscle.

Table 6.1 summarizes several of the target nerves for brachial plexus blockade at the interscalene region. Each nerve is traced from its origin at the root level and motor responses associated with nerve stimulation are described.

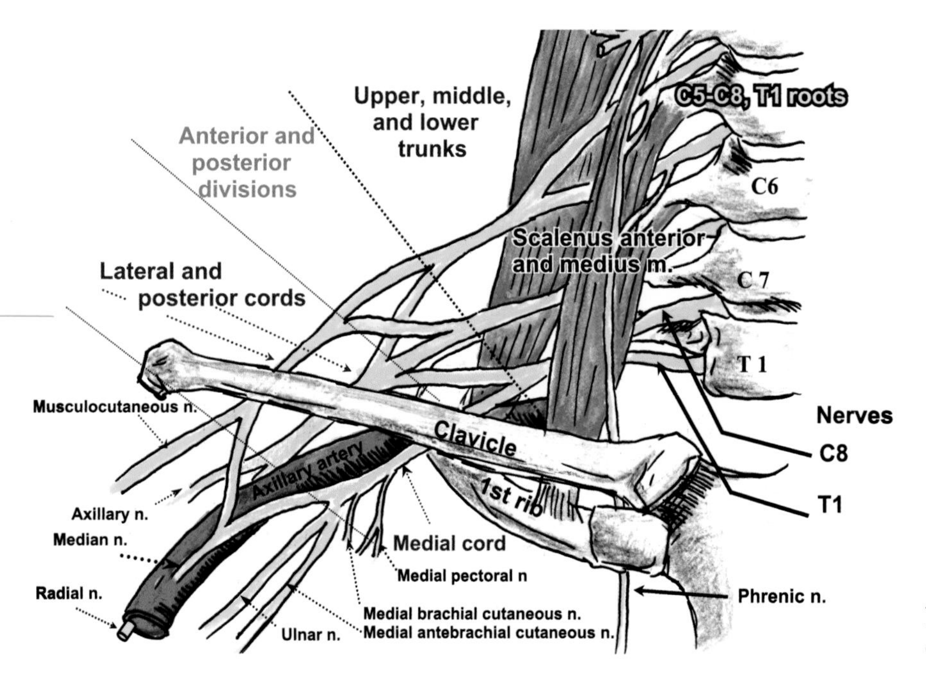

Figure 6.2. Anatomy of the brachial plexus.

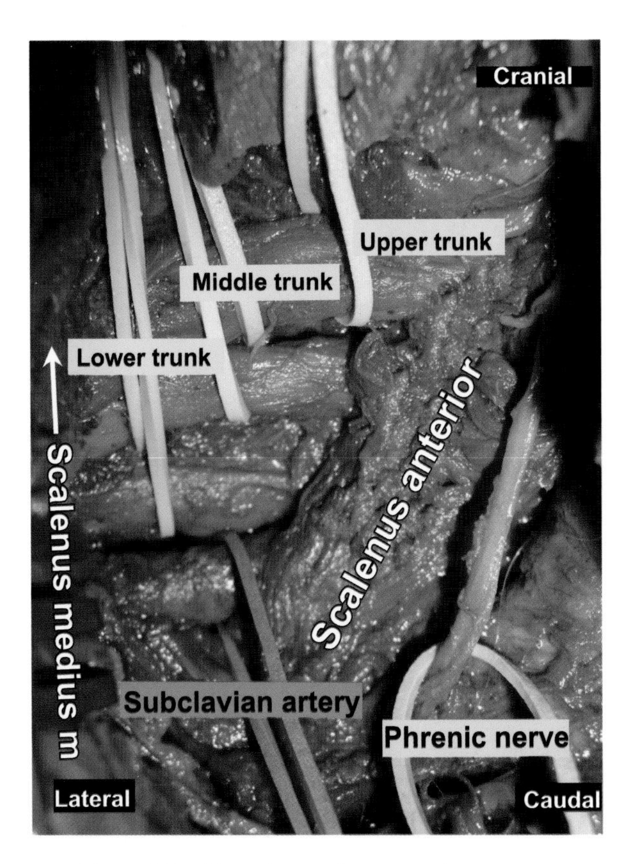

Figure 6.3. Dissection at the interscalene groove.

Table 6.1. Target nerves of the interscalene block: origin and motor response associated with nerve stimulation.

Movement	Nerve	Cord	Division	Trunk	Root
Arm abduction	Suprascapular			Upper	C5, C6
Arm abduction	Axillary	Posterior	Posterior	Upper	C5, C6
Elbow flexion	Musculocutaneous	Lateral	Posterior and anterior	Upper	C5, C6
Extension (dorsiflexion) of elbow, wrist, hand, and fingers	Radial	Posterior	Posterior Posterior	Upper Middle	C5, C6 C7
Latissimus dorsi twitch	Thoracodorsal	Posterior	Posterior	Middle	C7
Forearm pronation and wrist flexion	Median (lateral head)	Lateral Medial	Anterior Anterior and posterior Anterior	Upper Middle Lower	C5, C6 C7 C8, T1
Thumb flexion and opposition (flexion middle and ring finger)	Median	Medial	Anterior	Lower	C8, T1
Thumb flexion and opposition	Anterior interosseous	Medial	Anterior	Lower	C8, T1
Fifth finger flexion and opposition, ulnar deviation of wrist	Ulnar	Medial	Anterior	Lower	C8, T1

Specific segmental dermatomal and myotomal distribution of the brachial plexus is discussed and illustrated in Chapter 5. Nerves that are purely sensory are not included in the table.

6.2. Patient Positioning and Surface Anatomy

6.2.1. Patient Positioning

The main surface landmark (sternocleidomastoid muscle) used for this block can be accentuated by asking the patient to reach for the ipsilateral knee and by rotating the head approximately 45° to the nonoperative side. The head should also be slightly elevated, and the patient should be instructed to take a deep breath (contraction of the scalenus muscles accentuates the interscalene groove).

6.2.2. Surface Anatomy (Figure 6.4)

- Sternocleidomastoid (SCM) muscle
  The lateral border of its clavicular head is a landmark for palpating the interscalene groove
- Interscalene groove
  To locate this groove, first place the tip of the index finger at the posterior edge of the clavicular head of the SCM at the level of C6 (at the cricoid cartilage). Moving posteriorly, the first groove encountered will be that between the SCM and SAM muscles, while the second groove felt is that of the interscalene groove, between the SAM and the SMM muscles. Following this groove inferiorly to the first rib will allow palpation of the scalene muscle attachments and the medially positioned subclavian arterial pulse.

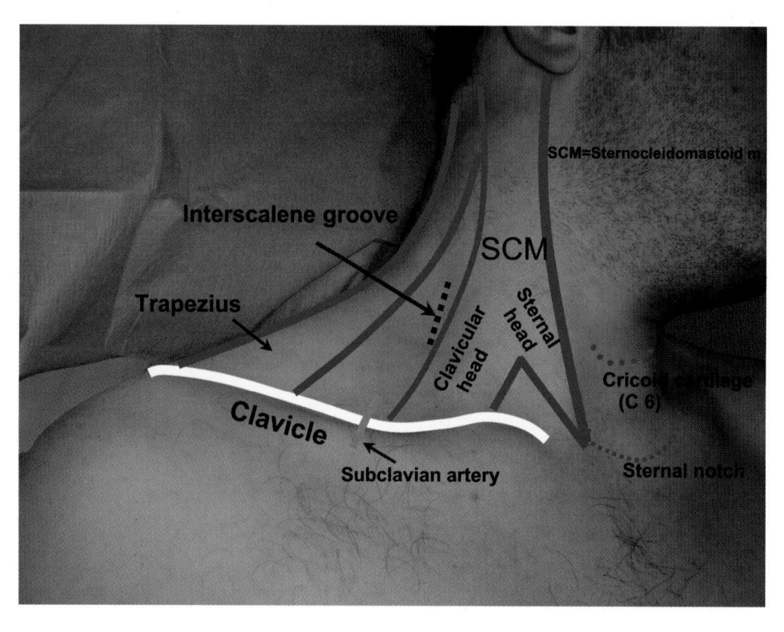

Figure 6.4. Surface anatomy for the interscalene block.

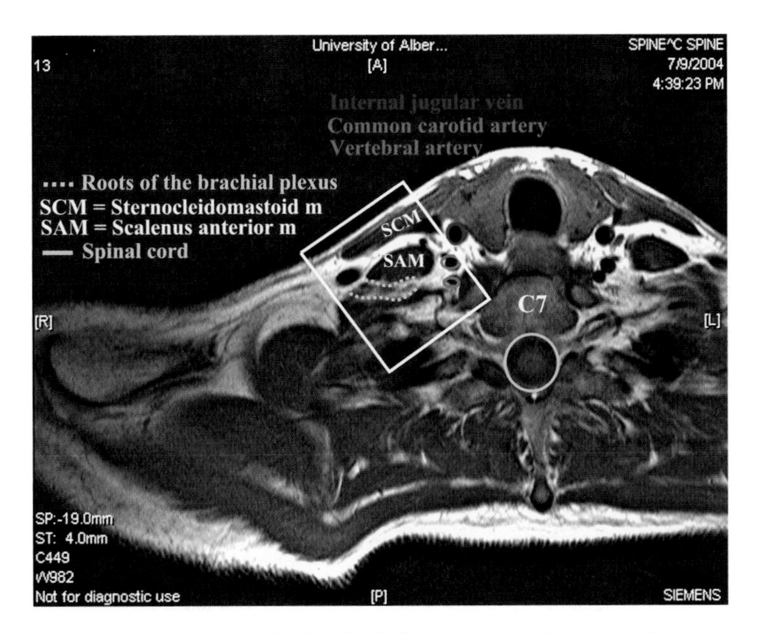

Figure 6.5. MRI depicting the brachial plexus roots in the interscalene groove.

6.3. Sonographic Imaging and Needle Insertion Technique

The trunks of the plexus are clearly shown in both the magnetic resonance imaging (MRI) scan (Figure 6.5) depicting the interscalene level and its corresponding ultrasound image (Figure 6.6).

Prepare the needle insertion site and skin surface with an antiseptic solution. Prepare the ultrasound probe surface by applying a sterile adhesive dressing to it prior to needling as discussed earlier (see Chapters 3 and 4).

6.3.1. Scanning Technique

- A high-frequency linear (10–15 MHz; 38 mm) transducer is often optimal to delineate the complex arrangements of the superficial structures in this region.

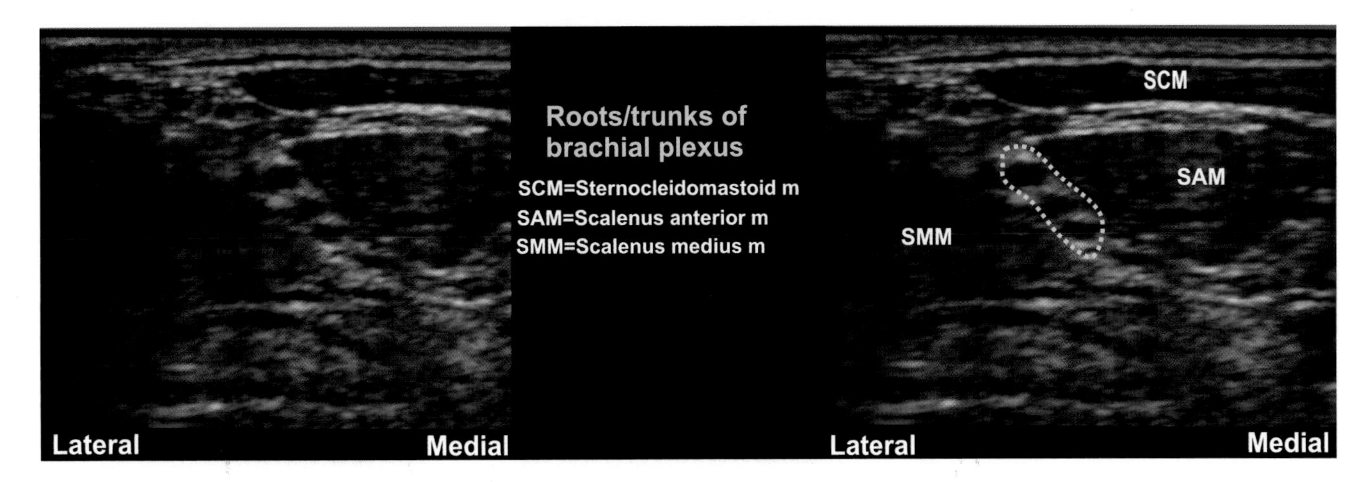

Figure 6.6. Ultrasound image using a linear probe at the interscalene groove. The nerve roots/trunks appear as hypoechoic nodules between scalenus medius and anterior muscles.

- The required depth of penetration is usually within 2 to 3 cm.
- The Doppler can be of great assistance if the subclavian artery is used initially as a landmark for plexus (trunks/divisions) identification at the supraclavicular region, with subsequent tracing in a cephalad direction (a traceback approach is described later in this section and in Chapter 4).
- Two scanning techniques are recommended for interscalene brachial plexus imaging: (1) proximal to distal scan beginning at the cricoid cartilage level (C6) with movement from anterior and medial to posterior and lateral towards the interscalene groove; and (2) distal to proximal scan from supraclavicular to interscalene locations (traceback approach). Clearly, there is considerable overlap between scanning techniques as emphasis is placed on dynamic scanning, whether it is scanning from proximal to distal, distal to proximal, medial to lateral, or vice versa. However, some sort of systematic (i.e., easy and reproducible) approach is best, in the author's opinion, to enhance learning and training.

6.3.1.1. *Cricoid Cartilage Approach*

- With the probe placed transversely over the SCM at the level of the cricoid cartilage (C6), scan laterally toward the interscalene groove. Once there, move the probe distally and proximally to capture the plexus.
- Notice how the SAM changes: smaller proximally above C6 and larger distally. Also notice the hypoechoic nerve roots as they emerge from the intervertebral foramina.
- It may be difficult to visualize the neural structures in the interscalene region, and therefore it may be beneficial to scan the neck inferiorly to the supraclavicular region to identify the nerve structures (hypoechoic, often seen as a cluster like a bunch of grapes; see below).

6.3.1.2. *Traceback Approach* (also see Chapter 4; Figure 6.7)

- The probe is positioned in a coronal oblique plane at the lateral aspect of the upper border of the clavicle.
- While maintaining contact with the clavicle, the probe is moved medially until the pulsating subclavian artery becomes visible (Doppler can be of great assistance).
- Next, the probe is adjusted to place the subclavian artery in the center of the ultrasound screen. The brachial plexus (trunks/divisions) can be seen in short axis as a tightly enclosed cluster (i.e., a honeycomb) superior and lateral to the subclavian artery.
- The image can be adjusted to obtain the clearest picture by tilting the probe anteriorly or posteriorly.
- From this point, the angle is maintained and the plexus is traced in a cephalad direction (to the level of the cricoid cartilage at C6) along the interscalene groove. There should now be a clear image of the neural structures on the ultrasound screen, in a transverse view, deep to the sternocleidomastoid muscle and between the scalenus anterior and medius muscles.

6.3.2. Sonographic Appearance (12+MHz Probe)

- At the level of the cricoid cartilage and deep to the sternocleidomastoid muscle:
  - The common carotid artery appears circular while the internal jugular vein (when present here), which is superolateral to the artery, appears flatter in shape; both are anechoic.
  - The nerve/plexus structures are located posterolateral to the vessels.
- At the interscalene groove in the short-axis view (Figures 6.6 and 6.7):
  - If using a traceback approach, the cluster or honeycomb image will change to become multiple (usually 3) distinct round or oval dark (hypoechoic) masses as the probe is traced cephalad.

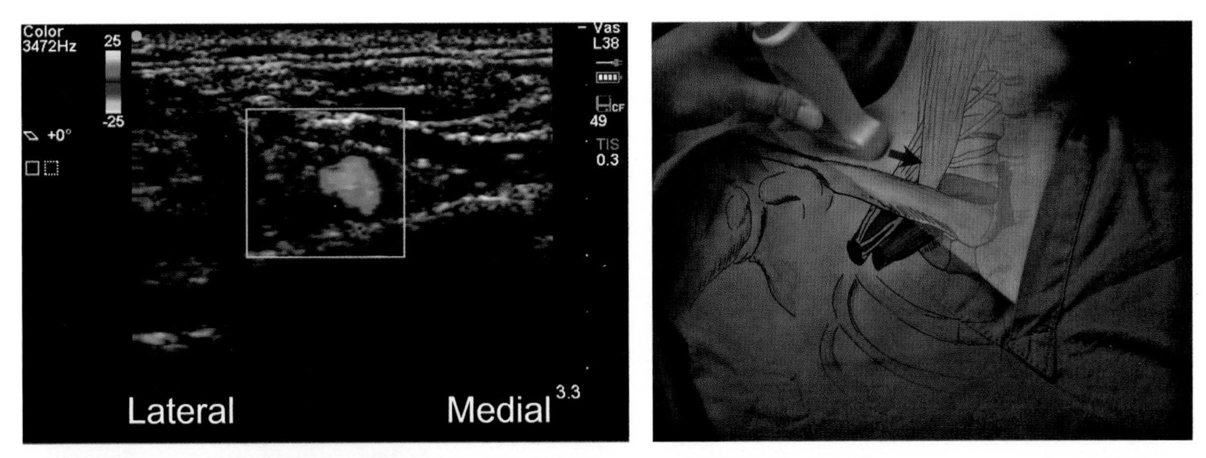

1. Locate the subclavian artery

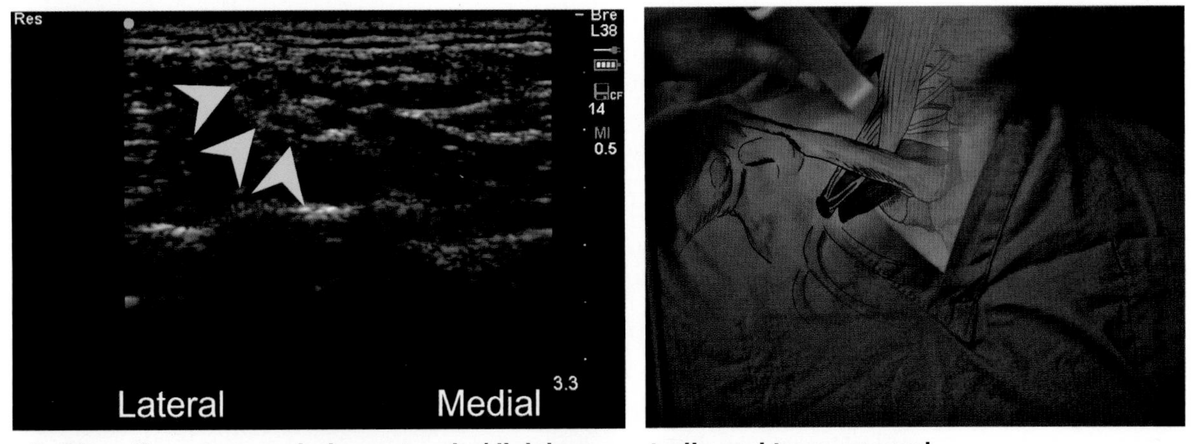

2. Place the artery and plexus trunks/divisions centrally and trace upward

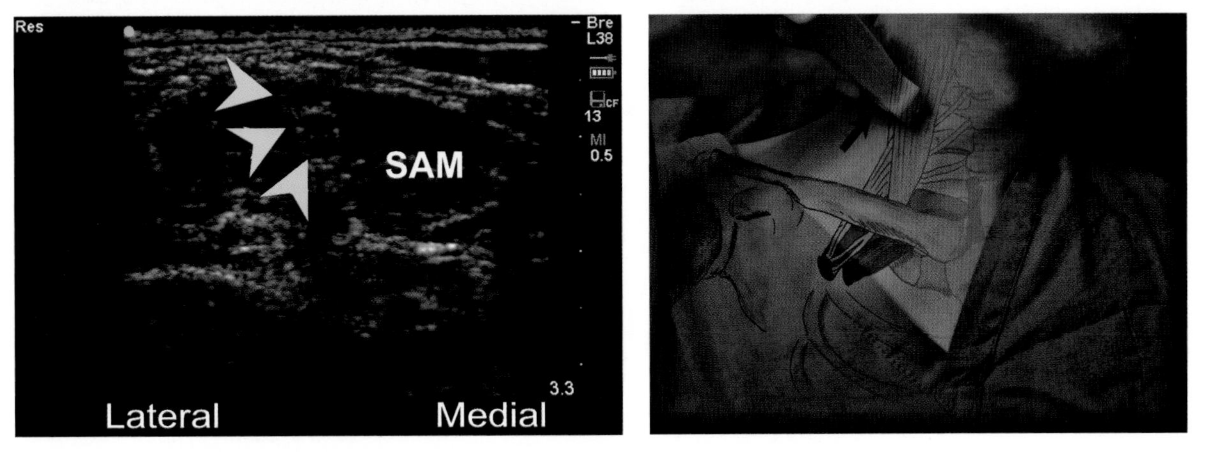

3. Title the probe upwards and downwards to obtain the best view

Figure 6.7. Traceback approach to locate the brachial plexus at the interscalene level. The plexus is first located next to the pulsating subclavian artery at the supraclavicular region before scanning cephalad towards the interscalene level.

- The sternocleidomastoid muscle is triangular and superficial overlying the internal jugular vein (again, if present) and common carotid artery—the structures are clearly distinct with the vessels being very dark (anechoic) and the artery appearing pulsatile.
- Lateral to the vessels and posterior to the sternocleidomastoid muscle lies the scalenus anterior muscle, and more posterolaterally, the scalenus medius and posterior muscles appear as a single mass.
- The hyperechoic image between the lining around the muscles is presumably the fibrous tissue of the interscalene sheath.
- Brachial plexus trunks and/or roots in a sagittal oblique section are visualized as three (usually; this is highly variable depending on the scan level) round or oval-shaped hypoechoic structures, sometimes with few internal punctate echoes, lying between the scalenus anterior and medius muscles.
- If the ultrasound field of view is large:
  - The hypoechoic C6 transverse process may be seen with an acoustic shadow effect beyond the level of the common carotid artery and directly medial to the scalenus medius (if seen at this high position in the neck).
  - The vertebral artery and vein may be seen deep to the plexus and anterior to the C6 transverse process. Occasionally, the vertebral vessels may only be seen at the C7 level as they are housed inside the transverse process at and above C6.
- In the long-axis plane, the plexus appears hypoechoic and tubular in structure with occasional internal fibrillar echoes; the mean diameter of each trunk is 2.5 mm. This view is often difficult to obtain.

- At the bottom of the interscalene groove in the supraclavicular fossa (Figure 6.7):
  - The pulsatile subclavian artery is anechoic and found centrally with this view; it can be confirmed by Doppler.
  - Plexus trunks/divisions generally appear superolateral to the subclavian artery as a tightly enclosed grapelike cluster, or honeycomb, of usually three or more (i.e., divisions may be captured) hypoechoic nodules interwoven with what appears to be a hyperechoic fascicular membrane.
  - The most medial structure visible is often the first rib (if seen), which is depicted as a bright white line under the subclavian artery.
  - The lung pleura (if seen) is often seen as a hyperechoic line with a hyperechoic shadow underneath (air artifact), particularly with respiration.
  - With medial movement of the probe, the oval-to-round subclavian vein may be seen inferomedial to the artery, appearing larger than the artery and slightly more echoic; the scalenus anterior muscle lies between the artery and vein.

6.3.3. Needle Insertion Technique

- Begin with local anesthetic infiltration of skin.
- Use a 3.5- to 5-cm 22-ga insulated block needle (if using nerve stimulation).
- Out-of-plane (OOP; short-axis) approach [Figure 6.8(A,B)]
  - Note that the ultrasound-guided approach is slightly different from the classic interscalene approach as traditionally the needle is placed perpendicular to the skin, whereas with OOP needling it is angled somewhat caudally toward the ultrasound plane.
  - It is important to line up the site of needle insertion at the skin with the nerve target, so place the probe with the target in the middle of the ultrasound screen to ensure a needle insertion at the probe's midline will direct the needle accurately.
  - With the clinician standing cephalad to the probe, place the initial needle puncture site cranial to the probe (in short axis to the plexus) and at a distance equal to the depth of the middle trunks [e.g., 2 cm; Figure 6.8(A); see Chapter 4 for a description of the walk down technique].
  - Angle the needle incrementally in a stepwise fashion similar to ultrasound-guided internal jugular vein catheterization.

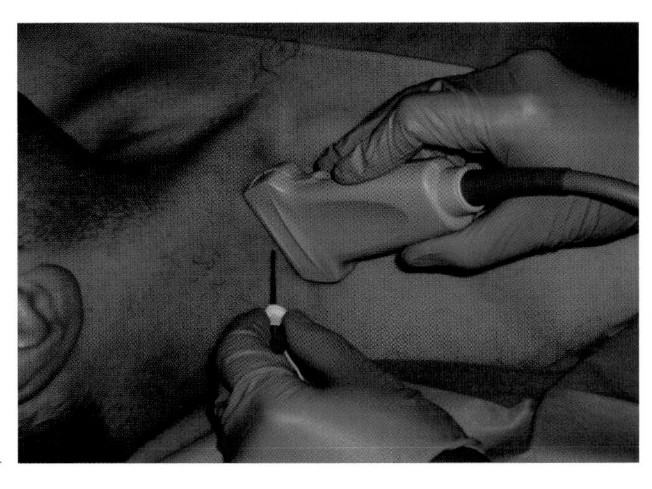

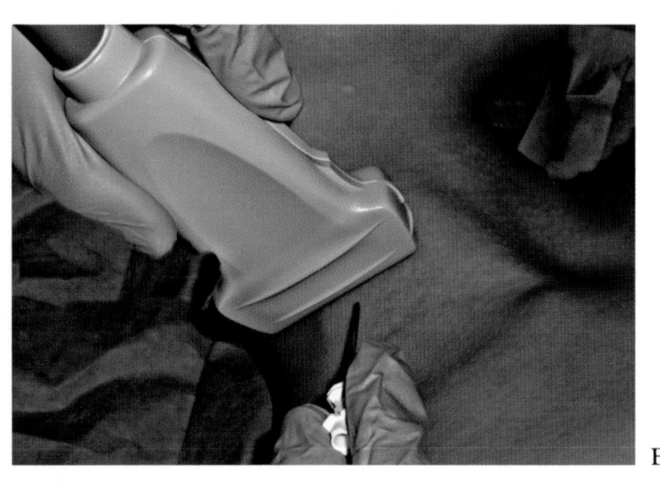

A B

Figure 6.8. Needling technique using a linear probe and an out-of-plane needle alignment with the needle either (A) cephalad to the probe or (B) caudad to the probe.

        - Start with an angle of 10° to the skin to localize the tip well with ultrasound as a bright dot, then withdraw the needle to the point where the needle tip disappears on the ultrasound screen.
        - Re-insert the needle caudally in a walk down manner, until the required depth is reached and the needle tip is seen in close proximity to the nerves.
        - If the initial puncture site is the same distance from the probe as the nerve target is deep to the skin, the approximate final angle of insertion will be 45°, based on trigonometry.
    - Avoid angling the needle more than 45° as the needle may insert too deep and directly towards the spinal cord.
    - The objective is to place the needle tip in between the scalenus anterior and medius muscles.
    - An alternative approach involves needle insertion inferior to the probe which approximates the classic interscalene technique (Figure 6.8(B)). Again, care must be taken to avoid spinal cord injury.
- In-plane (IP; long-axis) method
    - With the probe aligned to view the plexus in short axis, the needle may be moved from lateral to medial and will first penetrate the scalenus medius muscle before landing in the interscalene groove (Figure 6.9).

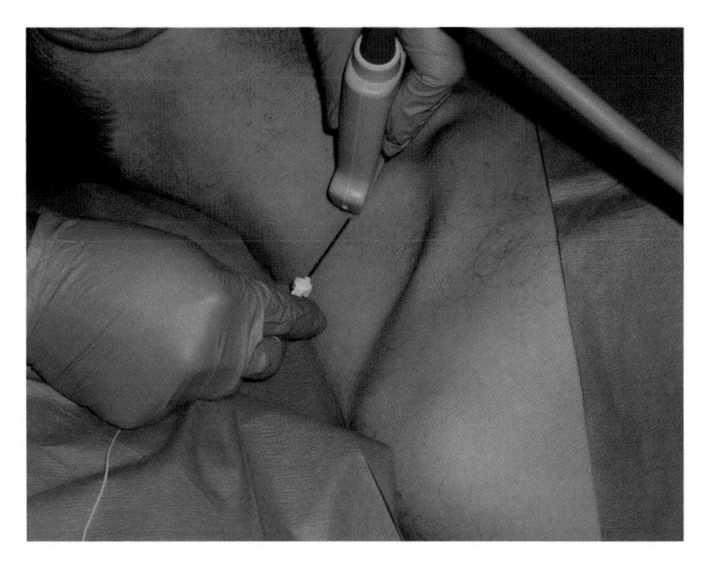

Figure 6.9. Needling technique using a linear probe and an in-plane needle alignment.

- For both IP and OOP approaches, scanning prior to needling will determine the angle, required trajectory distance, and vertical depth of needle penetration.
- The needle should usually be inserted to a maximum depth of 3 cm, but 2 cm may be sufficient in slim individuals.

6.4. Nerve Stimulation

- Applying an initial current of 0.8 mA (2 Hz, 100–300 μs) is sufficient for stimulation of the plexus (usually at a depth of 2–3 cm), and the current is reduced to aim for a threshold current of 0.4 mA (100–200 μs) before injection after obtaining the appropriate motor response.
- Equal success has been achieved when any of the appropriate muscle responses is elicited as a positive stimulating test. Palpation of the muscle may confirm the response. See Table 6.2 for correct responses and recommended adjustments with other common responses. Many responses will be eliminated with ultrasound guidance.

Table 6.2. Responses and recommended needle adjustments for use during nerve stimulation at the interscalene level.

Correct Response to Nerve Stimulation

Twitches elicited from the upper and middle trunks (pectoralis, deltoid, biceps brachii muscles), middle and lower trunks (triceps, forearm, or hand muscles) with current intensity of at least 0.4 mA (100–300 μs) verifies stimulation of the brachial plexus.

Other Common Responses and Needle Adjustment

- Muscle twitch from electrical stimulation
  - Neck (anterior scalene or sternocleidomastoid)
    - *Explanation*: Needle usually anteromedial to plexus
    - *Needle Adjustment*: Withdraw needle to subcutaneous tissue and reinsert in a 10 to 20° more posterior angle
  - Diaphragm (phrenic nerve)
    - *Explanation*: Needle plane is too anterior
    - *Needle Adjustment*: Withdraw needle to subcutaneous tissue and reinsert in a 15° more posterior angle
  - Scapula (thoracodorsal nerve to serratus anterior muscle)
    - *Explanation*: Needle tip is too posterior and deep to brachial plexus
    - *Needle Adjustment*: Withdraw to subcutaneous tissue and reinsert in a more anterior plane
  - Trapezius (accessory nerve)
    - *Explanation*: Needle tip too posterior to plexus
    - *Needle Adjustment*: Withdraw to subcutaneous tissue and reinsert in a more anterior plane
- Bone contact
  - Needle stops a depth of 1 to 2 cm (transverse process of cervical vertebrae or first rib), without twitches
    - *Explanation*: Needle shaft angle is too posterior and touching anterior tubercles
    - *Needle Adjustment*: Withdraw to subcutaneous tissue and reinsert in a 15° more anterior angle
- Vascular puncture
  - Most commonly carotid artery puncture; seen as arterial blood aspiration
    - *Explanation*: Needle angle and tip anterior to plexus
    - *Needle Adjustment*: Withdraw completely for pressure treatment and reinsert tip 1 to 2 cm posterior

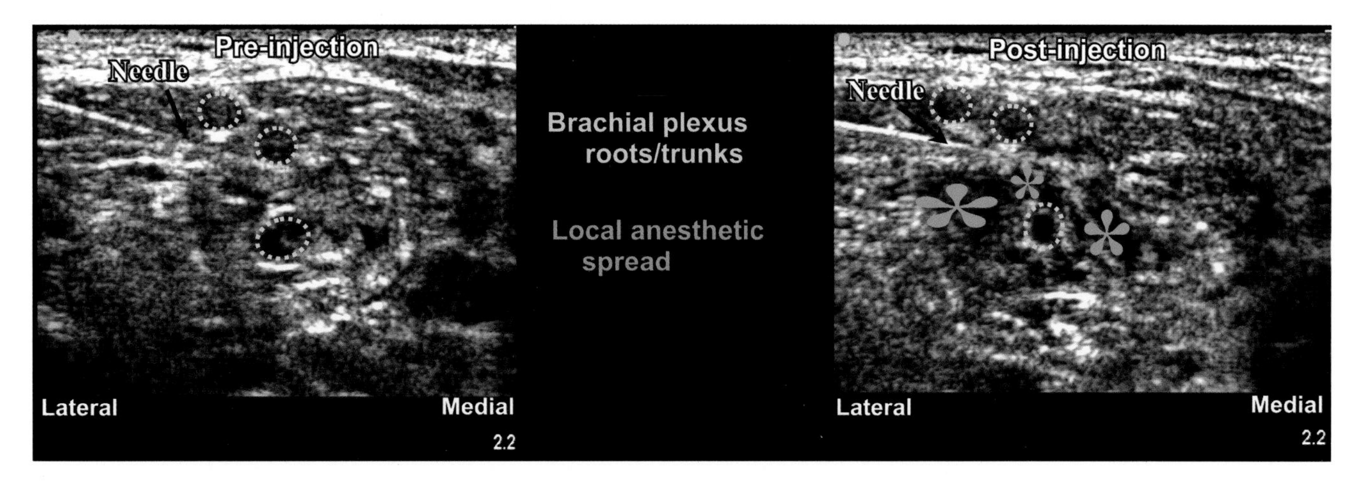

Figure 6.10. Local anesthetic application to the roots/trunks of the brachial plexus at the interscalene level.

- Avoid diaphragmatic or trapezius twitches, as they are associated with cervical plexus stimulation; a diaphragmatic response indicates that the phrenic nerve is being stimulated and that the needle is too anterior.
- Despite the fact that subarachoid injection can occur even when the threshold current is >0.4 mA, it is advisable to avoid injecting when stimulation occurs at less than 0.4 mA.
- The most commonly observed mistake is placement of the needle too anterior to the optimal skin insertion site. However, not infrequently the needle may be placed too posteriorly.

6.5. Local Anesthetic Application

- Nerve stimulation is recommended to confirm the identity of the nerve structures prior to the injection of local anesthetic.
- Performing a test dose with dextrose 5% in water (D5W) is recommended prior local anesthetic application to visualize the spread and confirm nerve localization (see Chapter 4 sidebar).
- Deposit local anesthetic in the midst of the neural structures so that it spreads to surround the nerves circumferentially.
- Local anesthetic distention in this compartment can be seen by ultrasound as a hypoechoic (fluid) expansion resulting in separation of the two scalene muscles (Figure 6.10).

Clinical Pearls

- The patient's movements can be problematic as any slight movement of the head may completely change the image of the plexus and make tracking the needle tip very difficult. Thus, it is important to maintain the patient's head steady and immobile during the procedure.
- It is advisable to insert the needle tangentially on each side of the nerves and not to directly contact the nerves.
- Local anesthetic spread should be seen as circumferential spread around the nerve structures within the interscalene groove and not within the scalene muscles.

Suggested Reading and References

Chan VW. Applying ultrasound imaging to interscalene brachial plexus block. Reg Anesth Pain Med 2003;28:340–343.

De Andres J, Sala-Blanch X. Ultrasound in the practice of brachial plexus anesthesia. Reg Anesth Pain Med 2002;27:77–89.

Sheppard DG, Lyer RB, Fenstermacher MJ. Brachial plexus: demonstration at US. Radiology 1998;208:402–406.

Soeding PE, Sha S, Royse CE, Marks P, Hoy G, Royse AG. A randomized trial of ultrasound-guided brachial plexus anaesthesia in upper limb surgery. Anaesth Intensive Care 2005;33:719–725.

Tsui BC, Finucane BT. The importance of ultrasound landmarks: a "traceback" approach using the popliteal blood vessels for identification of the sciatic nerve. Reg Anesth Pain Med 2006;31:481–482.

Yang WT, Chui PT, Metreweli C. Anatomy of the normal brachial plexus revealed by sonography and the role of sonographic guidance in anesthesia of the brachial plexus. AJR Am J Roentgenol 1998;171:1631–1636.

7 Supraclavicular Block

Ban C.H. Tsui

The supraclavicular block targets the trunks and/or divisions of the brachial plexus (Figure 7.1), depending on the location of the injection site and the patient's anatomy. The location of the needle puncture is usually at the midpoint of the clavicle, just cephaloposterior to the subclavian artery. The greatest concern when using this technique is pneumothorax as the cupula of the lung lies just medial to the first rib, not far from the plexus. The risk of pneumothorax is greater on the right side as the cupula of the lung is higher on that side. The risk is also greater in tall, thin patients. Ultrasound imaging will likely increase the utilization of this block as one can visualize the subclavian artery, the first rib, the pleura, and the block needle as it advances towards the plexus.

7.1. Clinical Anatomy

- Trunks of the brachial plexus (upper, middle, and lower) course through the supraclavicular fossa and separate into *divisions*, after passing through the groove between the scalenus anterior and medius muscles (anterior and middle scalene muscles), above the first rib with the subclavian artery on the medial side (Figures 7.2 and 7.3).

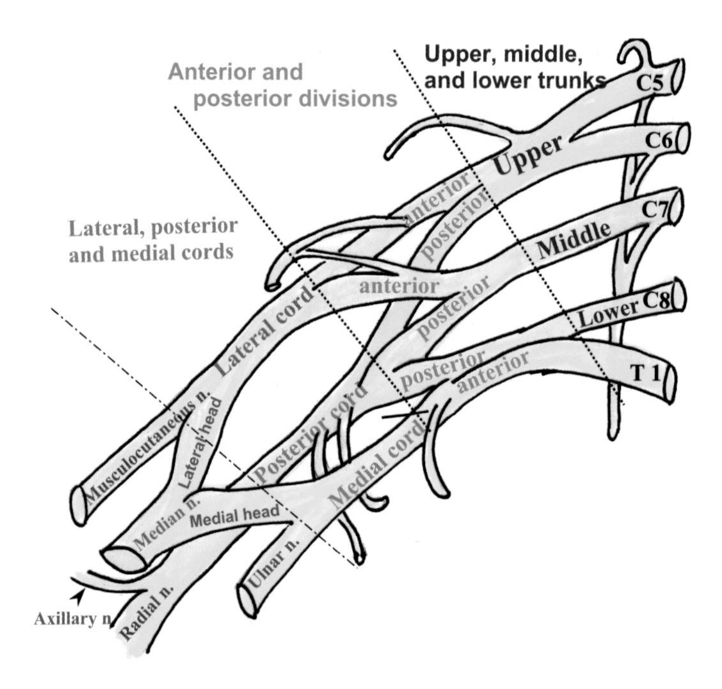

Figure 7.1. Supraclavicular block targets the trunks/divisions of the brachial plexus.

- The right and left subclavian arteries arise from the brachiocephalic trunk and the aortic arch, respectively; both arteries course cephalad anteromedial to the brachial plexus and then turn laterally over the first rib to become the axillary artery.
- The first rib is flat, broad and tilts as it curves posteriorly and laterally.
- The clavicular head of the sternocleidomastoid muscle inserts into the medial third of the clavicle, just medial to the plexus and the insertion point of the anterior scalene muscle into the first rib.
- The external jugular vein lies superficial to the sternocleidomastoid muscle at a more cephalad location to where the muscle divides into its sternal and clavicular heads, and then passes deep to the muscle layer to join the subclavian vein transversely under the clavicle.

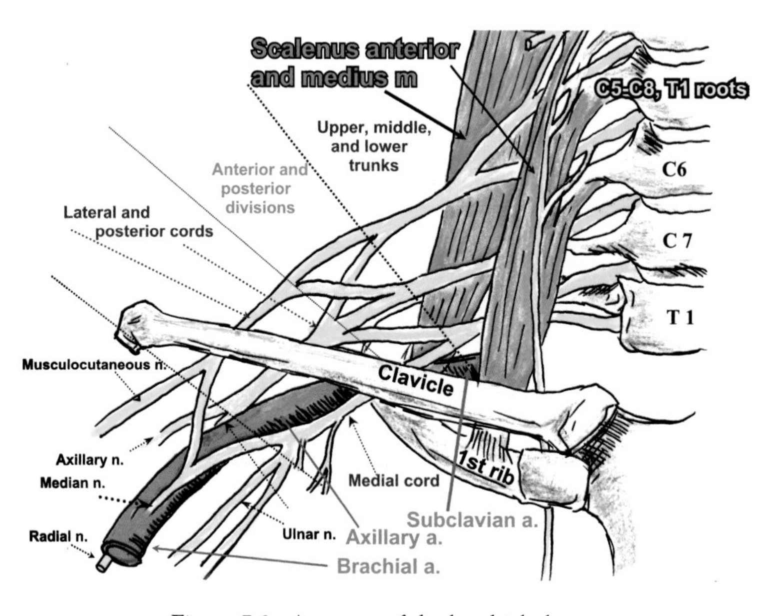

Figure 7.2. Anatomy of the brachial plexus.

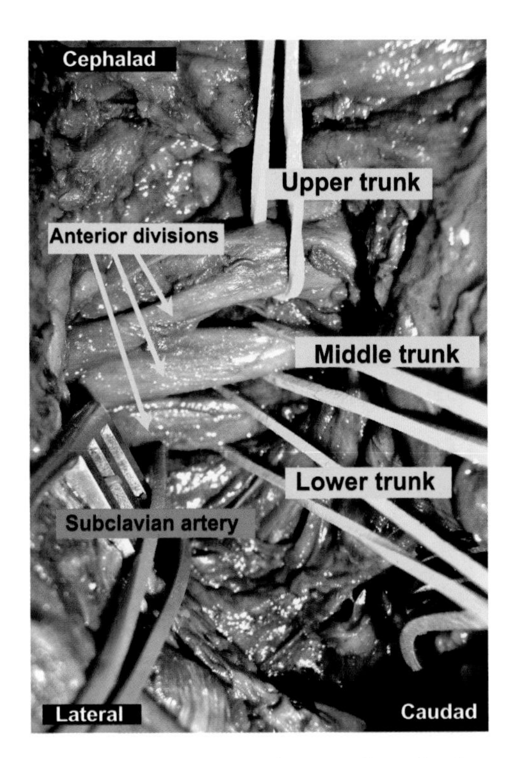

Figure 7.3. Dissection at the supraclavicular fossa.

- Immediately medial to the first rib, and about 1 to 2 cm from the posterior aspect of the plexus, is the cupula (apex) of the lung.

Table 7.1 summarizes the target nerves for the supraclavicular brachial plexus blockade. Each nerve is traced from its origin at the root level and the appropriate motor response

Table 7.1. Target nerves of the supraclavicular block: origin and motor responses associated with nerve stimulation.

Movement	Nerve	Cord	Division	Trunk	Root
Arm abduction	Suprascapular[a]			Upper	C5, C6
Arm abduction	Axillary	Posterior	Posterior	Upper	C5, C6
Elbow flexion	Musculocutaneous	Lateral	Posterior and anterior	Upper	C5, C6
Extension (dorsiflexion) of elbow, wrist, hand, and fingers	Radial	Posterior	Posterior	Upper	C5, C6
			Posterior	Middle	C7
Latissimus dorsi twitch	Thoracodorsal	Posterior	Posterior	Middle	C7
Forearm pronation and wrist flexion	Median (lateral head)	Lateral	Anterior	Upper	C5, C6
		Medial	Anterior and posterior	Middle	C7
			Anterior	Lower	C8, T1
Thumb flexion and opposition (flexion middle and ring finger)	Median	Medial	Anterior	Lower	C8, T1
Thumb flexion and opposition	Anterior interosseous	Medial	Anterior	Lower	C8, T1
Fifth finger flexion and opposition, ulnar deviation of wrist	Ulnar	Medial	Anterior	Lower	C8, T1

[a]The suprascapular nerve may not be blocked during the supraclavicular block if the needle is placed at the level of the divisions rather than the trunks.

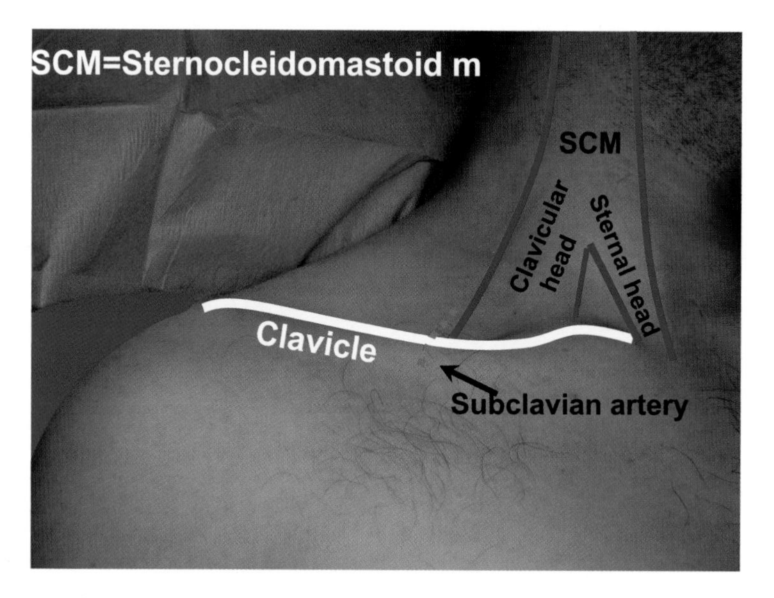

Figure 7.4. Surface anatomy for the supraclavicular block.

associated with nerve stimulation is described. Segmental dermatomal and myotomal distribution of the brachial plexus is discussed and illustrated in Chapter 5. Nerves that are purely sensory are not described in the above table.

7.2. Patient Positioning and Surface Anatomy

7.2.1. Patient Positioning

The patient is positioned supine with the head turned approximately 45° to the contralateral side.

7.2.2. Surface Anatomy (Figure 7.4)

- Clavicle
  - The needle insertion site is often at the midpoint of the clavicle with the conventional approach. The selected needle insertion site is often more lateral with the ultrasound-guided technique, as the probe is placed over the middle third of the clavicle, with the needle placed laterally.
  - However, there are many other ways to approach the brachial plexus.
- Clavicular head of sternocleidomastoid muscle
  - The plexus lies posterolateral to the lateral point of the muscle insertion; however, it is not critical to find this landmark.
- Subclavian artery pulse serves as a reliable landmark as the plexus lies immediately cephaloposterior to the subclavian artery.

7.3. Sonographic Imaging and Needle Insertion Technique

The trunks/divisions of the plexus are shown in the magnetic resonance imaging (MRI) scan (Figure 7.5) depicting the supraclavicular fossa level, as well as the corresponding ultrasound image (Figure 7.6).

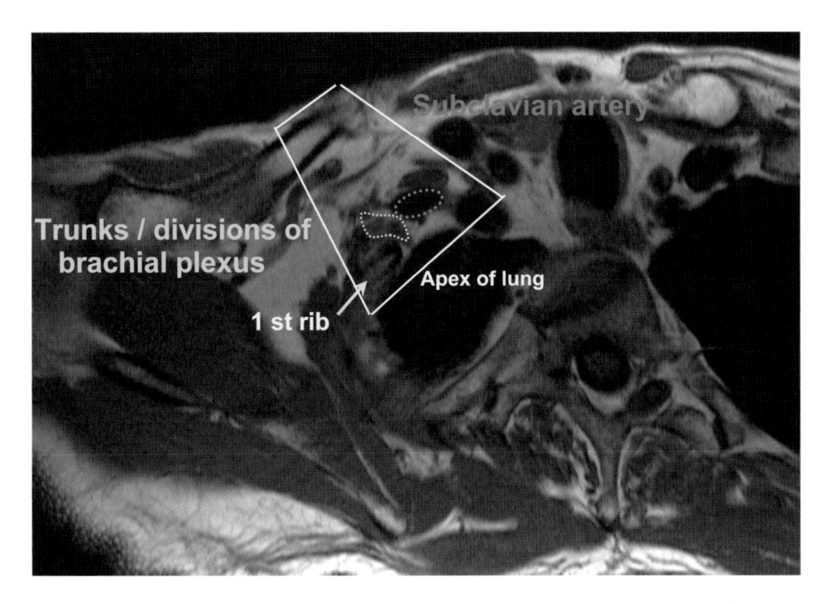

Figure 7.5. MRI image of the trunks/divisions in the supraclavicular fossa.

The major challenge with ultrasound imaging in this region is the presence of a bony prominence (clavicle) and curved soft tissue contour that can interfere with imaging of the brachial plexus in short-axis view. There is the potential for technical artifacts, such as anisotropy with the appearance of simulated hypoechoic images, which may distort the images and lead to false identification of nerves (see Chapter 3 for a discussion of anisotropy). Generally, the nerve structures are most visible when the angle of incidence is approximately 90° to the ultrasound beam. This is particularly obvious with pediatric patients, as it is often difficult to place the probe in the supraclavicular fossa while maintaining good skin contact and a beam–nerve axis angle of 90°. Use of a short footprint curved array probe can be very useful under such circumstances.

Prepare the needle insertion site and skin surface with an antiseptic solution. Prepare the ultrasound probe surface by applying a sterile adhesive dressing to it prior to needling as discussed earlier (see Chapters 3 and 4).

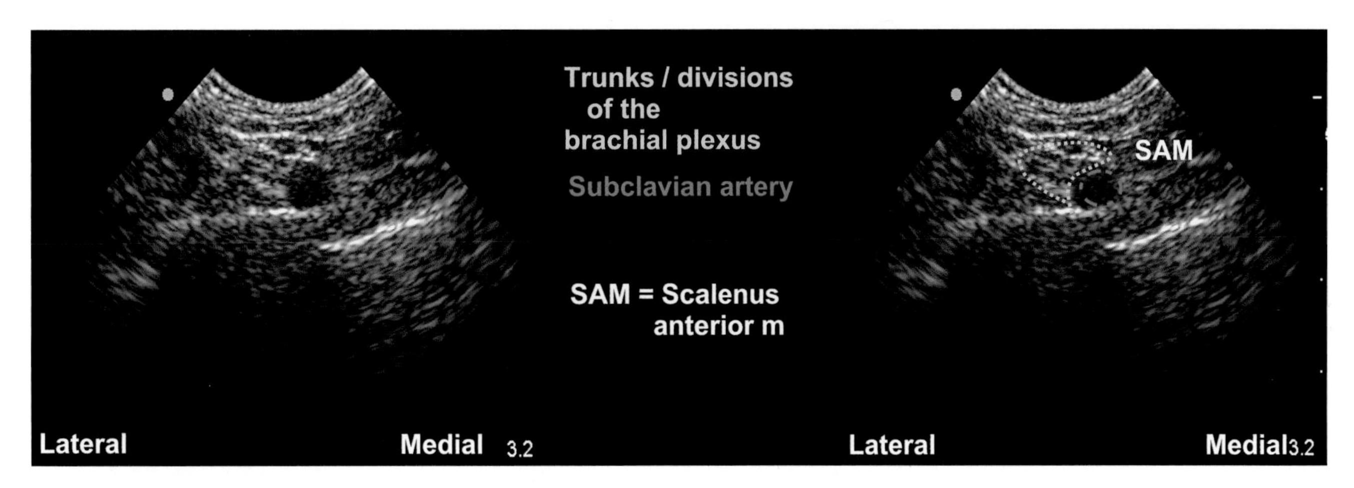

Figure 7.6. Ultrasound image using a curved probe at the supraclavicular fossa. The nerve trunks/divisions appear superior and lateral to the anechoic subclavian artery.

7.3.1. Scanning Technique

The required depth of penetration is usually within 1 to 2 cm.

- Despite the poor resolution with the low-to-moderate frequency of currently commercially available curved array probes (C11, TITAN, SonoSite, Inc., Bothell, WA, USA), a curved array probe with a small footprint is extremely useful in this compact area. Failure to maintain good skin-to-probe contact, or have a 90° beam-to-nerve incidence angle can result in an anisotropy effect and alter the appearance of the nerve (see Chapter 3).
- The probe is first placed in a coronal oblique plane at the lateral end of the upper border of the clavicle. It is then moved medially until an image of the subclavian artery appears on screen. Some dorsal and ventral rotation of the probe may be necessary.
- With the subclavian artery in the middle of the screen, the plexus is located superolateral to the artery and the neurovascular structures are lying above the first rib.

Clinical Pearls

- The author generally uses a curved array probe (C11, 8–5 MHz, TITAN, SonoSite, Inc., Bothell, WA, USA), to obtain reasonable image quality. It is important to point out those images obtained from curved linear array probes (C11) are far superior to those obtained by phased array probes (e.g., P10, 8–4 MHz, MicroMaxx, SonoSite, Inc., Bothell, WA, USA). The phased array transducer generally has a narrow near field which limits image resolution and clarity.
- Unless the patient is small, high-frequency probes (10–15 MHz) are preferred by Chan for the supraclavicular block in order to optimally view the plexus at its superficial location.

7.3.2. Sonographic Appearance (Figures 7.6 and 7.7)

- The subclavian artery is anechoic, hypodense, pulsatile, and round; its identity can be further confirmed by color Doppler.
- Trunks/divisions of the brachial plexus can be found superolateral to the subclavian artery in the ultrasound image plane; they are seen as a cluster of hypoechoic grapelike structures consisting of usually three (more as one moves distally) hypoechoic nodules.
- The outline of the grapelike structure is hyperechoic, likely representative of the fascicular lining/sheath.
- The first rib which lies medial and deep to the artery often appears as a hyperechoic linear structure with a hypoechoic shadow underneath.
- The lung pleura is often seen deep to the first rib as a hyperechoic line accompanied by a hyperechoic shadow underneath.
- Inferomedial to the subclavian artery, the anechoic, large and oval-to-round subclavian vein is sometimes seen. The anterior scalene anterior muscle lies between the artery and vein.

7.3.3. Needle Insertion Technique

- Infiltrate the skin with local anesthetic.
- Use a 3.5- to 5-cm, 22-ga needle (insulated if using nerve stimulation).
- Perform in-plane (IP) needling technique using a curved, small footprint probe or a linear probe (see Chapter 4):
  - The needle is inserted immediately above the clavicle, in a lateral to medial (the author finds a medial-to-lateral direction is often limited by the compact space) direction (Figure 7.8), and with a slightly cephalad angulation to avoid the lung.

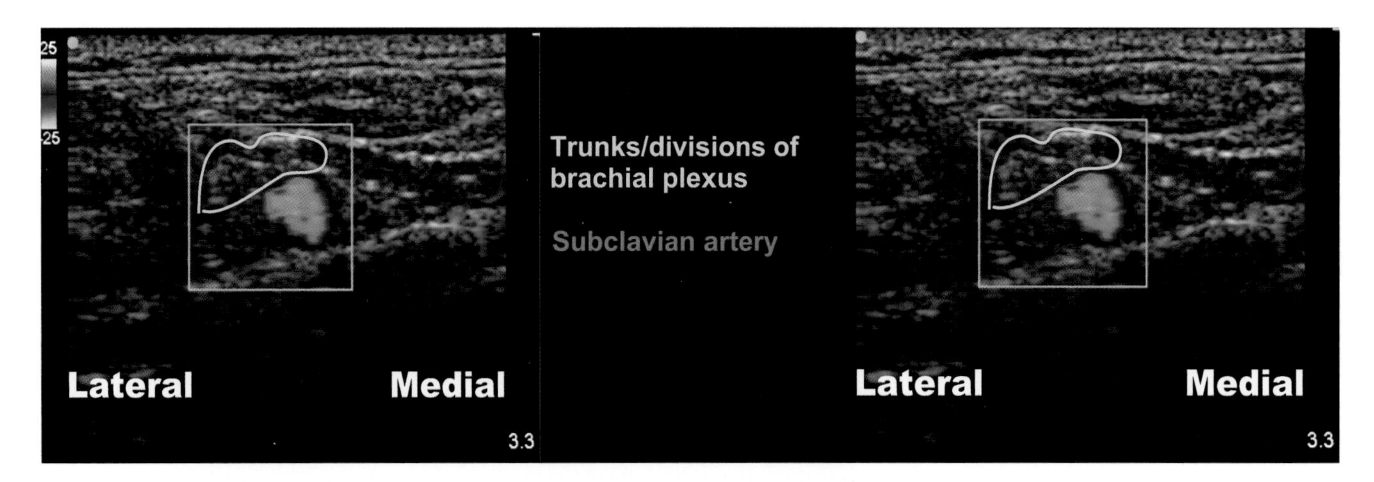

Figure 7.7. Ultrasound image using color Doppler to illuminate the subclavian artery.

Clinical Pearls

- To reduce the risk of pleural puncture, it is important to first identify and mark the distance of the first rib and pleura from the skin before needle insertion. It is also important to visually track needle movement in real-time during needle advancement in-plane with the ultrasound beam.
- If the nerve structures are not clearly visible when the probe is in the coronal oblique plane, slowly angle the probe more obliquely by moving the lateral end of the probe posteriorly. Remember that the brachial plexus is lateral and posterior to the subclavian artery, and this adjustment in the positioning of the probe can bring the nerve structures into view more clearly.

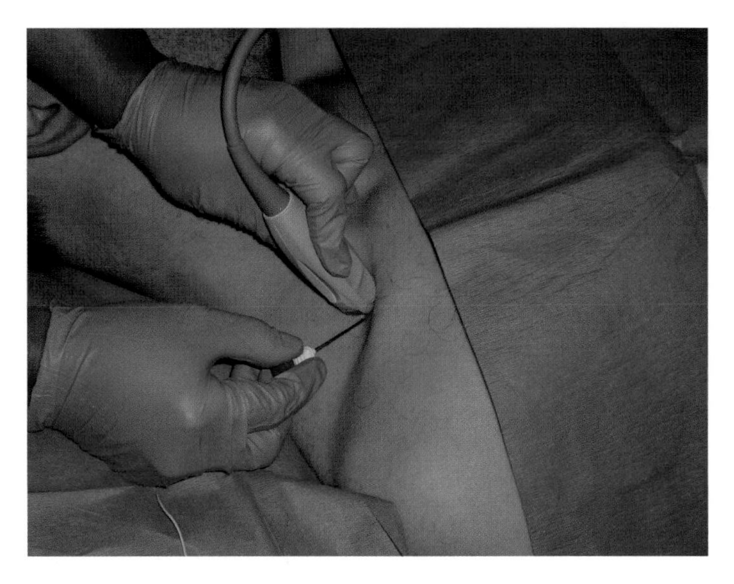

Figure 7.8. Needling technique using a curved probe and in-plane needle alignment.

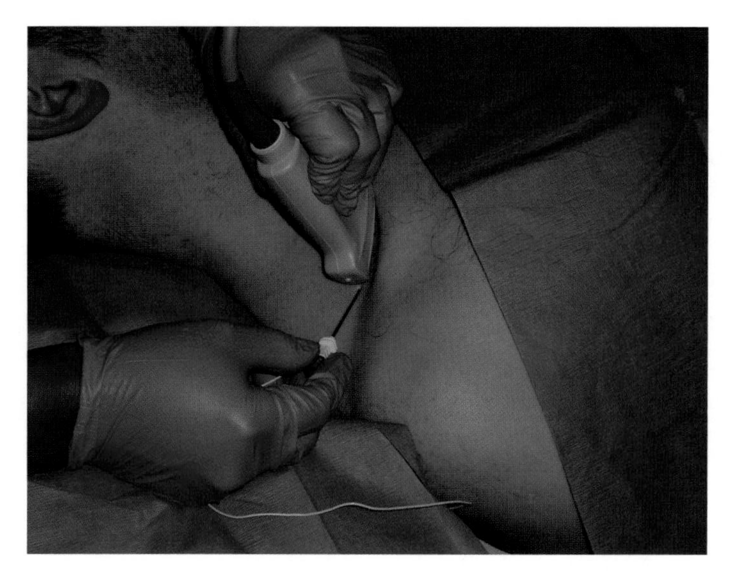

Figure 7.9. Needling technique using a linear probe and in-plane needle alignment.

- The IP approach facilitates clear visualization of the needle, which is important in order to avoid inadvertent pleural puncture. It will be important to observe the depth of needle insertion to ensure the needle is not too deep and therefore risking pleural puncture.
- The IP approach with lateral-to-medial needle insertion will ensure the needle approaches the nerve structures prior to reaching the subclavian artery (i.e., less chance of inadvertent vascular puncture).
- A drawback to this direction of needle insertion is that it aims towards the thorax and there is a real potential for pleural puncture unless the utmost care is taken to mark the skin–pleura distance prior to needle insertion.

Chan and colleagues (2003) suggest using a linear probe with an in-plane (IP) needling approach (Figure 7.9).

7.4. Nerve Stimulation

Because the vital structures, including the subclavian artery and pleura, are within centimeters of the brachial plexus, we strongly recommend ultrasound guidance to avoid the otherwise high risks of vascular puncture and pneumothorax. In our experience, ultrasound guidance can avoid such complications as long as an in-plane approach is used for observing the needle tip at all times. The nerve stimulation responses can be very useful for confirmation of needle proximity to the separate trunks. Table 7.2 is a guide for use with nerve stimulation technique during brachial plexus block at the supraclavicular location.

7.5. Local Anesthetic Application

Nerve stimulation should be used to confirm needle placement prior to local anesthetic injection (see Table 7.2).

Table 7.2. Responses and needle adjustments for use with nerve stimulation at the supraclavicular level.

Correct Response to Nerve Stimulation

The correct responses are similar to those observed when using the interscalene approach. At this location, the brachial plexus is starting to divide from trunks into anterior and posterior divisions. Twitches of pectoralis, deltoid, biceps (upper trunk), triceps (upper/middle trunk), forearm (upper/middle trunk), and hand (lower trunk) muscles with current intensity of 0.4 mA (100–300 μs) are acceptable. Distal responses (hand or wrist flexion or extension) are best to confirm placement within the fascia.

Other Common Responses and Needle Adjustment

- Muscle twitch from electrical stimulation
  - Diaphragm (phrenic nerve)
    - *Explanation*: Very unlikely as the needle plane is too anterior
    - *Needle Adjustment*: Withdraw needle to the subcutaneous tissue and reinsert in a 15° more posterior angle
- Vascular puncture
  - Subclavian artery puncture; indicated with arterial blood withdrawal
    - *Explanation*: Needle tip is deep to the plexus
    - *Needle Adjustment*: Withdraw completely for pressure treatment and reinsert carefully while observing the needle tip at all times using in-plane approach
- Bone contact
  - Needle stops at a depth of 3 cm (first rib)
    - *Explanation*: Needle is inserted too deep and well beyond the plexus. However, this scenario is very unlikely with ultrasound guidance
    - *Needle Adjustment*: Withdraw to subcutaneous tissue and reinsert
- Pleural Contact
  - Needle tip seen beyond the white line (first rib) and a pocket is observed to form beyond the bright line
    - *Explanation*: Needle inserted too deep, traversed the plexus and subclavian artery and has entered the pleural space. However, it is very unlikely with ultrasound-guided technique
    - *Needle Adjustment*: Withdraw needle to subcutaneous tissue and reinsert if there is a strong clinical indication

---

Clinical Pearls

- Having good control over needle trajectory and visually tracking the needle tip are critical for a safe and successful ultrasound-guided supraclavicular block. Chan and colleagues (2003) recommend deferring this block procedure until reaching an intermediate level of competency and experience with ultrasound scanning and needling.
- Anesthesia of the lower trunk is required for hand surgery and it is advisable to inject local anesthetic immediately next to the inferior portion of the nerve cluster and as close to the first rib as possible.
- Local anesthetic injection in the superior portion of the nerve cluster may achieve satisfactory anesthesia in the arm, although it may be deficient in the hand.

- Performing a test dose with dextrose 5% in water (D5W) is recommended prior to local anesthetic application to visualize the spread and confirm nerve localization (see Chapter 4 sidebar).
- In our experience, it is best to deposit local anesthetic next to the nerve structures in the supraclavicular window immediately lateral to the subclavian artery on top of the first rib. Injection in this location will often lift the nerve structures superiorly away from the first rib and subclavian artery.

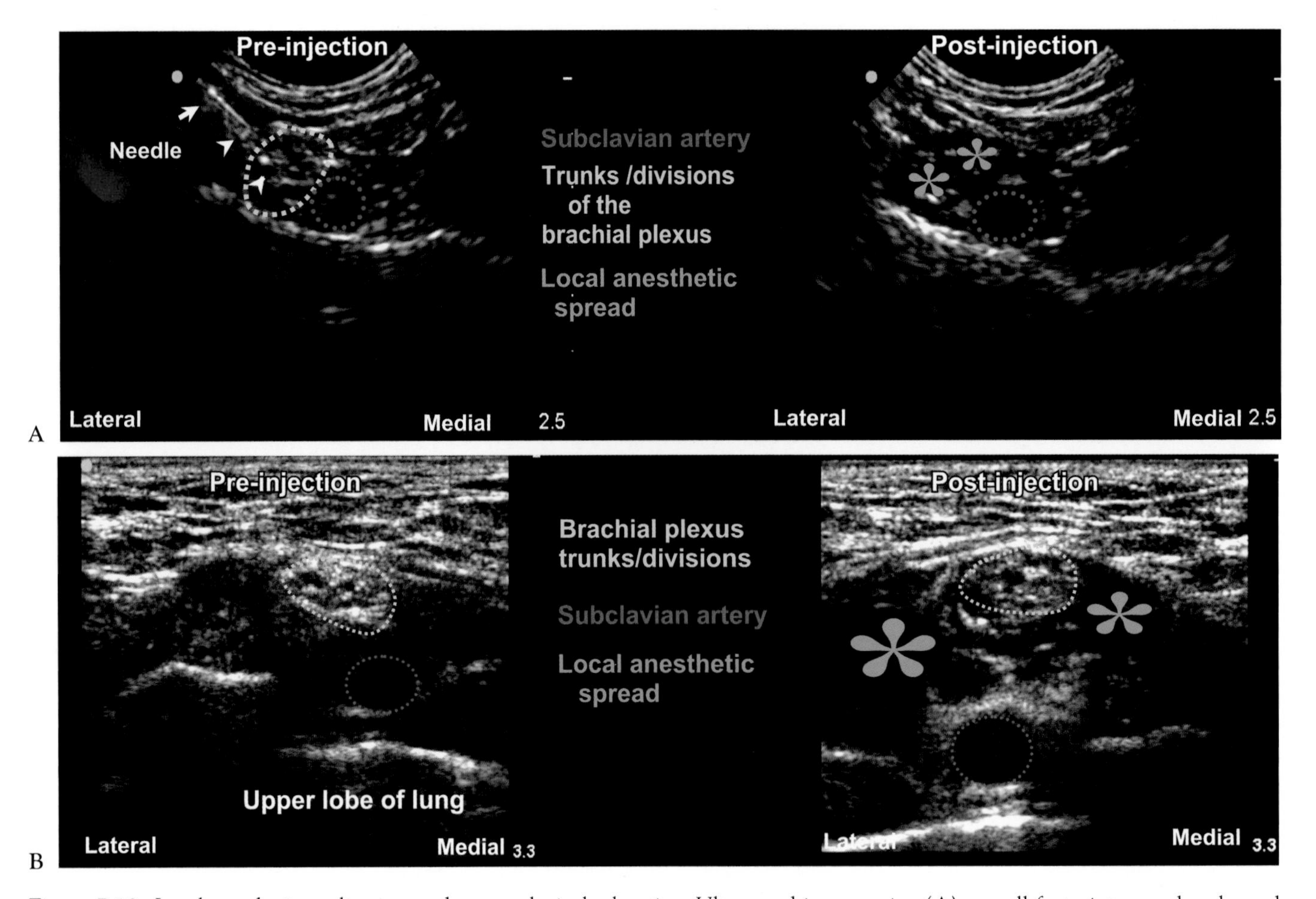

Figure 7.10. Local anesthetic application at the supraclavicular location. Ultrasound images using (A) a small footprint curved probe and (B) a linear probe.

- The hypoechoic spread of local anesthetic appears to surround the nerves on the ultrasound screen [Figure 7.10(A,B)].
- If the spread of anesthetic seems inadequate for the whole plexus, stop halfway through and reposition the needle prior to injecting the remaining solution.

Suggested Reading and References

Arcand G, Williams SR, Chouinard P, Boudreault D, Harris P, Ruel M, Girard F. Ultrasound-guided infraclavicular versus supraclavicular blook. Anesth Analg 2005;101:886–890.

Beach ML, Sites BD, Gallagher JD. Use of a nerve stimulator does not improve the efficacy of ultrasound-guided supraclavicular blocks. J Clin Anesth 2006;18:580–584.

Chan VW, Perlas A, Rawson R, Odukoya O. Ultrasound-guided supraclavicular brachial plexus block. Anesth Analg 2003;97;1514–1517.

De Andres J, Sala-Blanch. Ultrasound in the practice of brachial plexus anesthesia. Reg Anesth Pain Med 2002;27:77–89.

Kapral S, Krafft P, Eibenberger K, Fitzgerald R, Gosch M, Weinstabl C. Ultrasound-guided supraclavicular approach for regional anesthesia of the brachial plexus. Anesth Analg 1994;78:507–513.

Tsui BC, Twomey C, Finucane BT. Visualization of the brachial plexus in the supraclavicular region using a curved ultrasound probe with a sterile transparent dressing. Reg Anesth Pain Med 2006;31:182–184.

Williams SR, Chouinard P, Arcand G, et al. Ultrasound guidance speeds execution and improves the quality of supraclavicular block. Anesth Analg 2003;97:118–152.
Yang WT, Chui PT, Metreweli C. Anatomy of the normal brachial plexus revealed by sonography and the role of sonographic guidance in anesthesia of the brachial plexus. AJR Am J Roentgenol 1998;171:1631–1636.

8 Infraclavicular Block

Ban C.H. Tsui

Ultrasound-guided infraclavicular block targets the cords of the brachial plexus (Figure 8.1), generally where they surround the second part of the axillary artery at the level of the coracoid process (Figure 8.2). The infraclavicular approach can block the musculocutaneous and axillary nerves more consistently than the axillary block because these two nerves often branch off high in the axilla and are often missed with the axillary block. However, multiple injections are often required for both the infraclavicular and axillary blocks. As compared to blocks at more proximal locations, the infraclavicular block has the advantage of having a reduced risk of inadvertently blocking the phrenic nerve or stellate ganglion. This block is indicated for forearm, elbow, and hand surgery.

In the past, numerous techniques were developed with modifications to best localize the nerves and avoid vessel and pleural punctures. Ultrasound may essentially eliminate the need for arduous development of needle puncture sites and insertion trajectories as real-time guidance will address these issues.

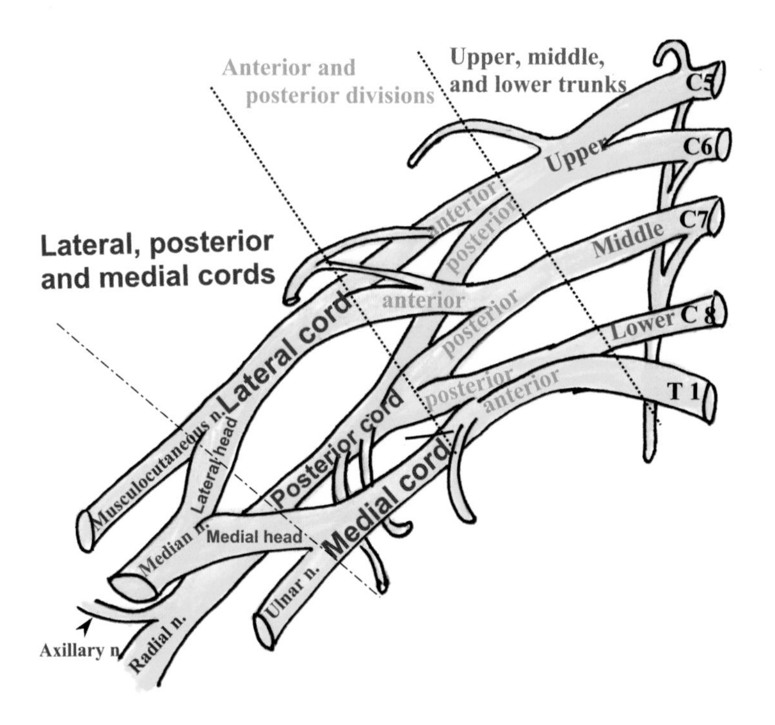

Figure 8.1. Infraclavicular block targets the divisions/cords of the brachial plexus.

8.1. Clinical Anatomy

- The *infraclavicular fossa* is formed by the pectoralis minor and major muscles anteriorly, the ribs medially, the clavicle and the coracoid process superiorly, and the humerus laterally.
- The brachial plexus courses inferolaterally through this fossa behind the clavicle and into the axilla.
- The plexus lies immediately lateral to subclavian vessels and not far from the apex of the lung.

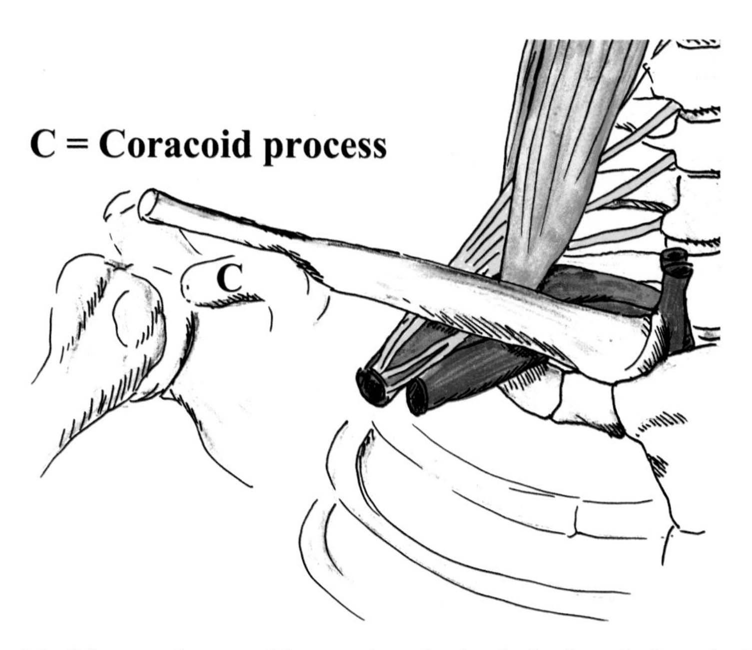

Figure 8.2. Schematic diagram of the main bony landmarks for the infraclavicular block.

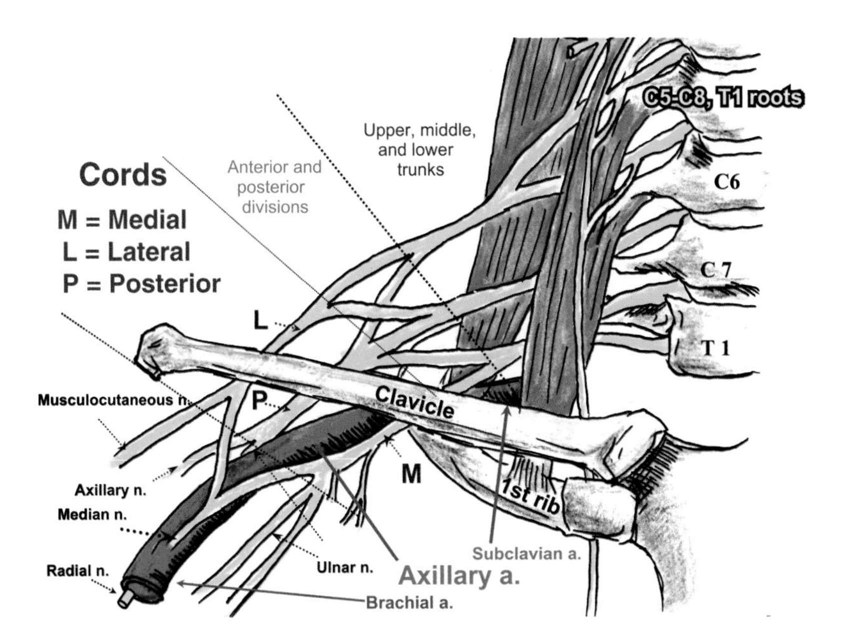

Figure 8.3. Cords of the brachial plexus form beyond the clavicle and below the coracoid process. They are named for their location relative to the axillary artery.

- The *divisions* of the plexus are formed at or above the level of the clavicle and enter the infraclavicular fossa to continue distally to form the *cords*; the terminal nerves have yet to branch (Figure 8.3).
- Below the coracoid process, the plexus lies approximately 2 to 4 cm deep to the skin and the pectoralis major muscle, with the lateral cord being most superficial.
- As the plexus reaches the lateral border of the pectoralis minor muscle, just distal to the deltopectoral groove (fossa) and lateral to the coracoid process, it lies deeper and the cords surround the third part (the part beyond the pectoralis minor muscle) of the axillary artery (Figure 8.4). Here the cords are named according to their relationship to the

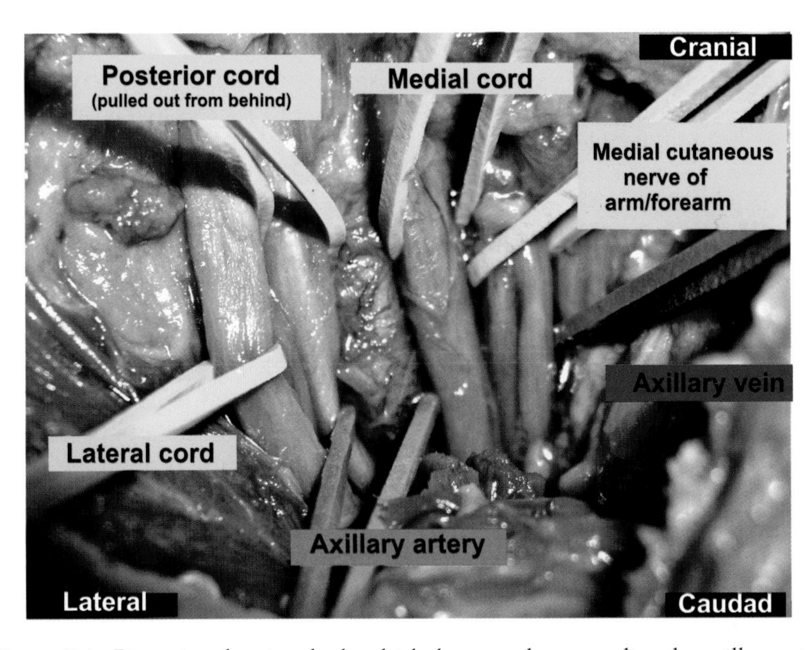

Figure 8.4. Dissection showing the brachial plexus cords surrounding the axillary artery.

Table 8.1. Target nerves of the infraclavicular block: origin and motor response associated with nerve stimulation.

Movement	Nerve	Cord	Division	Trunk	Root
Arm abduction	Axillary	Posterior	Posterior	Upper	C5, 6
Elbow flexion	Musculocutaneous	Lateral	Posterior and anterior	Upper	C5, 6
Extension (dorsiflexion) of elbow, wrist, hand, and fingers	Radial	Posterior	Posterior Posterior	Upper Middle	C5, 6 C7
Latissimus dorsi twitch	Thoracodorsal	Posterior	Posterior	Middle	C7
Forearm pronation and wrist flexion	Median (lateral head)	Lateral Medial	Anterior Anterior and posterior Anterior	Upper Middle Lower	C5, 6 C7 C8, T1
Thumb flexion and opposition (flexion middle and ring finger)	Median	Medial	Anterior	Lower	C8, T1
Thumb flexion and opposition	Anterior interosseous	Medial	Anterior	Lower	C8, T1
Fifth finger flexion and opposition, ulnar deviation of wrist	Ulnar	Medial	Anterior	Lower	C8, T1

axillary artery (lateral, posterior, and medial): the lateral cord of the plexus often lies superior and lateral, the posterior cord lies posterior, and the medial cord lies inferior and medial to the axillary artery.

- It is important to realize that there is a great deal of individual anatomical variation in cord location around the artery.
- The axillary vein is commonly medial to the axillary artery in the midclavicular region (medial aspect of the infraclavicular fossa) and becomes inferior (caudad) to the artery when it moves more laterally at the level of the coracoid process.

Table 8.1 summarizes the target nerves for the infraclavicular brachial plexus blockade. Each nerve is traced from its origin at the root level and the motor response associated with nerve stimulation is described. Segmental dermatomal and myotomal innervation by the brachial plexus is also discussed and illustrated in Chapter 5. Nerves that are purely sensory are not described in the table.

8.2. Patient Positioning and Surface Anatomy

8.2.1. Patient Positioning

The patient is supine with the head turned approximately 45° contralaterally and the arm is placed by the side to identify the anatomical landmarks. The coracoid process can be palpated just medial to the head of the humerus. It is common to perform the block with the patient's elbow flexed and the hand resting on the abdomen. It may be, however, more advantageous to keep the patient's elbow flexed and the arm abducted and externally rotated. This maneuver can render the cords taut and bring them to a more superficial location, thus accentuating their ultrasonographic appearance. Stretching the cords also brings the nerves closer around the axillary artery, which may facilitate local anesthetic spread around the nerves.

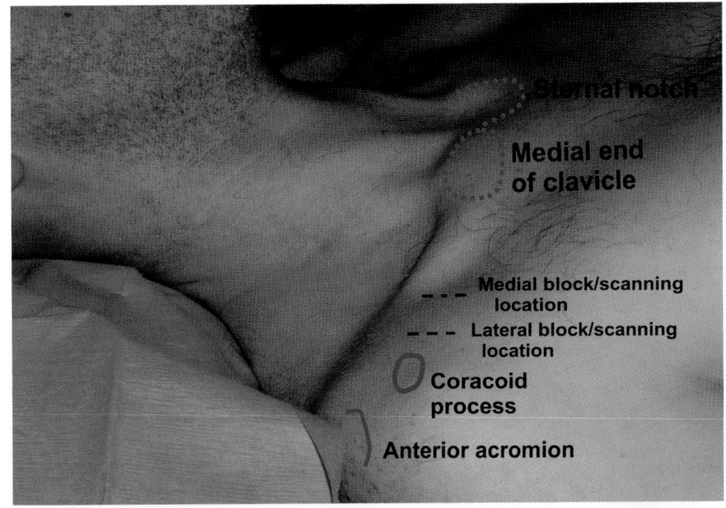

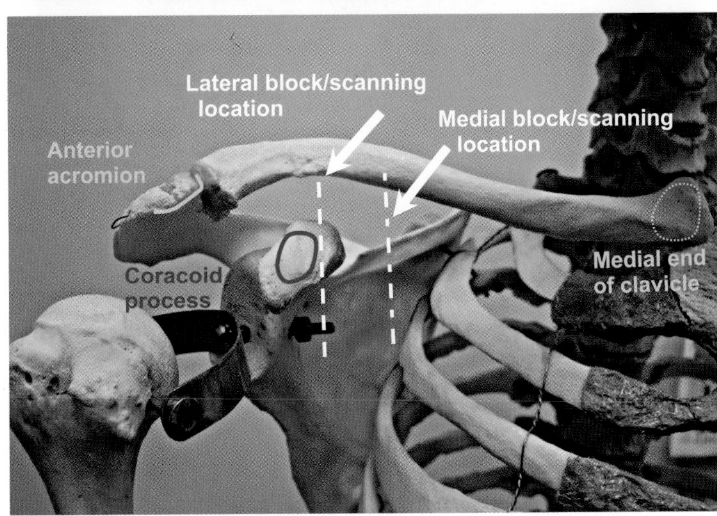

Figure 8.5. (A) Surface anatomy and (B) skeleton model of main landmarks for the infraclavicular block.

8.2.2. Surface Anatomy [Figure 8.5(A,B)]

- Medially
  - Sternal notch and sternoclavicular joint
  - Medial end of the clavicle
- Laterally
  - Anterior aspect of acromion (palpate scapular spine and follow it to the acromion; differentiate from the mobile humerus)
  - Coracoid process medial and inferior to acromioclavicular joint

8.3. Sonographic Imaging and Needle Insertion Technique

Anatomical details of the cords of the brachial plexus in the infraclavicular region are shown in the magnetic resonance imaging (MRI) scan (Figure 8.6) and the corresponding ultrasound image [Figures 8.7(A,B)].

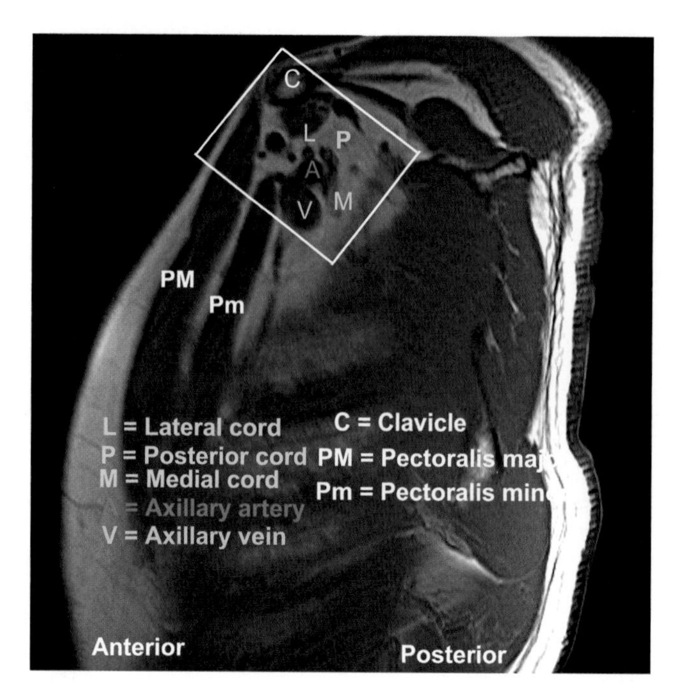

Figure 8.6. MRI image of a transverse/sagittal plane at the lateral infraclavicular block location.

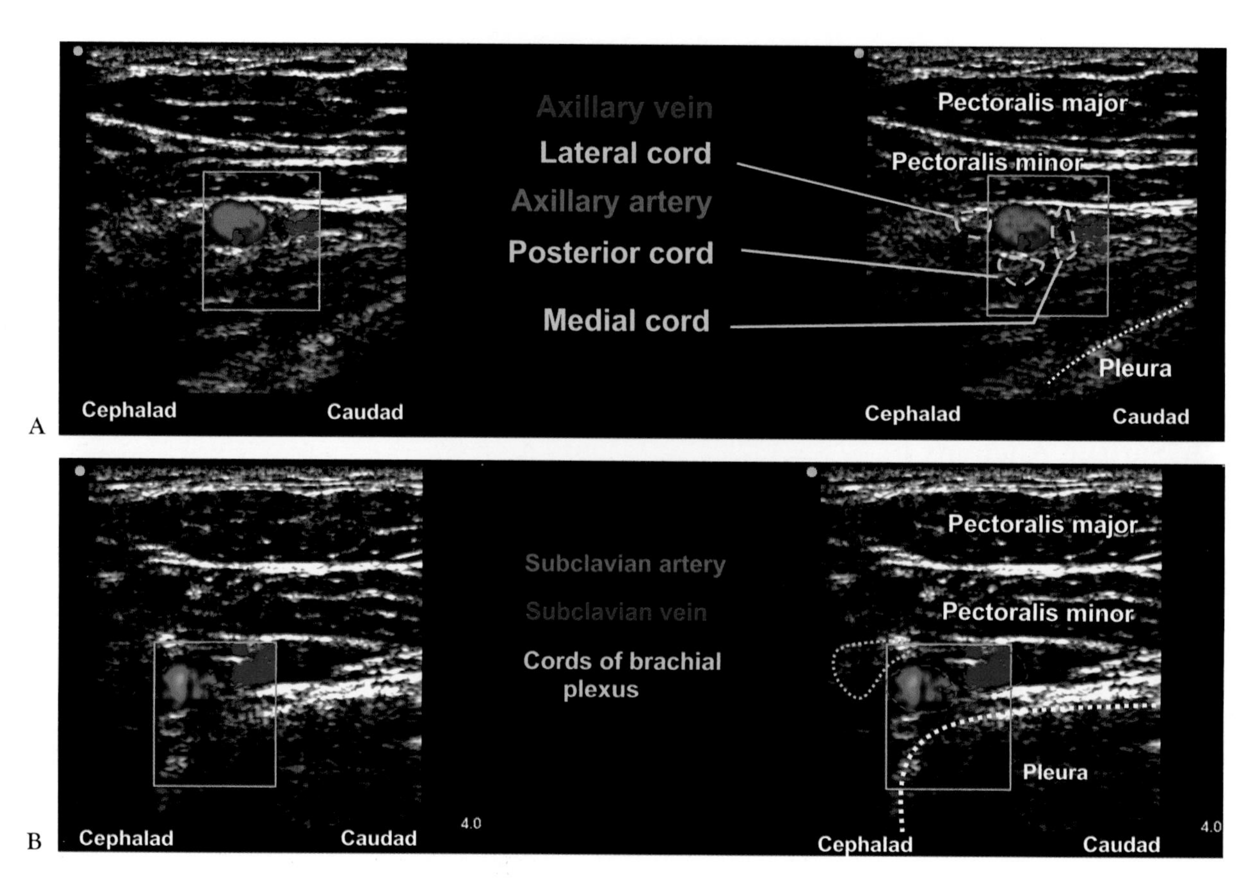

Figure 8.7. Ultrasound images using a linear probe at the infraclavicular level. (A) The image was taken at the lateral location and illustrates the brachial plexus cords surrounding the axillary artery. (B) The medial block location near the subclavian artery, vein, and the pleura.

Prepare the needle insertion site and skin surface with an antiseptic solution. Prepare the ultrasound probe surface by applying a sterile adhesive dressing to it prior to needling as discussed earlier (see Chapters 3 and 4).

8.3.1. Scanning Technique

As vascular puncture and pneumothorax are the most likely complications of this block, it is advisable to use color Doppler to identify the vessels (axillary artery and vein and cephalic vein), particularly if the neural structure is in doubt. It is also important to identify the pleural cavity.

- A linear or curved lower frequency transducer (4–7 MHz) is required for the lateral approach due to the relatively deep location; higher frequencies may be suitable for more medial probe placement.
- The required depth of penetration is usually within 3 to 4 cm, but can be deeper depending on the size of the pectoralis muscle layers.
- At the coracoid process (lateral location; Figure 8.8):
  - Immediately medial and inferior to the coracoid process, position the probe in a parasagittal plane and capture the best possible short-axis view of the nerve structures and axillary vessels (a curved probe is shown in this figure as an alternative to the linear probe as shown in Figures 8.9 and 8.10).
- At the midpoint between the anterior acromion and sternal notch (medial location):
  - The cords of the brachial plexus and the vessels are superficial (usually within 1–2 cm from the skin surface) and are located immediately anterior to the pleura. It is important to note the skin to pleura distance to avoid inadvertent pleural puncture.

Approach

The blind technique described by Borgeat and colleagues (2001), with a lateral angulation of the needle towards the emergence of the axillary artery in the axillary fossa, from a medial puncture site, localized the median nerve well (at the center of the emergence of the terminal nerves from the plexus) and resulted in all five terminal nerves being blocked effectively. The tangential angle and short bevel of the needle presumably helped prevent vascular puncture, which is a common complication with these blocks. This approach would be well suited to ultrasound, with the probe at the lateral site and an OOP needling approach from medial to lateral with an insertion site at the medial location (Figure 8.9). Despite this, the in-plane (IP) approach at a lateral coracoid location (Figures 8.8 and 8.10) may allow better visibility of the needle shaft and tip with this block.

8.3.2. Sonographic Appearance

- Parasagittal plane at the lateral coracoid infraclavicular region (immediately medial and inferior to the coracoid process) with linear probe [Figure 8.7(A)]:
  - The coracoid process is the most cephalad structure and appears, if seen, hypoechoic with hypoechoic shadowing beneath.

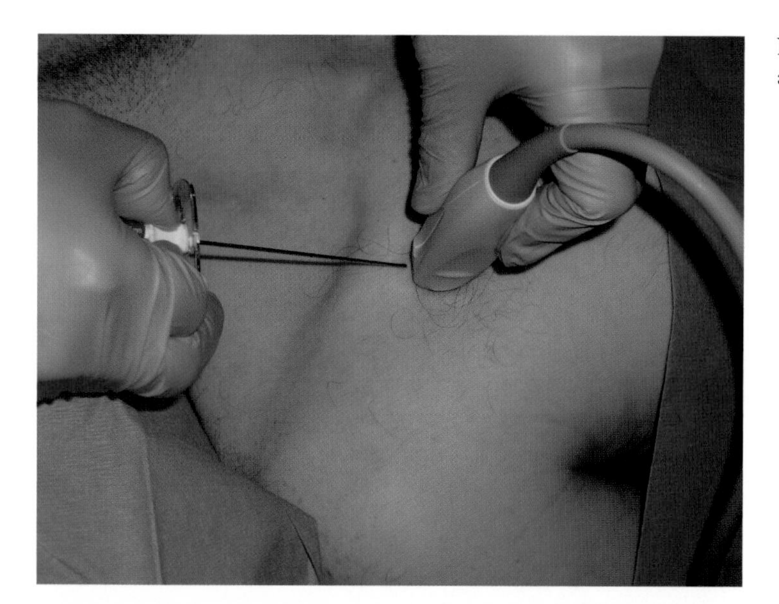

Figure 8.8. Needling technique using a curved probe and an IP needle alignment.

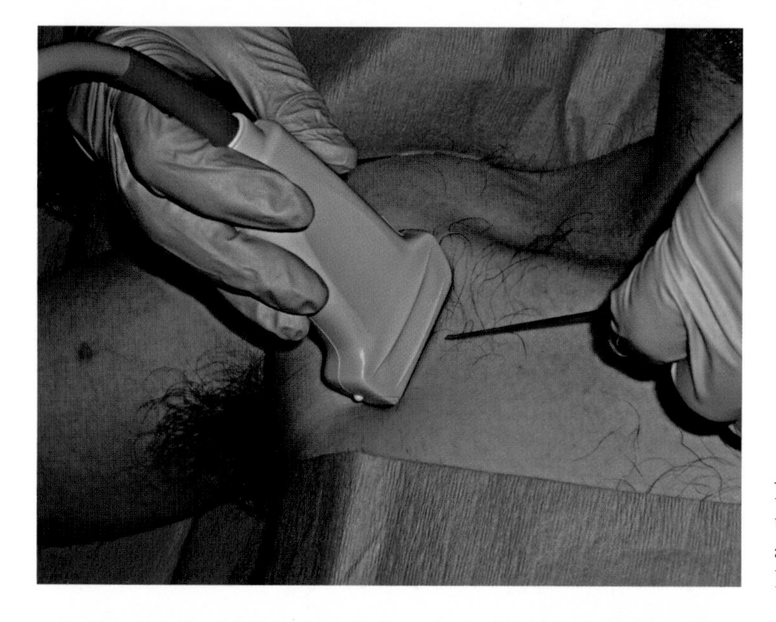

Figure 8.9. Needling technique using a linear probe at the lateral location (caudal to the coracoid process) with a needle placed in OOP alignment at the medial location.

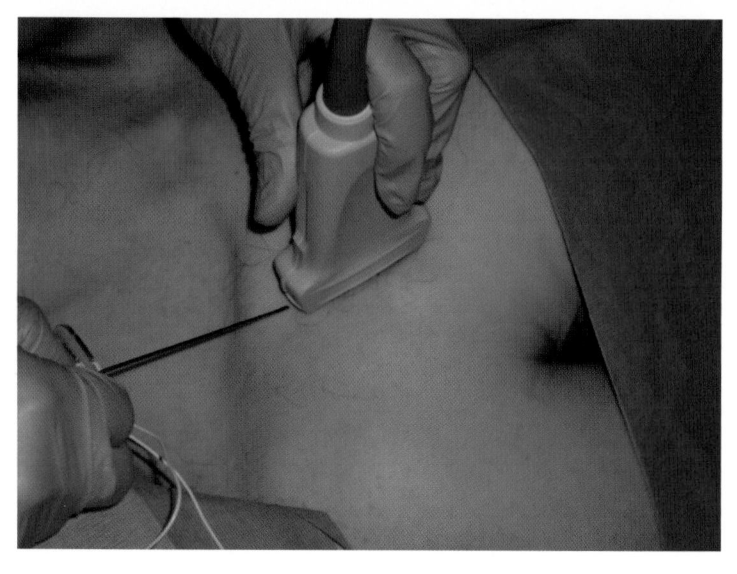

Figure 8.10. Needling technique using a linear probe at the lateral location with IP needle alignment.

- The pectoralis major and minor muscles are separated by a hyperechoic lining (perimysium); the pectoralis major lies superficial and lateral to the pectoralis minor.
- The pectoralis minor muscle is superficial to the axillary neurovascular bundle (approximately 4–5 cm deep); the large axillary vein lies medial and caudad to the artery, with cords of the plexus surrounding the artery.
- The lateral and posterior cords of the plexus are often readily visualized as hyperechoic oval structures; the medial cord may not be readily identified because it lies between the axillary artery and vein. However, the medial cord can be posterior or even slightly cephalad to the axillary artery [between the 6 and 9 o'clock position in Figure 8.7(A)].
- The deep aspect of the image may show an underlying rib (second or third).

- Parasagittal plane at the medial location—(at midpoint of line between anterior acromion and jugular notch) with linear probe [Figure 8.7(B)]:
  - The cords of the plexus are seen as a group of hypoechoic nodules, lying cephalad and lateral to the subclavian artery.
  - The subclavian vein lies anteromedial and the cephalic vein lies superficial to the subclavian artery; the veins may appear irregularly shaped and less hypoechoic than the artery or they may be hard to visualize.
  - The pleural cavity, sloping posteriorly, may appear hyperechoic due to an air artifact and is found inferior and posterior to the hyperechoic first rib.
  - As stated above, because the plexus and vessels are superficial and immediately anterior to the pleura at this location, it is important to mark the skin to pleura distance before needle advancement to avoid inadvertent pleural puncture.

8.3.3. Needle Insertion Technique

Here we address both an in-plane (IP) needling approach with the needle and probe placed at the lateral block location and an out-of-plane (OOP) approach with the probe at the lateral and the needle at the medial block location. The latter allows for a more shallow insertion angle, but will not provide as good a view as an IP technique (see Chapter 4 for details on needling technique). Despite this, the tangential approach of the needle to the plexus during the medial approach may help reduce puncture complications. Ultimately, operator experience and patient body habitus will determine the choice of ultrasound-guided infraclavicular block approaches.

- Use a 5- to 8-cm 18- to 22-ga insulated needle, if using nerve stimulation, for single-injection technique in the lateral coracoid location, and no more than 5 cm for blockade in the medial location; but an 8-cm 18- to 20-ga needle for catheter placement.
- Aim to place the needle and local anesthetic posterior to the axillary artery next to the posterior cord (spread from this location is most optimal for complete block success) for the lateral location.
- Both the in-plane (IP) and out-of-plane (OOP) approaches are appropriate for ultrasound-guided infraclavicular block.
- A modified Borgeat technique for ultrasound-guided block involves an OOP needle alignment with the probe in the parasagittal plane at the lateral probe location (distal to the coracoid process). The needle insertion point is 2 to 3 cm medial to the probe and the needle is inserted in a medial-to-lateral direction (Figure 8.9).
  - The patient's elbow is flexed, and the arm is abducted and externally rotated.
  - The puncture site is within the mid/upper aspect of the pectoralis major muscle, with the needle OOP to the probe.
  - A shallow needle insertion angle is used initially to localize the needle tip on the screen; then the needle is incrementally angled to a 45° to 60° angle to the skin and directed towards the emergence of the axillary artery at the axillary fossa (see description of the incremental walk down OOP technique in Chapter 4).

    - The subclavian artery can be palpated above the clavicle and medial to the needle insertion point; this helps confirm the insertion site is lateral to the lung apex.
- Alternatively, the parasagittal lateral IP approach for coracoid block can be utilized (Figure 8.10):
    - The patient's arm is abducted, with the palm of hand on the abdomen or, with external rotation of the arm, placed behind the head.
    - The block needle is inserted cephalad to the probe and advanced caudally or inferiorly at approximately 45° to 60° from the ultrasound probe axis. After passing through the pectoral muscles, the needle will first contact the lateral cord [10–11 o'clock position in Figure 8.7(A)].
    - It is desirable to move the needle deeper to reach a point posterior to the axillary artery in order to contact the posterior cord.
    - Aim to position the needle tip immediately posterior to the axillary artery prior to local anesthetic injection.

Clinical Pearls

- With the medial infraclavicular approach, the plexus and vessels are superficial and immediately anterior to the pleura at this location, so it is important to limit the insertion depth and angle of the needle to avoid inadvertent pleural puncture.
- With the lateral infraclavicular approach, an acoustic shadow is commonly observed posterior to the axillary artery. This acoustic artifact can be distinguished from the nerve structures by changing the scanning angle or using nerve stimulation.
- It may be difficult to track the needle because of the steep angle of penetration with the lateral coracoid approach. The needle tip position may be identified by angling the needle; for example, if the needle tip is placed too deep (posterior) to the axillary artery, tilting the needle anteriorly will lift up the axillary artery, that is, push the artery more anteriorly.

8.4. Nerve Stimulation

Table 8.2 is a guide for use with nerve stimulation during infraclavicular brachial plexus blockade. At the fairly distal lateral/coracoid infraclavicular block location, the musculocutaneous nerve is often spared because it splits from the brachial plexus at approximately this point. This nerve may also be selectively blocked in this location, without blockade of the cords. Obtaining an elbow flexion response (without pronation) may indicate needle proximity to the musculocutaneous nerve rather than near the cords and additional maneuvers should be made to target the cords.

Clinical Pearl

Nerve stimulation in the infraclavicular region may not always be reliable. A successful block depends ultimately on adequate local anesthetic spread even without a nerve stimulating current of 0.5 mA or less.

Table 8.2. Responses and recommended needle adjustments for use during nerve stimulation at the infraclavicular location.

Correct Response from Nerve Stimulation
Distal responses (hand or wrist flexion or extension) are best for surgery of the elbow and below.

Other Common Responses and Necessary Needle Adjustment

- Muscle twitches from electrical stimulation
  - Pectoralis (adduction of arm)
    - *Explanation*: Needle tip is too shallow
    - *Needle Adjustment*: Advance needle deeper
  - Deltoid (axillary nerve stimulation)
    - *Explanation*: Needle tip is too inferior
    - *Needle Adjustment*: Withdraw needle to subcutaneous tissue and reinsert slightly more superiorly
  - Biceps (musculocutaneous nerve)
    - *Explanation*: Needle tip is too superior
    - *Needle Adjustment*: Withdraw needle to subcutaneous tissue and reinsert slightly more inferiorly
- Vascular puncture
  - Cephalic vein (seen as blood withdrawal when needle appears to be placed superficially)
    - *Explanation*: Cephalic vein is superficial to the plexus and the subclavian artery and vein
    - *Needle Adjustment*: Withdraw needle and redirect carefully while observing the needle tip at all times using in-plane approach
  - Subclavian artery/vein puncture (seen as blood aspiration)
    - *Explanation*: Artery and vein are next to the plexus
    - *Needle Adjustment*: Withdraw needle completely and reinsert carefully while observing the needle tip at all times using in-plane approach; if the blood is venous, the needle tip is likely too caudal
- Bone contact
  - Needle stops at rib
    - *Explanation*: Needle is inserted too deep and has passed the plexus and subclavian artery. However, it is very unlikely with ultrasound-guided technique.
    - *Needle Adjustment*: Withdraw needle to subcutaneous tissue and reinsert
- Pleural—more risk with medial locations of needle insertion
  - Needle observed to pass beyond the white line (rib), with a pocket forming
    - *Explanation*: Needle inserted too deep, past the plexus and subclavian artery and entering into pleural space. However, it is very unlikely with ultrasound-guided technique
    - *Needle Adjustment*: Withdraw to subcutaneous tissue and reinsert

8.5. Local Anesthetic Application

We recommend using nerve stimulation to confirm nerve identity prior to local anesthetic injection.

- Performing a test dose with dextrose 5% in water (D5W) is recommended prior to local anesthetic application to visualize the spread and confirm nerve localization (see Chapter 4 sidebar).
- Our preliminary experience suggests that local anesthetic deposited posterior to the axillary artery with cephalad and caudad spreading will result in consistent surgical anesthesia in the hand when performing the block in the lateral position.
- A hypoechoic fluid collection is often observed (Figure 8.11 illustrates the solution near the posterior cord) and this will accentuate imaging of adjacent nerve structures.
- If local anesthetic spread is deemed inadequate to surround all the cords, stop halfway through and reposition the needle prior to applying the remaining injectate.

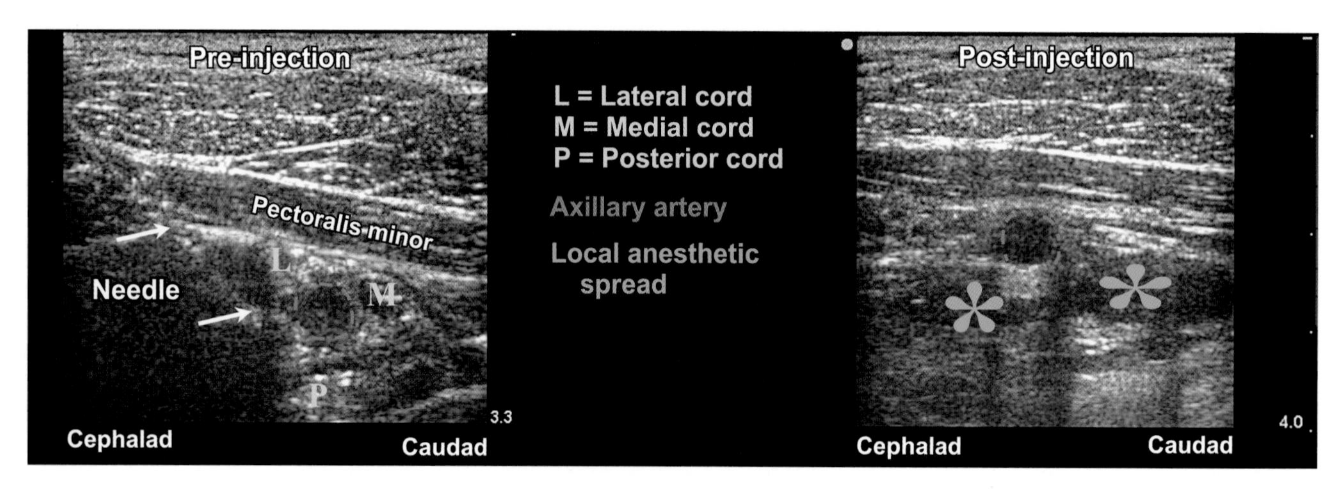

Figure 8.11. Local anesthetic application near the posterior cord.

Suggested Reading and References

Arcand G, Williams SR, Chouinard P, et al. Ultrasound-guided infraclavicular versus supraclavicular block. Anesth Analg 2005;101:886–890.

Borgeat A, Ekatodramis G, Dumont C. An evaluation of the infraclavicular block via a modified approach of the Raj technique. Anesth Analg 2001;93:436–441.

De Andres J, Sala-Blanch X. Ultrasound in the practice of brachial plexus anesthesia. Reg Anesth Pain Med 2002;27:77–89.

Kapral S, Jandrasits O, Schaberinig C, et al. Lateral infraclavicular plexus block vs. axillary block for hand and forearm surgery. Acta Anaesthesiol Scand 1999;43:1047–1052.

Porter JM, McCartney CJ, Chan VW. Needle placement and injection posterior to the axillary artery may predict successful infraclavicular brachial plexus block: a report of three cases. Can J Anesth 2005;52:69–73.

Raj PP, Montgomery SJ, Nettles D, Jenkins MT. Infraclavicular brachial plexus block—a new approach. Anesth Analg 1973;52:897–904.

9

Axillary Block

Ban C.H. Tsui

The nerves targeted for the axillary block course distally with the axillary artery and vein along the humerus from the apex of the axilla (Figure 9.1). This block is useful for surgery of the elbow, forearm, and hand. The ulnar, median, and radial nerves are the primary targets; the musculocutaneous nerve often leaves the plexus (via the lateral cord) proximal to this point and may be blocked separately at a different location or at midhumeral locations (where it enters the coracobrachialis muscle diagonally). The three terminal nerves (radial, ulnar, and median) can also be blocked effectively using ultrasound guidance at more distal regions within the upper arm (see Chapter 10).

9.1. Clinical Anatomy

- The axilla has an *apex* (between the first rib, clavicle, and base of coracoid process), a *base* (axillary fascia), and is bordered by 4 *walls—anterior* (pectoralis major and minor), *posterior* (latissimus dorsi, teres major, and subscapularis), *medial* (serratus anterior), and *lateral* [intertubercular (bicipital) groove of humerus].
- The neurovascular bundle is located within the internal bicipital sulcus, between the flexor and extensor musculature (Figure 9.1), and lies approximately 1 to 2 cm below the skin at its most proximal axillary location.
- Beyond the clavicle and at the lower border of the pectoralis minor muscle the cords diverge into their terminal branches (Figure 9.2).

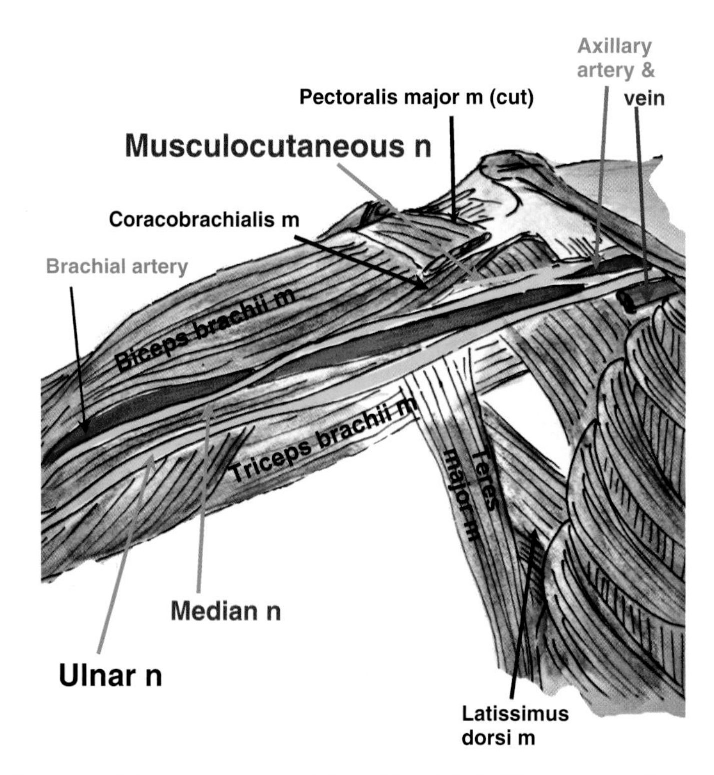

Figure 9.1. Anatomy of the target nerves of the axillary block. The ulnar, median, and radial (not shown as it lies in a posterior plane) nerves travel with the brachial artery beyond the axilla, and the musculocutaneous nerve leaves the plexus and penetrates the coracobrachialis muscle at the superior aspect of the axilla.

- The axillary artery has three parts separated by the pectoralis minor muscle: the first part is medial, the second part posterior, and the third part lateral to the muscle.
- The axillary artery becomes continuous with the brachial artery at the lower border of the teres major muscle.
- Relative to the third part of the axillary artery, the usual course of the terminal nerves is: the median nerve is anterior and lateral; the ulnar nerve is posterior and medial; the

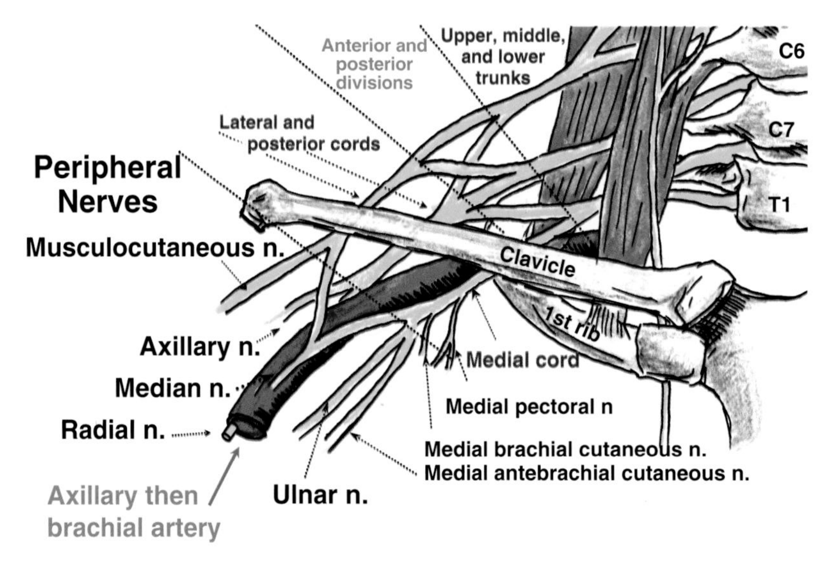

Figure 9.2. Anatomy of the brachial plexus.

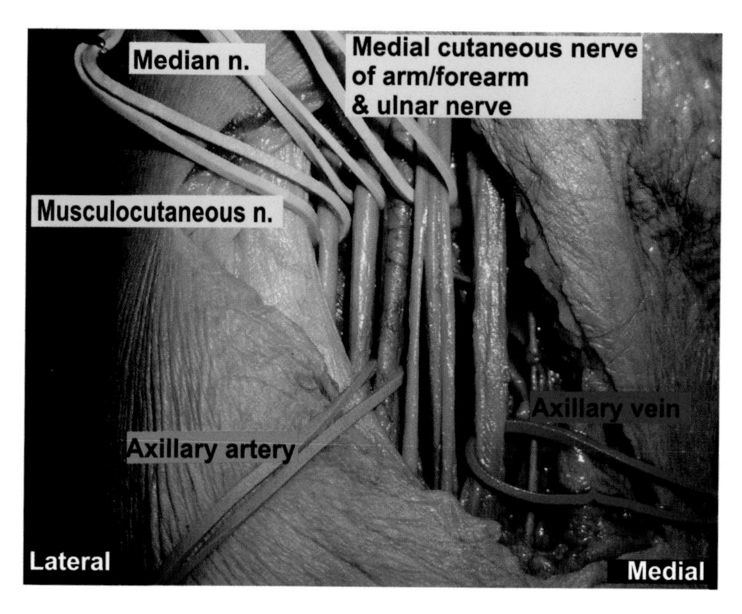

Figure 9.3. Dissection showing the peripheral nerves immediately distal to the axilla.

musculocutaneous nerve is anterior and lateral; and the radial nerve is posterior and lateral (Figures 9.2 and 9.3).
- The axillary vein is usually medial to the third part of the axillary artery.
- Anatomical variations of the neurovascular structures are commonly observed; for example, it is common to find more than one axillary vein.

Table 9.1 summarizes the target nerves for the axillary brachial plexus blockade; please note that the musculocutaneous nerve must be blocked separately (see Chapter 10). Each nerve is traced from its origin at the root level and the motor response associated with nerve

Table 9.1. Target nerves of the axillary block: origin and motor responses associated with nerve stimulation.

Movement	Nerve	Cord	Division	Trunk	Root
Elbow flexion	Musculocutaneous[a]	Lateral	Posterior and anterior	Upper	C5, C6
Extension (dorsiflexion) of elbow, wrist, hand, and fingers	Radial	Posterior	Posterior Posterior	Upper Middle	C5, C6 C7
Latissimus dorsi twitch	Thoracodorsal	Posterior	Posterior	Middle	C7
Forearm pronation and wrist flexion	Median (lateral head)	Lateral Medial	Anterior Anterior and posterior Anterior	Upper Middle Lower	C5, C6 C7 C8, T1
Thumb flexion and opposition (flexion middle and ring finger)	Median	Medial	Anterior	Lower	C8, T1
Thumb flexion and opposition	Anterior interosseous	Medial	Anterior	Lower	C8, T1
Fifth finger flexion and opposition, ulnar deviation of wrist	Ulnar	Medial	Anterior	Lower	C8, T1

[a]The targets of the axillary block are the terminal nerves of the upper extremity and branches at the cord level of the brachial plexus. The musculocutaneous nerve may not be blocked if the injection does not spread to the proximal location where it branches.

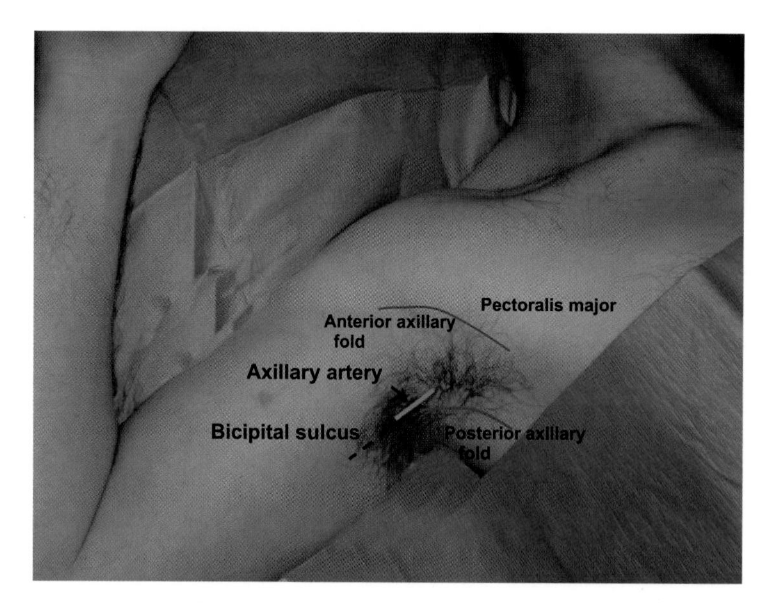

Figure 9.4. Surface anatomy for the axillary block.

stimulation is described. Nerves that are purely sensory are not included in the above table. Segmental dermatomal, myotomal, and osteotomal innervation of the brachial plexus is discussed and illustrated in Chapter 5.

9.2. Patient Positioning and Surface Anatomy

9.2.1. Patient Positioning

The patient is positioned supine with the arm abducted at 70° to 80° and externally rotated, the elbow flexed at 90°, and the dorsum of the hand facing the table.

9.2.2. Surface Anatomy (Figure 9.4)

- Anterior axillary fold
  - Formed by the pectoralis major muscle
  - Palpating the axillary artery just deep to the insertion of this muscle will identify the optimal site of needle insertion if attempting to block the musculocutaneous nerve
- Posterior axillary fold
  - Formed by the latissimus dorsi and teres major muscles
  - The lower part of the axillary artery can be palpated anterior to this fold on the medial side of the arm; trace this pulse to a proximal location for an optimal block for targeting all the nerves
- Bicipital sulcus
  - A groove between the tendons of the biceps and triceps brachii muscles

9.3. Sonographic Imaging and Needle Insertion Technique

The terminal nerves of the brachial plexus are shown in Figure 9.5 and the corresponding magnetic resonance imaging (MRI) scan (Figure 9.6) at the axillary level.

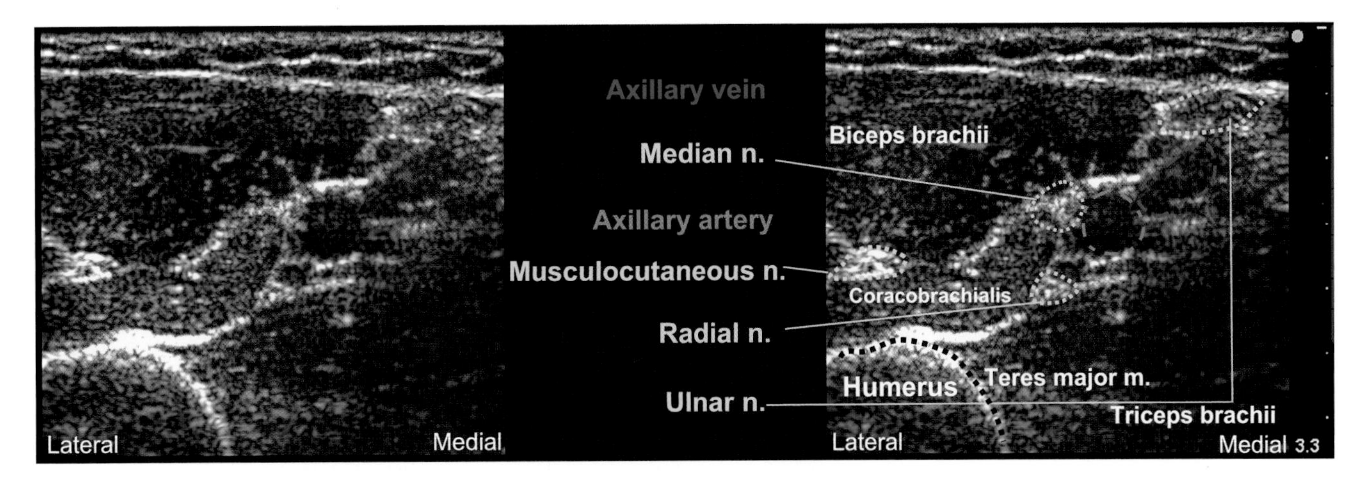

Figure 9.5. Ultrasound image using a linear probe just distal to the axilla and transverse to the nerves.

Prepare the needle insertion site and skin surface with an antiseptic solution. Prepare the ultrasound probe surface by applying a sterile adhesive dressing to it prior to needling as discussed earlier (see Chapters 3 and 4).

9.3.1. Scanning Technique

- High-frequency, linear probes are generally recommended (10–15 MHz) for imaging as the nerves are superficial (1–2 cm) below the skin.
- The vascular structures, including the pulse, are easily identified on palpation and Doppler will not add additional information with respect to the artery location. Despite this, Doppler may be able to distinguish the artery from the nerves as some small nerves appear on ultrasound to be pulsating.
- The most proximal location at the apex of the axilla may be the best for viewing all the terminal branches of the brachial plexus.

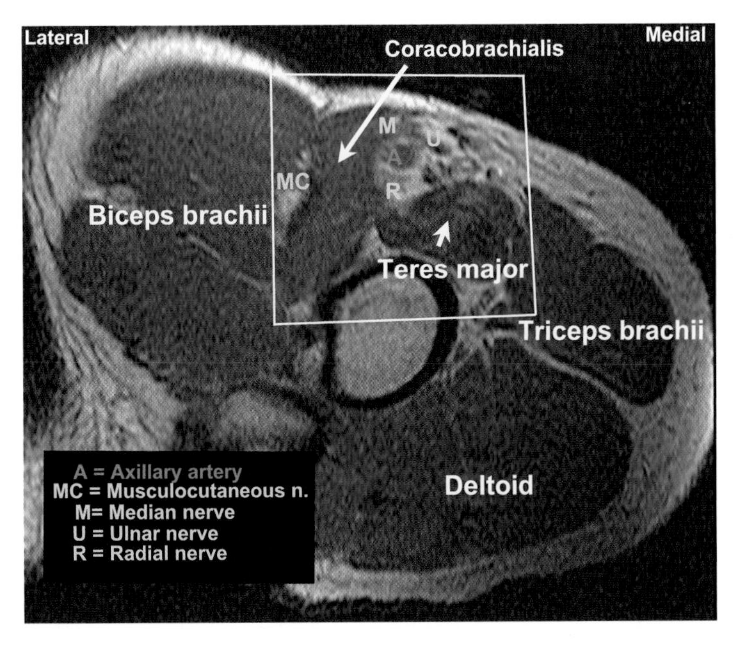

Figure 9.6. MRI image of the axillary block location.

- The probe is positioned perpendicular to the anterior axillary fold and in cross-section to the humerus at the bicipital sulcus (and at the level of the axillary pulse) to capture the transverse, or short-axis, view of the neurovascular bundle.

Clinical Pearls

- Applying light to moderate probe pressure may help to spread the nerves apart with the median nerve moving towards the biceps muscle.
- Probe pressure should be partially reduced to visualize the axillary vein(s); otherwise it may collapse.
- Move the probe proximally and distally in the axilla to identify the location of the median, ulnar, and radial nerves and the location at which they are closest together; this is the optimal location for ultrasound-guided nerve block.
- The radial nerve is often the most difficult nerve to visualize because it is deep to the ulnar nerve. It may be beneficial to move the probe more medially to localize the radial nerve by scanning through the triceps muscle and posterior to the ulnar nerve.
- Particularly when using the in-plane approach, it is possible to reach the radial nerve by advancing the needle either above or below the axillary artery.

9.3.2. Sonographic Appearance (12 MHz, Linear Probe)

- Transverse cross-section (as seen in Figure 9.5)
  - The biceps and coracobrachialis muscles are seen on the left/lateral aspect (biceps being most superficial). The triceps are seen on the right/medial side, deeper than the biceps.
  - The anechoic and circular axillary artery lies in the middle and is adjacent to both the biceps and coracobrachialis.
  - The compressible anechoic axillary vein (two may be present) lies superficial (although there are many variants) between the median and ulnar nerves.
  - The axillary artery runs deep to the vein and is surrounded by the nerves.
  - The nerves appear round to oval in short-axis view with a honeycomb appearance of hypoechoic fascicles surrounded by hyperechoic connective tissue rims (epineurium).
  - The median nerve is often located superficial and between the artery and biceps muscle.
  - The ulnar nerve is usually located medial and superficial to the artery.
  - The radial nerve lies deep to the artery at the midline.
  - Clockwise: median, ulnar, radial, but there are many variations.
  - The musculocutaneous nerve is commonly located in the hyperechoic plane between the biceps and coracobrachialis muscles; it may appear round/oval or triangular or many times it is flat.

9.3.3. Needle Insertion Technique

A single-injection technique, within the axillary sheath, has been used to target the entire plexus, although this is usually not reliable because the local anesthetic spread is often limited. Thus, it is recommended to block each nerve separately.

- Use a 5-cm, 22-ga insulated needle if using nerve stimulation.
- Both in-plane (IP) and out-of-plane (OOP) needle approaches can be used for axillary block (see Chapter 4).

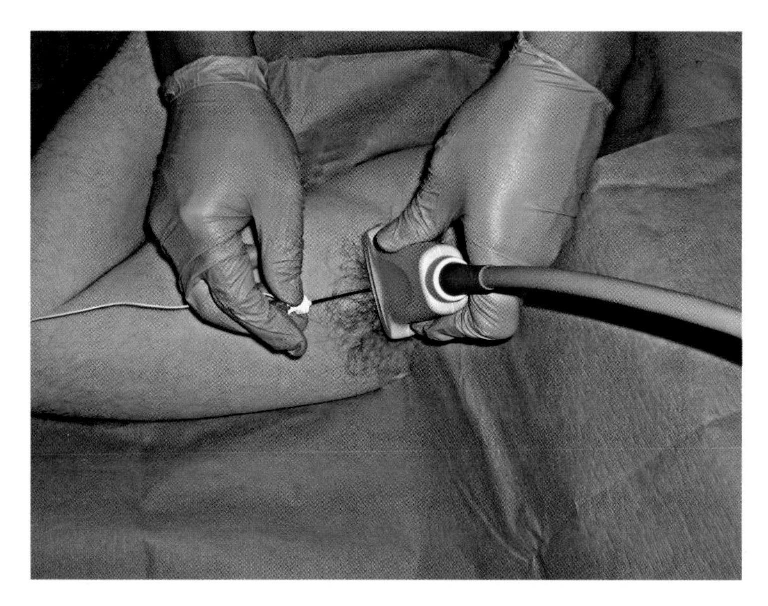

Figure 9.7. Needling technique using a linear probe and an out-of-plane (OOP) needle alignment.

- An OOP approach is similar to the traditional blind procedure with the needle distal and perpendicular to the probe placed in transverse axis to the nerves (Figure 9.7):
  - Place the needle 1 cm from the probe at a 30° to 45° angle from the skin and align the needle insertion site with the neurovascular bundle target (often associated with a fascial click upon sheath entry; see Chapter 4 for a description of the walk down approach using OOP needling).
- The IP approach involves inserting the needle at an acute angle (20°–30°) to the skin in a lateral to medial direction (Figure 9.8):
  - Typically, the block needle is advanced to first contact the median nerve, then it is crossed over the axillary artery to contact the ulnar nerve superficially and then finally the radial nerve somewhat deeper.
  - Alternatively, the sequence of nerves blocked can be changed to suit the surgical requirements.

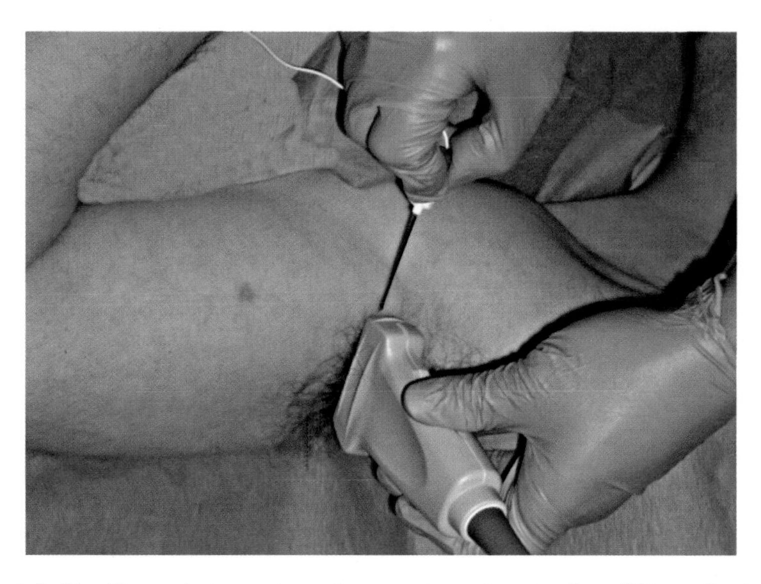

Figure 9.8. Needling technique using a linear probe with an in-plane (IP) needle alignment.

- For intercostobrachial and medial cutaneous nerve blocks, subcutaneous injections should be performed on the medial surface of the upper arm all the way from the biceps to triceps muscles.
- For musculocutaneous nerve block, often the best results will be from infraclavicular blockade (see Chapter 8); however, the nerve may also be blocked in a separate injection during the axillary approach, above the artery into the body of the coracobrachialis (with biceps twitch as nerve stimulation response), or at a midhumeral location (see Chapter 10 discussion of musculocutaneous nerve block in the midhumeral location).

9.4. Nerve Stimulation

Table 9.2 depicts the correct responses obtained for general axillary block as well as blockade for individual terminal nerves of the brachial plexus. Motor responses and their interpretations with recommended needling adjustments are included. Ultrasound may be of use to eliminate several of these traditional responses as the vessels and bone in relation to the needle are visible.

Table 9.2. Responses and recommended needle adjustments for use with nerve stimulation at the axillary location.

Correct Response from Nerve Stimulation
- Hand twitch with approximately 0.4 mA (median, radial, or ulnar nerve)
- For a higher success rate, multiple injections at each nerve are recommended:
  - Median nerve (C5–C8, T1; flexion of middle, index fingers, and thumb, and pronation and flexion of wrist; ulnar nerve (C7–C8, T1; flexion of ring and little fingers and ulnar deviation of wrist); radial nerve (C5–C8, T1; extension of fingers and wrist)

Other Common Responses & Necessary Needle Adjustment
- Muscle twitches from electrical stimulation
  - Upper arm (local twitches from biceps or triceps)
    - *Explanation*: Needle angle is too superior or inferior
    - *Needle Adjustment*: Withdraw completely and redirect accordingly
- Vascular puncture
  - Axillary artery with arterial blood in tubing
    - *Explanation*: Needle in lumen of axillary artery
    - *Needle Adjustment*: Inject two thirds of the local anesthetic posterior to the artery and one third anterior to the artery
  - Axillary venous blood in tubing
    - *Explanation*: Needle in lumen of axillary vein
    - *Needle Adjustment*: Redirect slightly more laterally or superiorly
- Paresthesia without motor response
  - Needle has contacted brachial plexus
    - *Explanation:* Stimulator, needle, or electrode malfunctioning
    - *Needle Adjustment*: None if typical distribution and transient (inject); withdraw if persistent
- Bone contact
  - Humerus (2–3 cm deep)
    - *Explanation*: Needle has advanced beyond plexus, too deep
    - *Needle Adjustment*: Withdraw to subcutaneous tissue and reinsert with an angle 20° to 30° more superior or inferior

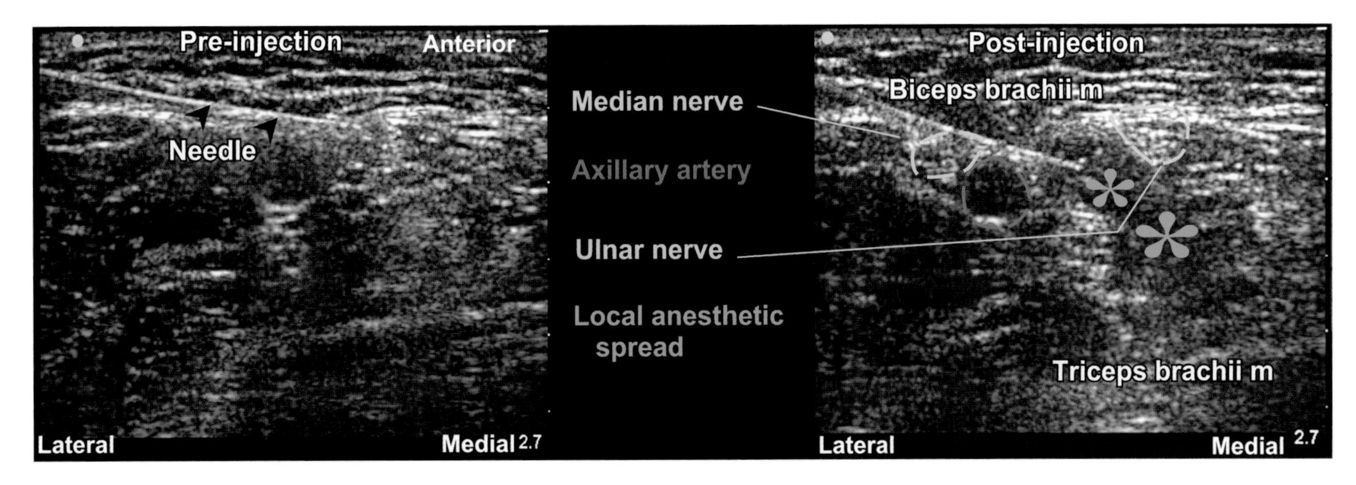

Figure 9.9. Local anesthetic application between the ulnar nerve and the axillary artery.

9.5. Local Anesthetic Application

It is recommended to confirm nerve identity with nerve stimulation prior to anesthetic injection. Tracing the nerves distally or proximally along their known path may be adequate in some cases.

- Performing a test dose with dextrose 5% in water (D5W) is recommended prior to local anesthetic application to visualize the spread and confirm nerve localization (see Chapter 4 sidebar).
- Experience has shown that a multiple injection technique, with injection around each individual nerve is the most reliable approach (10–15 mL at each nerve location); it may require less anesthetic but the minimum required dose/volume per nerve is not known at this time.
- A proper injection is indicated by fluid spread completely around the nerve structure (Figure 9.9 shows anesthetic injected between the ulnar nerve and axillary artery) and nerve movement away from the needle tip. Improper injection, for example, injection outside the sheath is indicated by a partial asymmetrical fluid expansion not immediately adjacent to the nerve structure.
- Nerve visualization often becomes more difficult after local anesthetic injection.

Suggested Readings and References

Chan VW, Perlas A, McCartney CJ, Brull R, Xu D, Abbas S. Ultrasound guidance improves success rate of axillary brachial plexus block. Can J Anesth 2007;54:176–182.

Kapral S, Jandrasits O, Schaberinig C, et al. Lateral infraclavicular plexus block vs. axillary block for hand and forearm surgery. Acta Anaesthesiol Scand 1999;43:1047–1052.

Retzl G, Kapral S, Greher M, Mauritz W. Ultrasonographic findings of the axillary part of the brachial plexus. Reg Anesth Pain Med 2001;92:1271–1275.

Schafhalyter-Zoppoth I, Gray AT. The musculocutaneous nerve: ultrasonic appearance for peripheral nerve block. Reg Anetsh Pain Med 2005;30:385–390.

Sites BS, Beach ML, Spence BC et al. Ultrasound guidance improves the successs rate of a perivascular axillary brachial plexus block. Acta Anaesthesiol Scand 2006;50:678–684.

Soeding PE, Sha S, Royse CE, Marks P, Hoy G, Rogyse AG. A randomized trial of ultrasound-guided brachial plexus anaesthesia in upper limb surgery. Anaesth Intensive Care 2005;33:719–725.

10

Selective Terminal Nerve Blocks of the Upper Extremity

Ban C.H. Tsui

10.1. Introduction

Peripheral nerve blocks in the upper extremity [Figure 10.1(A,B)] are particularly valuable as rescue blocks to supplement surgical anesthesia and to provide long-lasting selective analgesia in the postoperative period.

An exception to this is blockade of the musculocutaneous nerve when the axillary, or possibly infraclavicular, block is utilized for blocking the brachial plexus. This is due to the musculocutaneous nerve leaving the brachial plexus proximal to the popular axillary block location. Occasionally, it is possible to produce neural blockade of the terminal nerves in the periphery rather than targeting the entire brachial plexus. This approach may be favorable as the requirement for motor paralysis after surgery is reduced, which can be beneficial for postoperative discharge and rehabilitation. As well, single nerve blocks can allow lower doses of local anesthetic, thus reducing the risk of systemic toxicity.

For example, selective ulnar nerve blockade is indicated for hand surgery involving the fifth digit when tourniquet inflation is not required. Nevertheless, additional subcutaneous infiltration of local anesthetic around the intercostobrachial nerve at the medial aspect of the axilla has shown to be useful for reducing tourniquet pain if peripheral nerve blockade is the primary source of surgical anesthesia.

The radial, median, and ulnar nerves are traditionally blocked around the elbow or wrist. With the help of color Doppler, ultrasound can be used to clearly identify the nerves at many desirable locations as they are often situated near blood vessels. For instance, ultrasound-assisted ulnar nerve block on the medial aspect of the forearm is easier to perform (i.e., the area is less compact and the Doppler-illuminated adjacent ulnar artery is a good landmark) as opposed to blocking the ulnar nerve at the level of the medial epicondyle,

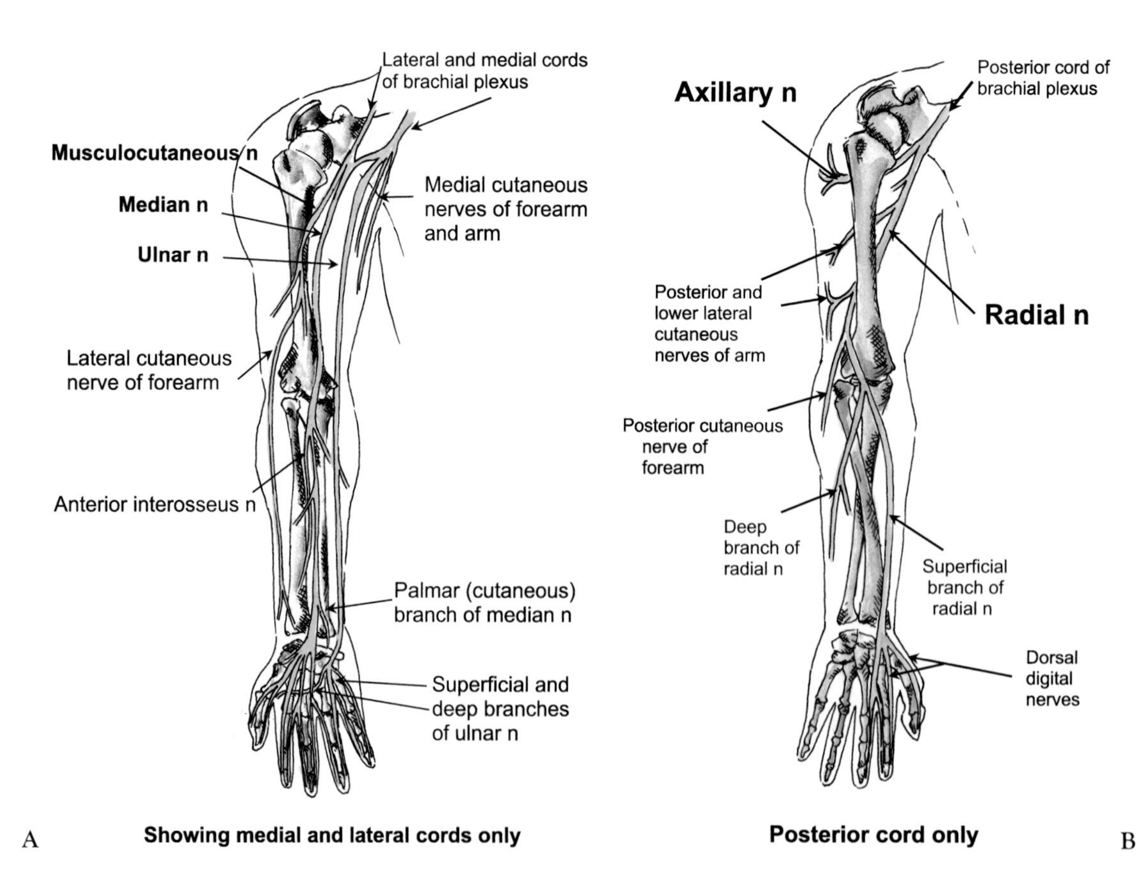

Figure 10.1. Peripheral nerves of the upper extremity. For ease of illustration, (A) shows the lateral and medial cords and their branches and (B) shows the posterior cord and its branches.

Table 10.1. Target peripheral nerves of the upper extremity blocks: origin and motor response associated with nerve stimulation.

Movement	Nerve	Cord	Division	Trunk	Root
Elbow flexion	Musculocutaneous	Lateral	Posterior and anterior	Upper	C5, C6
Extension (dorsiflexion) of elbow, wrist, hand, and fingers	Radial	Posterior	Posterior Posterior	Upper Middle	C5, C6 C7
Forearm pronation and wrist flexion	Median (lateral head)	Lateral Medial	Anterior Anterior and posterior Anterior	Upper Middle Lower	C5, C6 C7 C8, T1
Thumb flexion and opposition (flexion middle and ring finger)	Median	Medial	Anterior	Lower	C8, T1
Thumb flexion and opposition	Anterior interosseous	Medial	Anterior	Lower	C8, T1
Fifth finger flexion and opposition, ulnar deviation of wrist	Ulnar	Medial	Anterior	Lower	C8, T1

where there is an increased risk of ulnar nerve palsy (neuritis). Ultrasound-guided median nerve block is probably easier at the elbow as the sonographic appearance of the tendons at the wrist is subject to anisotropy, making it difficult to distinguish them from the nerve (see Chapter 3 for a description of anisotropy). In addition, blockade of the median nerve at the antecubital fossa rather than the anterior aspect of the wrist may reduce the chances of causing carpal tunnel syndrome.

In this chapter, we will focus on discussing the most commonly performed peripheral nerve blocks. Because ultrasound imaging during nerve block procedures at the wrist can be difficult without extensive experience (partly due to the anisotropic effect discussed above and in Chapter 3), the wrist blocks are not discussed at length in this text. In addition to this chapter's sections on anatomy, the reader is referred to Chapter 5 for more details of the segmental distribution of the upper extremity. Table 10.1 is an overview of many terminal motor nerves of the upper extremity and summarizes their origin from within the brachial plexus and the associated movements for use with nerve stimulation technique. The schematic diagram (Figure 10.2) of the brachial plexus can also be referred to for tracing the peripheral nerves to their root levels.

10.2. Radial Nerve Block at Lateral Aspect of Elbow

The radial nerve [Figure 10.1(B)] can be blocked successfully at the anterosuperior aspect of the lateral epicondyle of the humerus. To confirm the identity of the nerve with ultrasound, it can first be located proximally at the level of the spiral (radial) groove of the humerus where it lies immediately adjacent to the humerus and posteromedial to the deep brachial (profunda brachii) artery of the arm. Subsequent tracing of the nerve from this humeral location to the anterior radial location may then facilitate its precise localization.

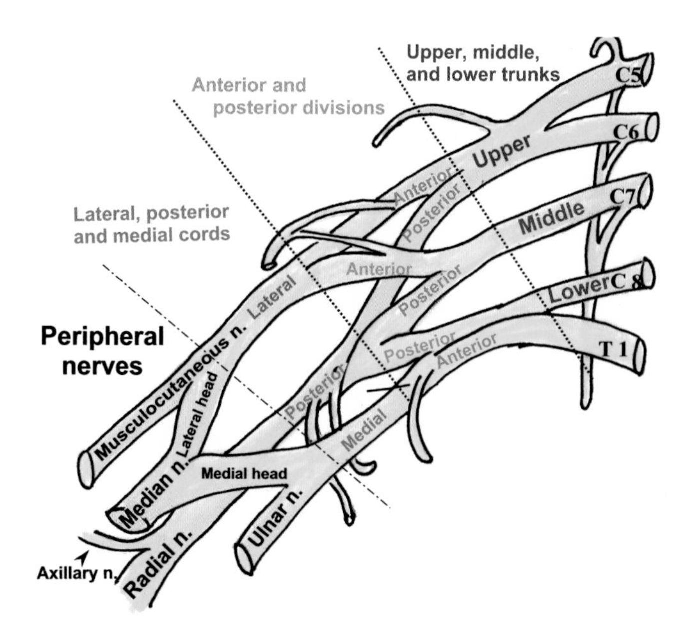

Figure 10.2. Peripheral nerves within the design of the brachial plexus.

10.2.1. Clinical Anatomy

- The nerve originates from C5 to C8 roots; innervates muscles which produce extension (dorsiflexion) of the wrist and digits.
- The radial nerve carries fibers from the upper and middle trunks and the posterior divisions and the posterior cord of the brachial plexus; it emerges from the posterior aspect of the plexus.

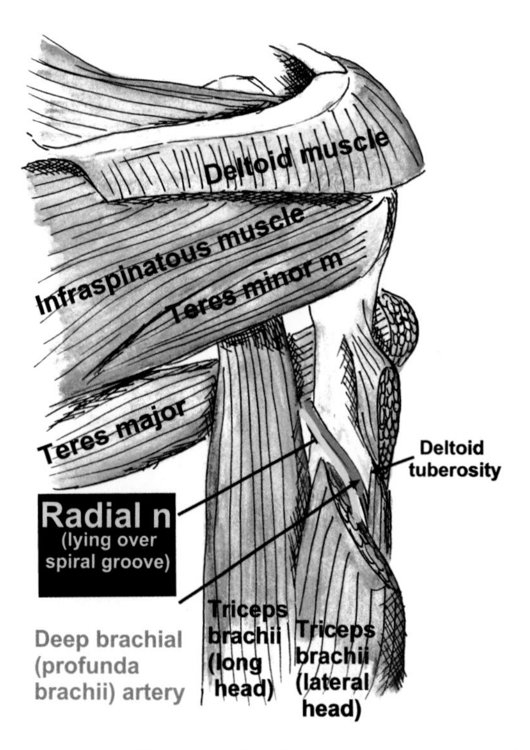

Figure 10.3. Radial nerve travels medial to the deep brachial artery and travels inferolaterally beyond the deltoid tuberosity along the spiral groove of the humerus.

- Its origin lies deep to the second and third parts of the axillary artery and it descends within the axilla across the subscapularis, teres major, and latissimus dorsi muscles (it lies on the insertion of this latter muscle).
- It then passes between the medial and lateral heads of the triceps, and descends obliquely across the posterior aspect of the humerus along the spiral (radial) groove at the level of the deltoid insertion (Figure 10.3). It travels posterior and medial to the deep brachial artery of the arm at this location.
- The nerve reaches the lateral margin of the humerus 5 to 7 cm above the elbow before crossing over the lateral epicondyle and entering the anterior compartment of the arm in a deep groove between the brachialis and brachioradialis muscles [Figure 10.4(A,B)] proximally and the extensor carpi radialis longus muscle distally.
- In front of the lateral epicondyle of humerus, the nerve divides and continues as the superficial radial (sensory) and the deep posterior interosseous (motor) nerves.

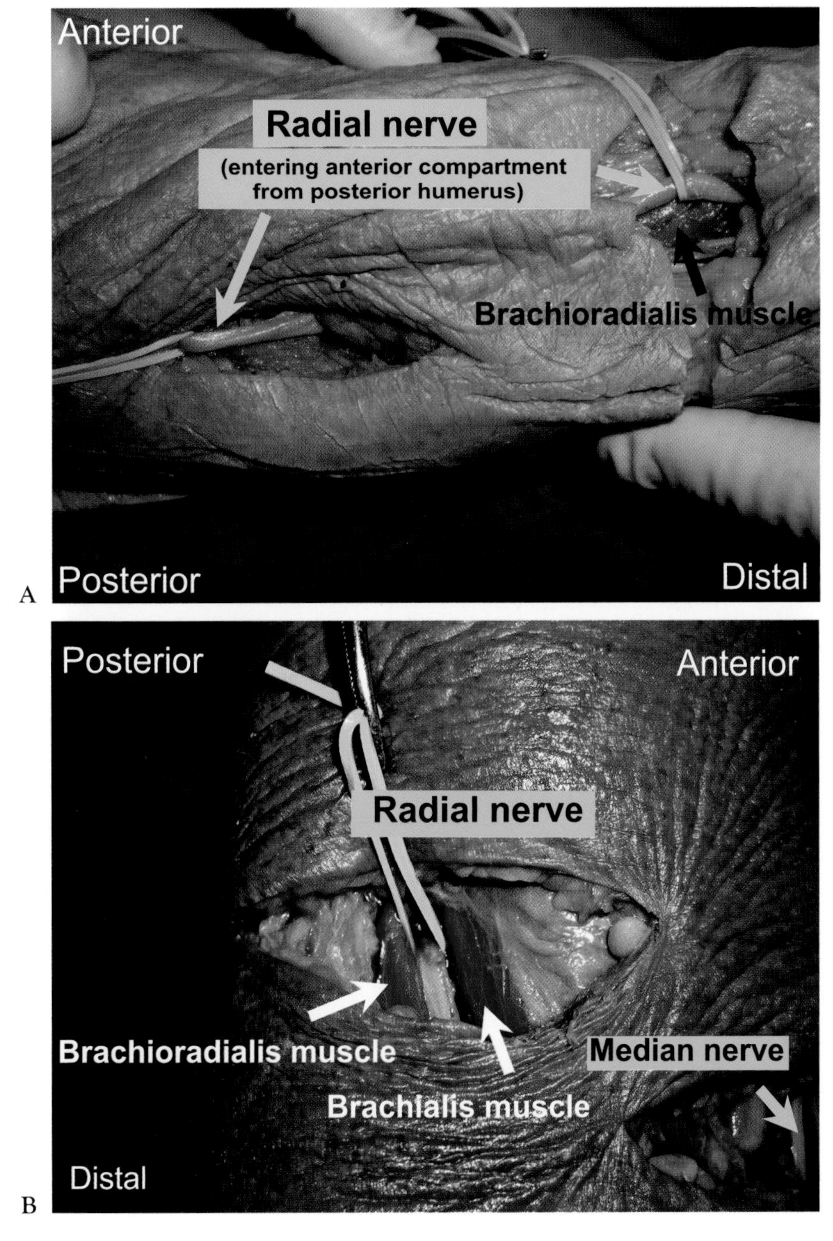

Figure 10.4. Dissections showing the radial nerve at the (A) lateral margin of the arm and (B) anterior compartment.

- The radial nerve supplies the posterior compartments of the arm and forearm, including skin and subcutaneous tissues. It also supplies skin on the posterior aspect of the hand laterally near the base of the thumb and the dorsal aspect of the index and the lateral half of the ring finger up to the distal interphalangeal crease.

10.2.2. Patient Positioning and Surface Anatomy

10.2.2.1. *Patient Positioning*

10.2.2.1.1. For Scanning at the Spiral Groove

The patient's arm should be internally rotated and placed across the abdomen with the hand on the opposite side of the body. The probe will be scanned from the posterior to anterior aspect of the arm with an oblique inferior angle (i.e., the same direction as the spiral groove of the humerus).

10.2.2.1.2. For Scanning at the Lateral Epicondyle

The patient's arm is slightly abducted and laterally rotated, with the elbow extended and the forearm resting on an arm board.

10.2.2.2. *Surface Anatomy* (Figures 10.5 and 10.6)

- Deltoid tuberosity: Internal rotation of the arm accentuates the posterior deltoid region and enables the operator to trace the deltoid muscle to its point of insertion on the tuberosity. The spiral groove lies just distal to the tubercle.
- Lateral epicondyle of the humerus: Palpate from proximal to distal along the lateral aspect of the humerus towards the elbow and feel the curvature of the lateral supracondylar crest proximal to the epicondyle.
- Biceps brachii muscle: Palpate the lateral border of the distal muscle belly. The radial nerve lies deep and lateral to this portion of the muscle.

10.2.3. Sonographic Imaging and Needle Insertion Technique

The relationships between the radial nerve and the posterior aspect of the humerus (at the spiral groove) and the lateral epicondyle are depicted with magnetic resonance imaging (MRI) in Figure 10.7(A,B). Both images can be used for reference with the ultrasound images [Figure 10.8(A,B)].

Prepare the needle insertion site and skin surface with an antiseptic solution. Prepare the ultrasound probe surface by applying a sterile adhesive dressing to it prior to needling as discussed earlier (see Chapters 3 and 4).

10.2.3.1. *Scanning Technique*

- A linear probe in the frequency range of 5 to 10MHz is suitable for scanning in most cases; a lower frequency probe is required for scanning in a region with a considerable amount of subcutaneous tissue.
- The depth of penetration is variable at both the spiral groove and above the lateral epicondyle at the elbow (often >2 to 3cm).
- For scanning the nerve at the spiral groove of the humerus, palpate the posterior aspect of the deltoid muscle down to the deltoid tubercle and position the probe in the transverse axis to the path of the radial nerve (see Figure 10.3).
- Once located at this level [using color Doppler if necessary; see Figure 10.8(A)], the nerve can be traced downward as it courses laterally and anteriorly towards the anterior surface of the lateral epicondyle (see Chapter 4 for details on the traceback approaches).
- Rotate the probe slowly to scan the nerve both in the longitudinal and transverse planes at the elbow for confirmation of its location.

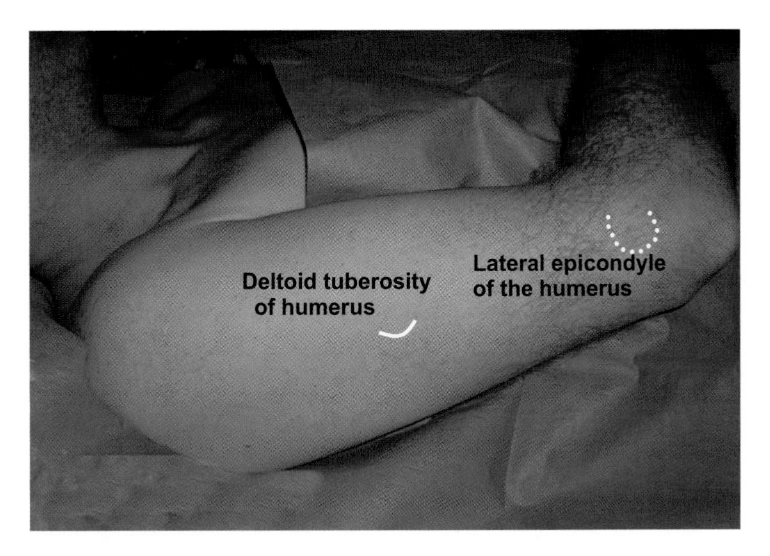

Figure 10.5. Surface anatomy for scanning at the spiral groove.

Clinical Pearls

- During ultrasound imaging at the spiral (radial) groove, the hyperechoic bone and adjacent nerve are usually obvious, lying on the posterior surface of the humerus, but additional verification using Doppler at the level of the deep brachial (profunda brachii) artery, immediately anterolateral to the nerve, may be useful to identify the radial nerve.
- To confirm the radial nerve at the anterior elbow, it can be easily traced proximally (back) and posteriorly to its location abutting the spiral groove of the humerus (see Figure 4.4).

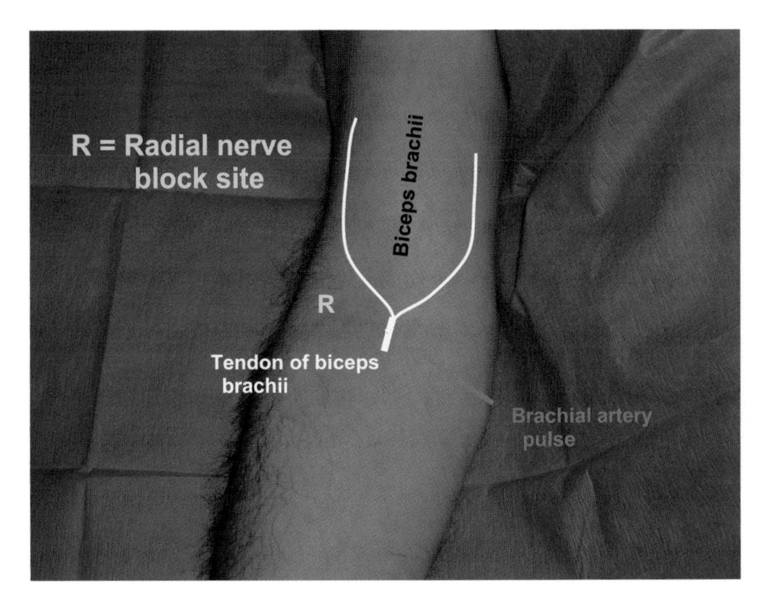

Figure 10.6. Surface anatomy for radial nerve blockade at the lateral humeral epicondyle.

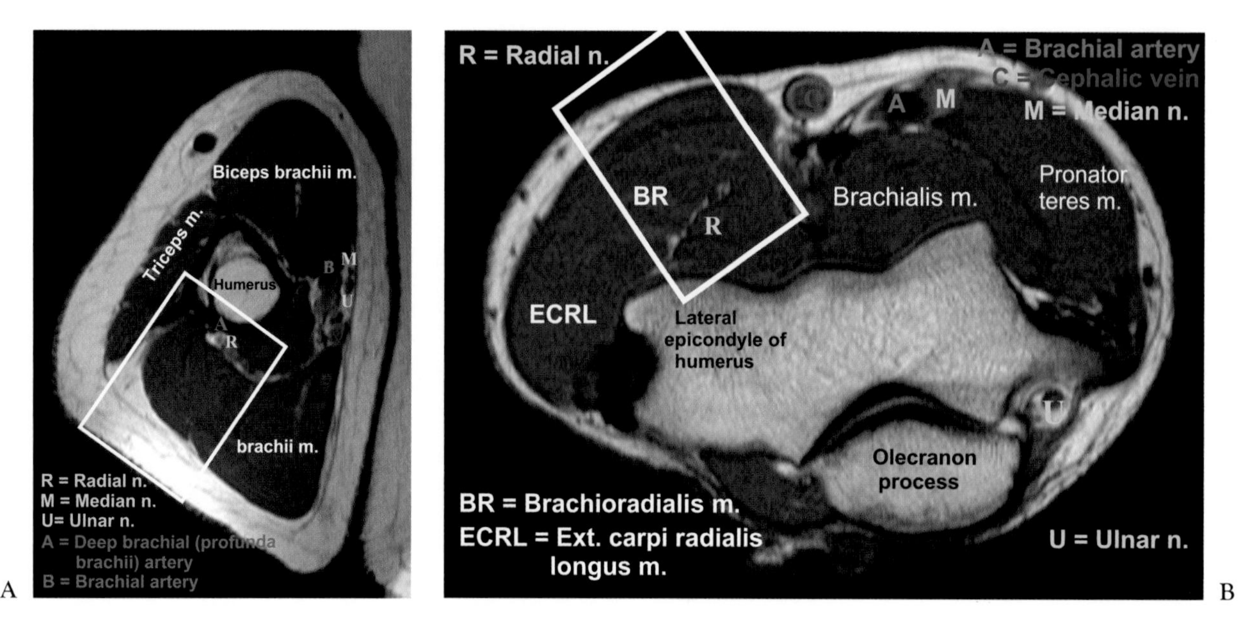

Figure 10.7. MRI images. (A) The radial nerve at the posterior aspect of the humerus and (B) the anterior aspect at the lateral epicondyle of the humerus.

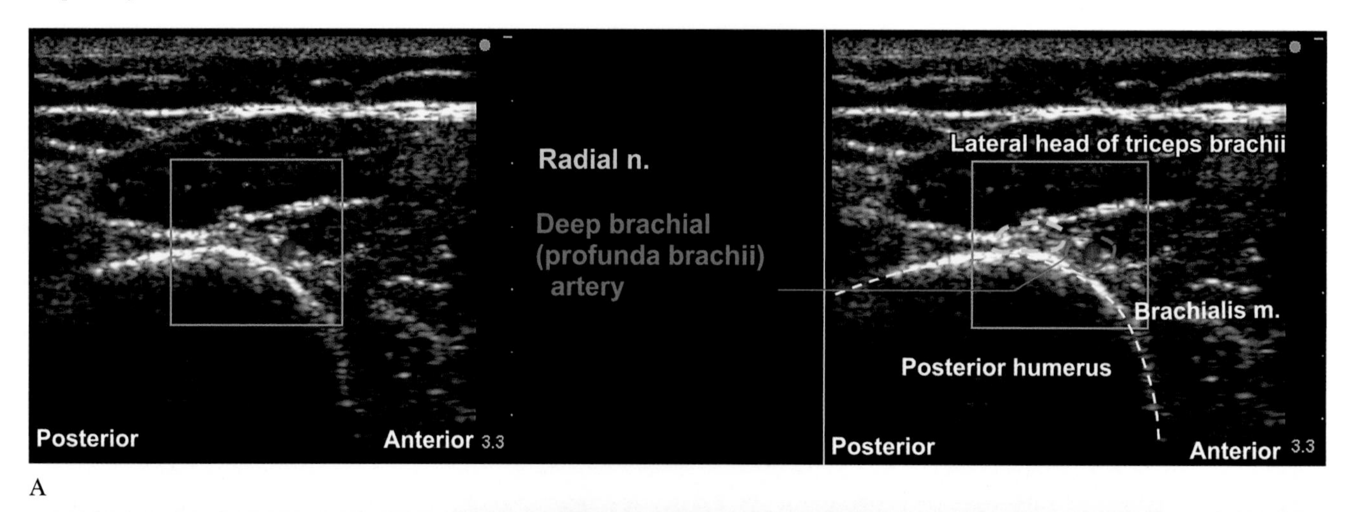

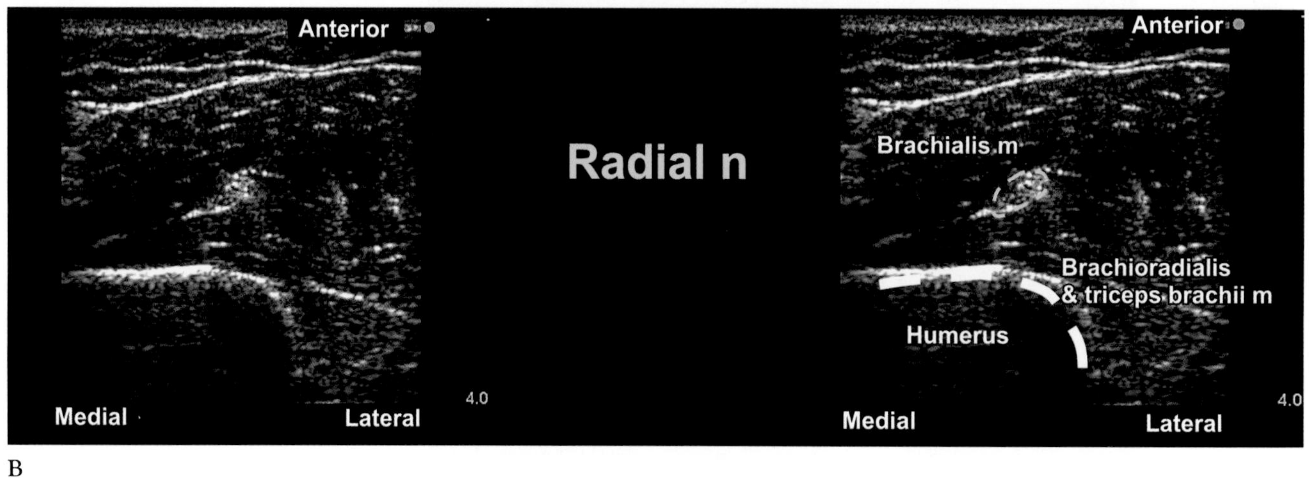

Figure 10.8. Ultrasound images using a linear probe at (A) the posterior humerus posteromedial to the deep brachial artery of the arm with color Doppler to confirm the artery position, and (B) as the nerve travels to the anterior compartment of the forearm anterior to the lateral epicondyle of the humerus.

10.2.3.2. *Sonographic Appearance*

10.2.3.2.1. At the Spiral Groove [Figure 10.8(A)]

- Superficially, bright subcutaneous tissue is apparent. The underlying triceps muscle appears hypoechoic with a curved hyperechoic border depicting the connective tissue.
- The humerus is quite superficial at this level and appears clearly demarcated as a hyperechoic oval shape with dark shadowing in its interior.
- The nerve appears oval and predominantly hyperechoic and is located in the posterior aspect of the humerus and immediately adjacent to the small, pulsatile deep brachial (profunda brachii) artery (as verified with Doppler).

10.2.3.2.2. Approaching the Anterior Compartment [Figure 10.8(B)]

- The anterior compartment of the forearm is approached from the anterior aspect of the lateral humeral supracondylar ridge. At this more distal location, the humerus has changed in shape and appears smaller and almost rectangular in cross-section.
- The hyperechoic radial nerve now lies at some distance from the humerus and is sandwiched between the brachialis and brachioradialis muscles; it remains oval in shape.

10.2.3.3. *Needle Insertion Technique*

- Use a 3.5- to 5-cm, 22-ga insulated needle if using nerve stimulation.
- Both in-plane (IP) and out-of-plane (OOP) needling (see Chapter 4) can be utilized for radial nerve block at the anterosuperior aspect of the lateral humeral epicondyle.
- The block needle is advanced to approach the target nerve on each side, preferably avoiding direct needle contact with the nerve.
- OOP approach (Figure 10.9)
  - The needle is inserted OOP to a transversely placed probe.

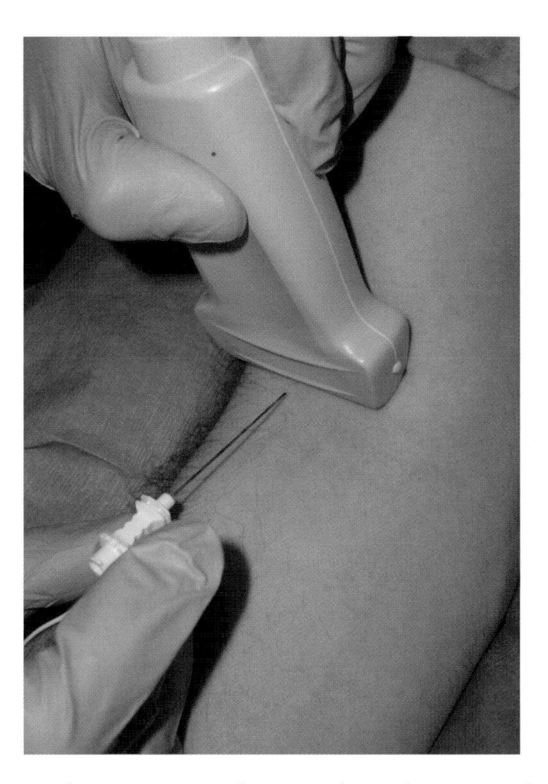

Figure 10.9. Needling technique using a linear probe with an out-of-plane (OOP) needle alignment.

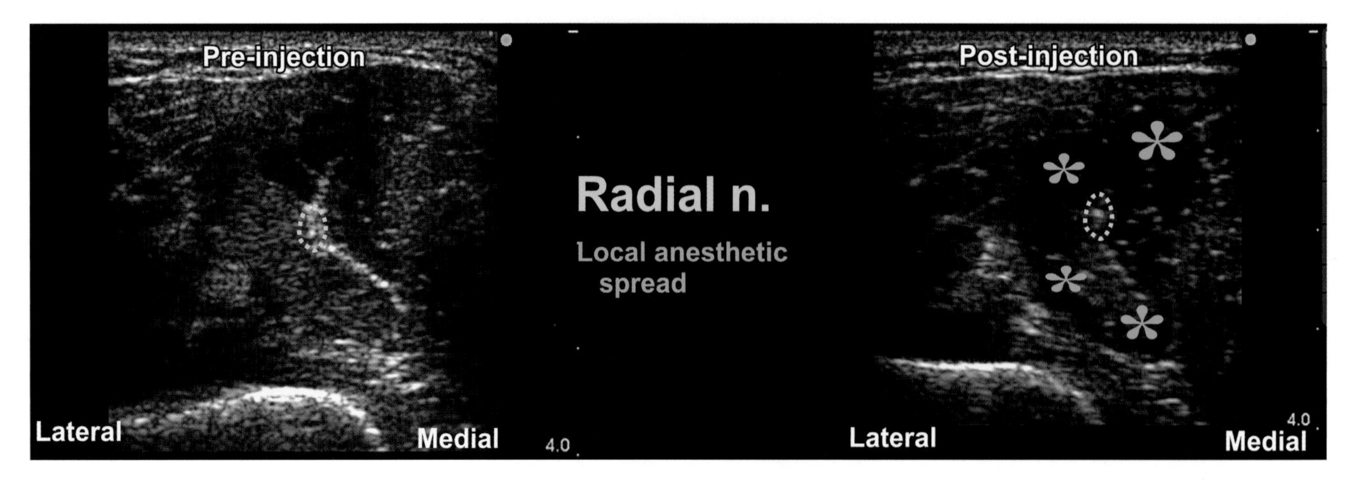

Figure 10.10. Local anesthetic application surrounding the radial nerve.

- In thin patients the nerve will be fairly superficial and the needle tip may be localized easily.
- A "walk down" approach (Chapter 4) can be used, especially if the patient has a significant amount of subcutaneous tissue and the nerve is deeper than usual.
  - Use an initial needle insertion site 2 to 3 cm distal to the probe.
  - Insert the needle with incrementally greater angles, starting initially at 10° to the skin in order to visualize the tip as a bright dot, and finally reaching an angle of approximately 45° to the skin with the needle tip at the deeper position.

10.2.4. Nerve Stimulation

- The correct motor response to nerve stimulation for radial nerve blockade at this location is extension (dorsiflexion) of the wrist and digits on the operative side.
- Needle contact with the humerus indicates that the needle is too deep, while deep needle penetration without bone contact indicates that the needle is too lateral to the humerus (beyond the bone).

10.2.5. Local Anesthetic Application (Figure 10.10)

- Performing a test dose with dextrose 5% in water (D5W) is recommended prior to local anesthetic application to visualize the spread and confirm nerve localization (see Chapter 4 sidebar).
- Aim to spread approximately 5 mL of local anesthetic around the nerve circumferentially.
- As the anesthetic is injected, an expanding area of hypoechogenicity can be seen surrounding the nerve and spreading to quite an extent within the surrounding tissues.

10.3. Median Nerve

Ultrasound guidance is usually more useful for localizing the median nerve at the antecubital fossa than at the wrist, because within this fossa the median nerve lies medial to the brachial artery and is easily distinguishable from it. Ultrasound guidance, however, is generally not as helpful when blocking the median nerve at the wrist, because this site is a very compact area with numerous tendons coursing alongside the nerve, making resolution with ultrasound poor and often difficult to interpret (i.e., anisotropy of the tendons can be significant; see Chapter 3, Figures 3.8 and 3.9) In addition, at the wrist, where the median nerve lies deep to the flexor retinaculum, there is always the potential risk of causing carpal tunnel syndrome due to a rise in pressure within the tunnel from the injectate. For these reasons, the elbow location for blocking the median nerve is the more logical choice.

10.3.1. Clinical Anatomy

The origin of the nerve can be reviewed in Figure 10.2 and Table 10.1, as well as in Chapter 5.

- The nerve originates from C5 to C8, T1; innervates muscles which produce flexion and opposition of the thumb, middle, and index fingers, and pronation and flexion of the wrist.
- The median nerve carries fibers from all roots and trunks of the brachial plexus; the *lateral head* of the nerve is mainly from the lateral cord; the *medial head* from the medial cord.
- The nerve descends initially along the medial aspect of the arm lateral to the brachial artery (continuation of the axillary artery); it then crosses the artery, usually anteriorly, at the midpoint of the arm at the insertion of the coracobrachialis muscle (Figure 10.11).
- The nerve crosses the elbow lying medially on the brachialis muscle and just medial to the brachial artery and vein (all of these medial to the biceps brachii tendon; Figure 10.12). The cross-sectional view at the antecubital fossa seen in Figure 10.13 illustrates its relationship to the artery, vein, and adjacent musculature.
- Passing deep to the bicipital aponeurosis and median cubital vein, the nerve divides between the two heads of the pronator teres, giving off the anterior interosseous nerve (supplies the flexor pollicis longus, pronator quadratus, and the lateral half of flexor digitorum profundus).
- Distal to the antecubital fossa, cutaneous sensory branches emerge and supply the palm, the palmar aspects of the first three digits, and the lateral half of the fourth digit. (Figure

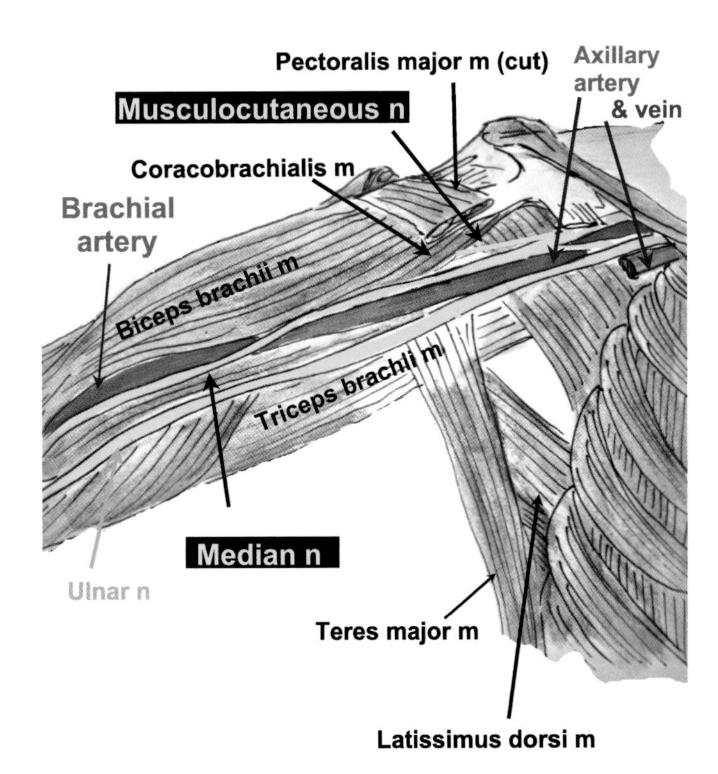

Figure 10.11. Peripheral nerves and vessels within the musculoskeletal anatomy in the upper extremity. The median nerve crosses the brachial artery in the midhumeral level. The musculocutaneous nerve departs from the other terminal nerves at the axillary location (or higher) and penetrates the coracobrachialis muscle at the upper arm.

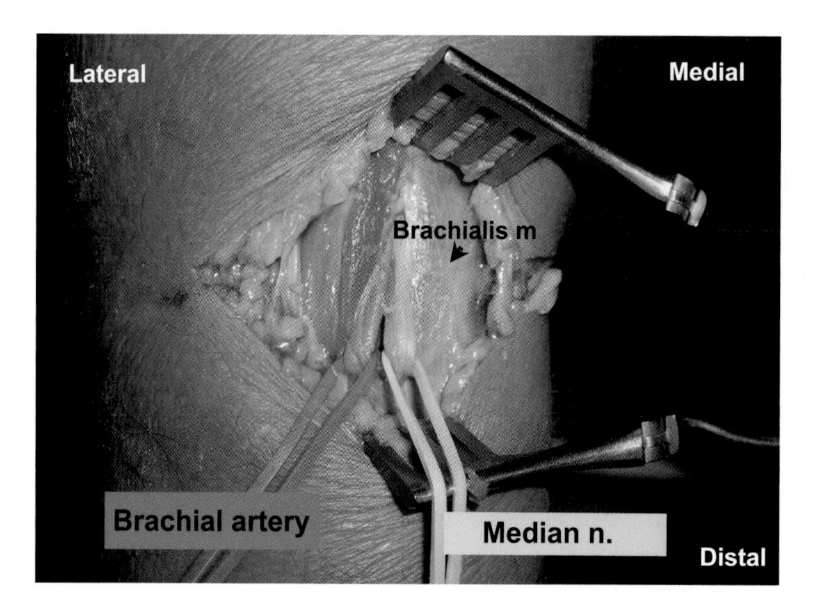

Figure 10.12. Dissection of the antecubital fossa.

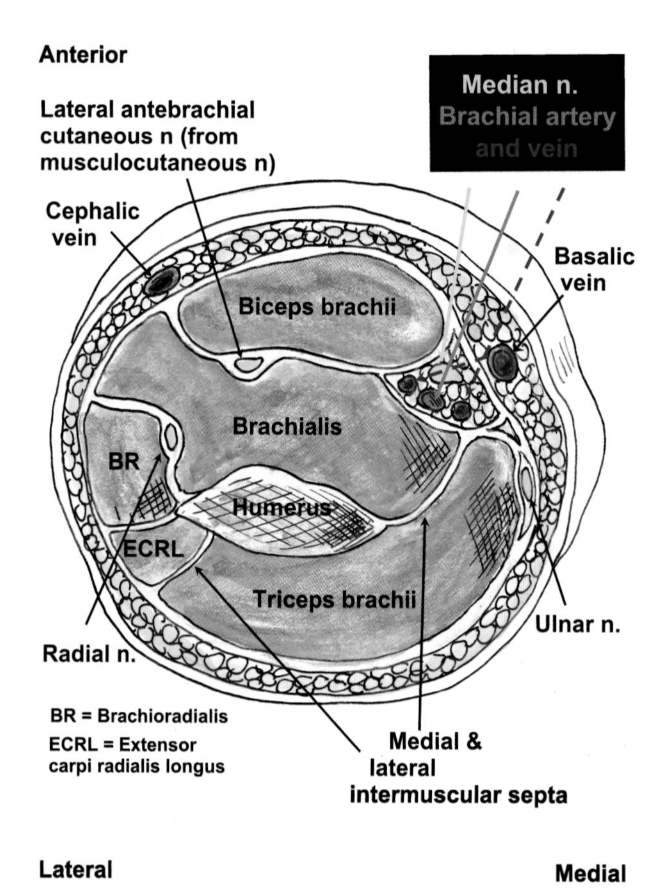

Figure 10.13. Cross-section at the antecubital fossa.

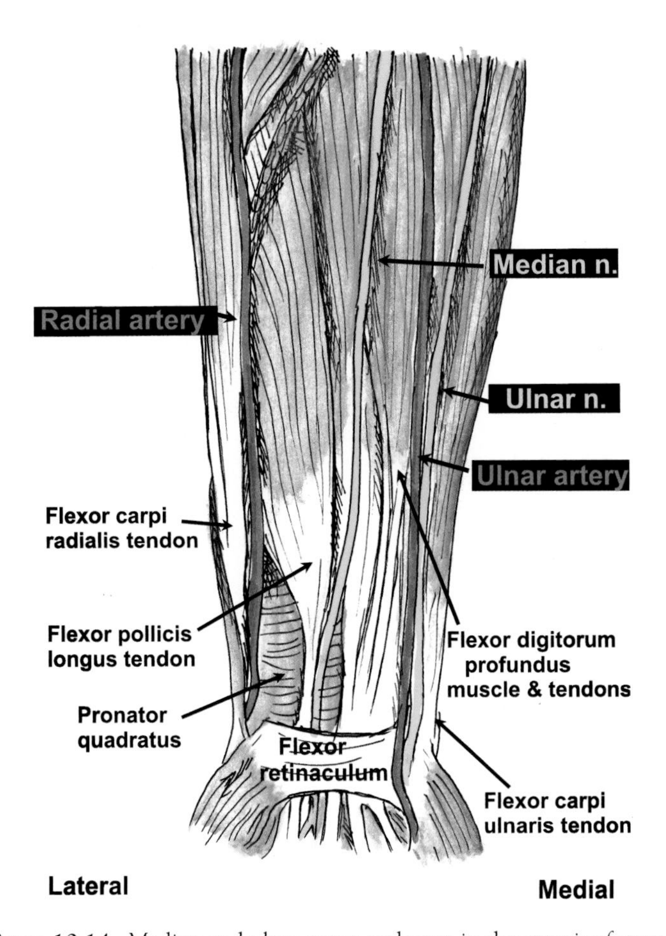

Figure 10.14. Median and ulnar nerve pathways in the anterior forearm.

10.1(A)) Generally, however, there may be some variation in terms of the overlap of cutaneous innervation from the ulnar nerve of the medial one and a half digits.

- At the most distal skin crease of the wrist, the nerve passes deep to the flexor retinaculum, and divides into medial and lateral branches (Figure 10.14).
- Through its innervation of the lateral two lumbricals it causes flexion of the metacarpophalangeal joints and extension of the interphalangeal joints of digits two and three.
- The median nerve supplies the thenar muscles, the lateral two lumbricals, and all the muscles in the anterior compartment of the forearm except the flexor carpi ulnaris, the deep head of the flexor pollicis brevis, and the medial half of the flexor digitorum profundus, which are supplied by the ulnar nerve.

10.3.2. Patient Positioning and Surface Anatomy

10.3.2.1. Patient Positioning

The patient's arm should be positioned next to the torso, with the elbow flexed and the hand free to allow a wrist or thumb flexion response elicited by nerve stimulation. A pillow placed by the patient's side under the forearm may provide support and stabilize the arm position.

10.3.2.2. Surface Anatomy (Figure 10.15)

- Medial
  - Medial epicondyle of the humerus

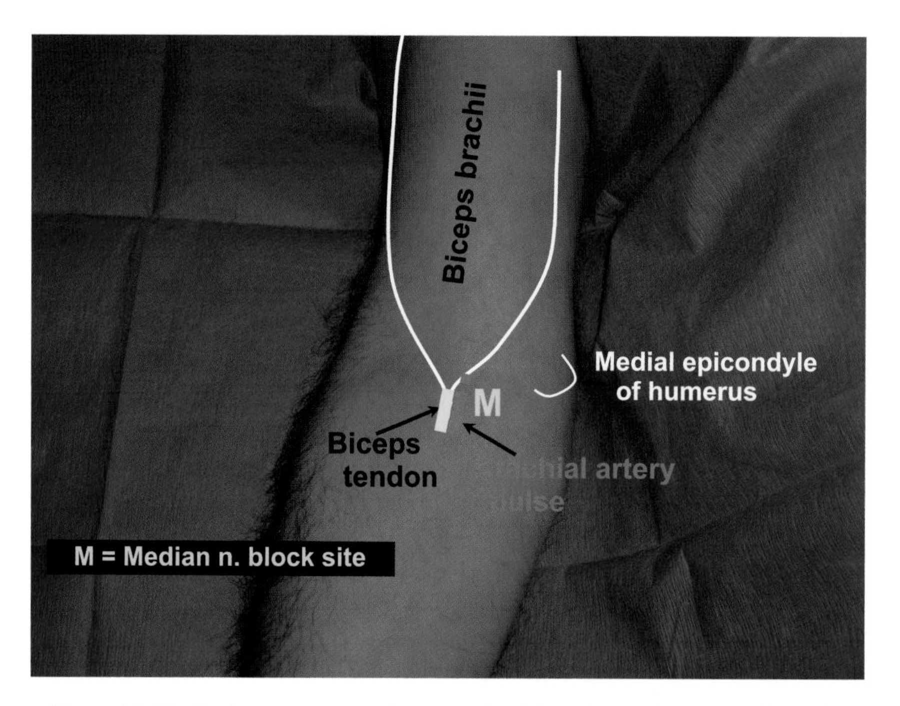

Figure 10.15. Surface anatomy at the antecubital fossa for median nerve blockade.

- Lateral
  - Brachial artery pulse: immediately medial to the biceps brachii tendon; it may be palpated best with the elbow extended
  - Biceps brachii tendon: lateral to the brachial artery and median nerve at the elbow and may be palpated best with slight elbow flexion or with resistance to elbow flexion

10.3.3. Sonographic Imaging and Needle Insertion Technique

The median nerve within the antecubital fossa is depicted with MRI in Figure 10.16, and can be used for reference when studying the ultrasound appearance (Figure 10.17) and sonographic imaging descriptions.

Prepare the needle insertion site and skin surface with an antiseptic solution. Prepare the ultrasound probe surface by applying a sterile adhesive dressing to it prior to needling as discussed earlier (see Chapters 3 and 4).

10.3.3.1. *Scanning Technique*

- A high-frequency (10–15 MHz) linear probe can be used in average-sized individuals, although lower frequency probes may be necessary in patients with excessive subcutaneous tissue.
- Scan to capture a transverse view of the nerve and artery and localize the artery on the lateral aspect of the nerve and medial to the biceps tendon. Color Doppler may be used for confirming the location of the artery and identifying the nerve on its medial aspect.

10.3.3.2. *Sonographic Appearance* (Figure 10.17)

- The median nerve can be identified as a hyperechoic, yet distinctly honeycomb structure, lying medial to the anechoic pulsatile brachial artery; it may have a peanut shape as it abuts the muscle tissue.
- The depth of penetration for the median nerve is typically 1 to 2 cm.

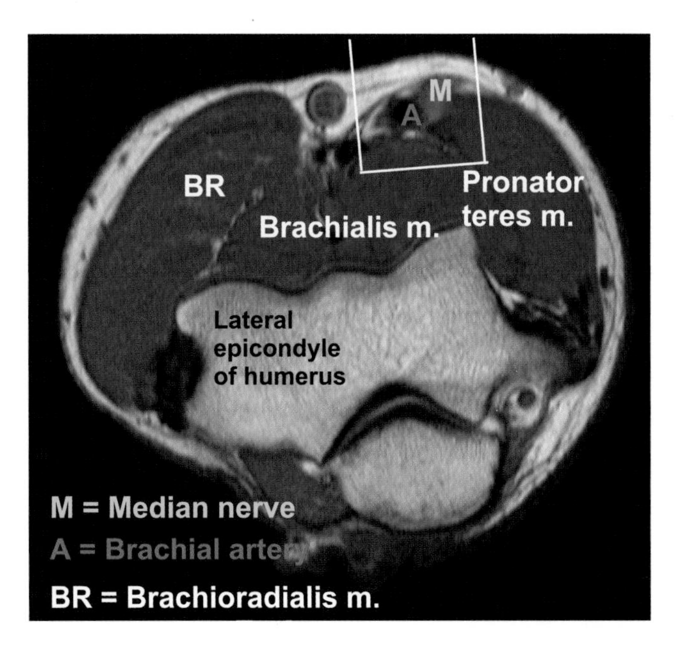

Figure 10.16. MRI image of the location immediately proximal to the antecubital fossa.

Clinical Pearls

Although not illustrated in detail within this text, the median nerve can be localized and blocked just proximal to the wrist; this location may allow the nerve to be distinguished from the tendons as well as the radial artery. The following are Chan's (2006) brief descriptions for median nerve blockade at the wrist (see Figure 3.5):

- The nerve can be found at the wrist (with flexor digitorum superficialis and palmaris longus tendons seen medially and the flexor carpi radialis tendon seen laterally) and traced proximally to verify its identity with the changing appearance of the tendons.
- More proximally, the median nerve will remain round/oval shaped in the transverse view, while the tendons become irregular in their margins (no longer oval; see Figure 3.6) and eventually disappear once they merge into their respective muscle bellies.
- The nerve lies deeper in this location than at the wrist.

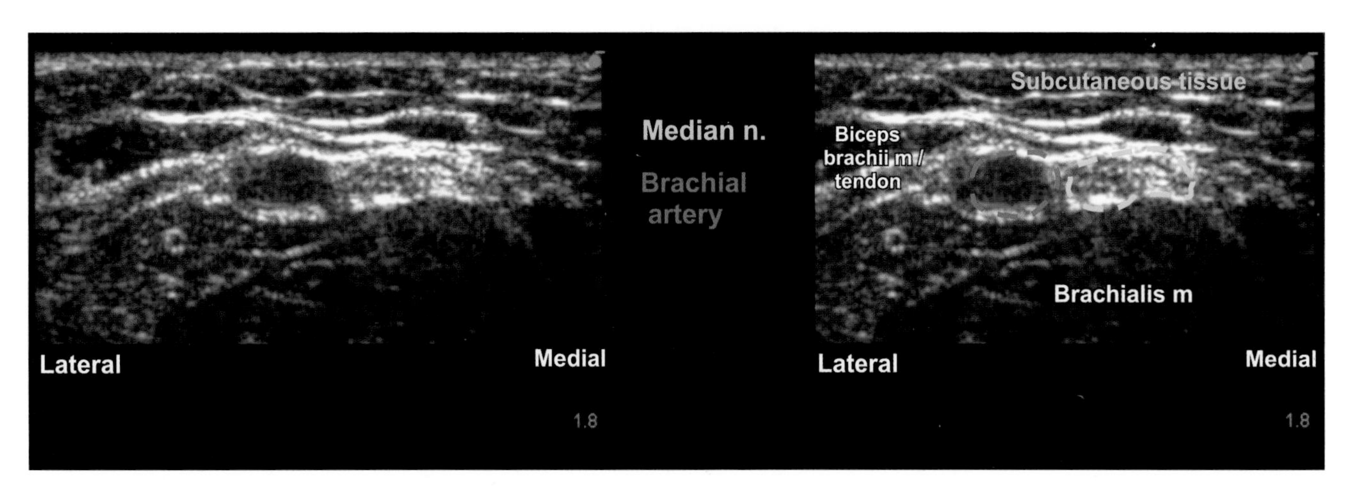

Figure 10.17. Ultrasound image of the anteromedial aspect of the elbow.

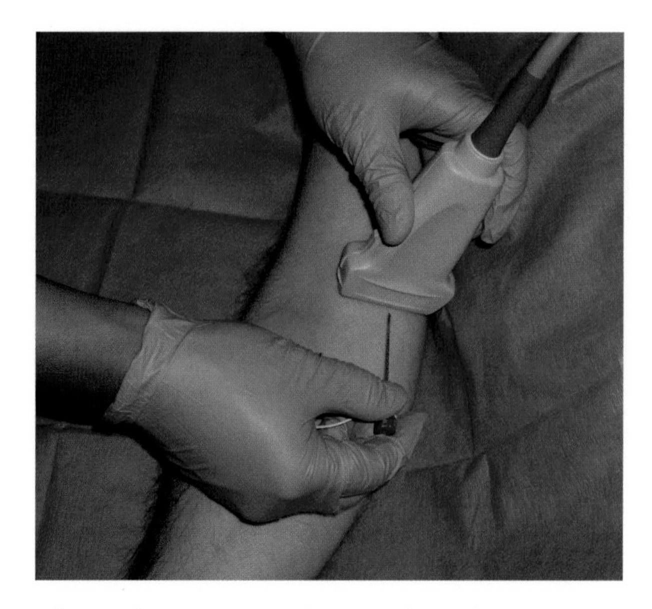

Figure 10.18. Needling technique using a linear probe and an out-of-plane (OOP) needle alignment.

- Deep to the neurovascular structures lies the musculature of the superior aspect of the elbow (pronator teres and brachialis) as a hypoechoic homogeneous mass with the classic "starry night" appearance.
- If the probe is moved medially from the nerve and artery, the medial supracondylar ridge of the humerus may be seen as a hyperechoic linear structure in the scan.

10.3.3.3. *Needle Insertion Technique*

- Use a 3.5- to 5-cm insulated needle if using nerve stimulation.
- Both needle alignments (IP and OOP) can be used for this block (see Chapter 4).
- OOP technique includes (Figure 10.18):
  - Adjusting the ultrasound image to have the nerve located in the middle of the screen.
  - Inserting the needle at the center of the transversely placed probe at a 45° to 60° angle. An incremental "walk down" technique may be used to improve the ability to track the needle (see Chapter 4).

10.3.4. Nerve Stimulation

- The optimal nerve stimulation response for median nerve blockade at the elbow location is any one of the following or a combination thereof: flexion and opposition of the thumb, middle and index fingers, flexion of the wrist, and pronation of the forearm.
- Blood aspirated into the tubing indicates brachial artery puncture and the needle should be reinserted after applying pressure to the puncture site; contact with the humerus indicates that the needle is too deep; localized contraction of the arm muscles (e.g., elbow flexion and/or forearm pronation) indicates stimulation of the local muscles and that the needle is also likely too deep.

10.3.5. Local Anesthetic Application

- Performing a test dose with D5W is recommended prior to local anesthetic application to visualize the spread and confirm nerve localization (see Chapter 4 sidebar).
- Aim to spread approximately 5 mL of local anesthetic around the nerve in a circular fashion in order to avoid nerve contact and obtain complete blockade.

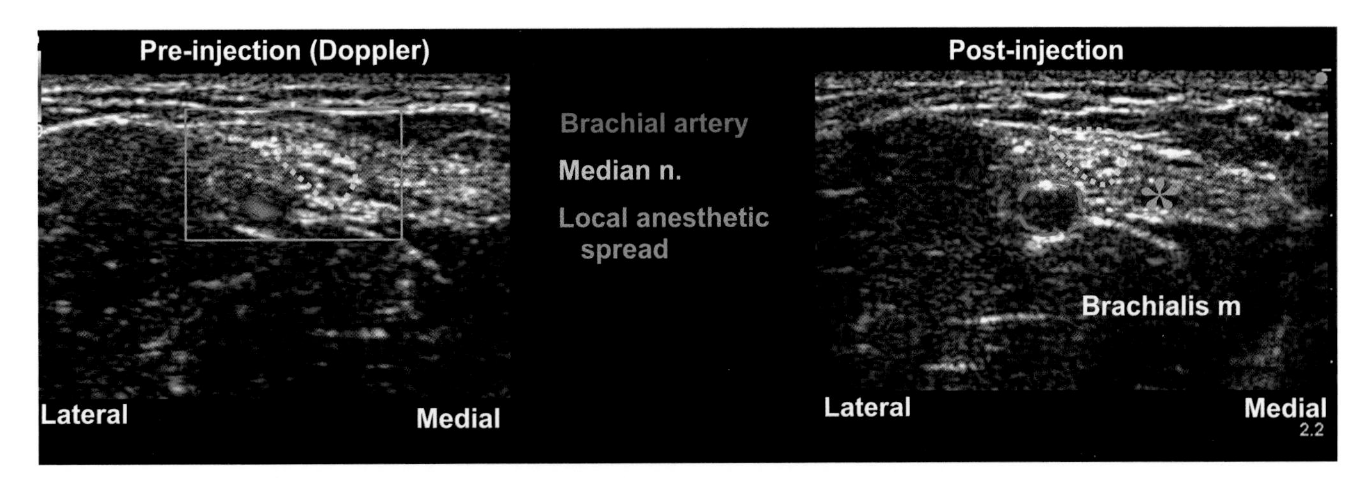

Figure 10.19. Local anesthetic application to the median nerve in the antecubital fossa.

- The local anesthetic will appear similar to what it does in other blocks, with the injectate appearing as an expanding area of hypoechogenicity surrounding the nerve. The injection will brighten the surrounding area and illuminate the nerve as compared to prior to the injection (Figure 10.19).

10.4. Musculocutaneous Nerve

The musculocutaneous nerve can be blocked at the axillary or the midhumeral level. During the axillary block, it is necessary to block the musculocutaneous nerve separately if complete surgical anesthesia is desired. If rescue analgesia is required only in a region which is innervated by the musculocutaneous nerve (e.g., anterior upper arm), the midhumeral block may be beneficial rather than repeating a more proximal brachial block with the larger volume of local anesthetic. The median and ulnar nerves can also be blocked in this midhumeral location but this text focuses on describing their blockade at the elbow and forearm, as these are newer sites amenable to ultrasound guidance.

10.4.1. Clinical Anatomy

Figure 10.20 illustrates the nerve's course throughout the upper arm. The segmental origin of the nerve can be reviewed in Figure 10.2 and Table 10.1 as well as in Chapter 5.

- The musculocutaneous nerve originates from the C5 to C7 roots; it innervates the muscles which mainly cause flexion of the arm and elbow (coracobrachialis, biceps brachii, and brachialis).
- This nerve is the continuation of the lateral cord of the brachial plexus, being formed from the anterior divisions of the upper and middle trunks at the lower border of pectoralis minor.
- It leaves the fascial sheath of the plexus approximately at the level of the coracoid process.
- Just distal (2–3 finger widths) to the intersection of pectoralis major and biceps brachii, the nerve pierces the coracobrachialis (approximately 70% rate of occurrence; see Figure 10.11 for illustration).
- Further along its course it leaves the coracobrachialis by passing between the muscle's two fused parts and comes to lie between the coracobrachialis and the short and long heads of the biceps brachii.
- Although it is difficult to observe under ultrasound, the nerve continues as the lateral cutaneous nerve of the forearm at the antecubital fossa and courses along the lateral aspect of the forearm, providing subsequent anterior and posterior branches.

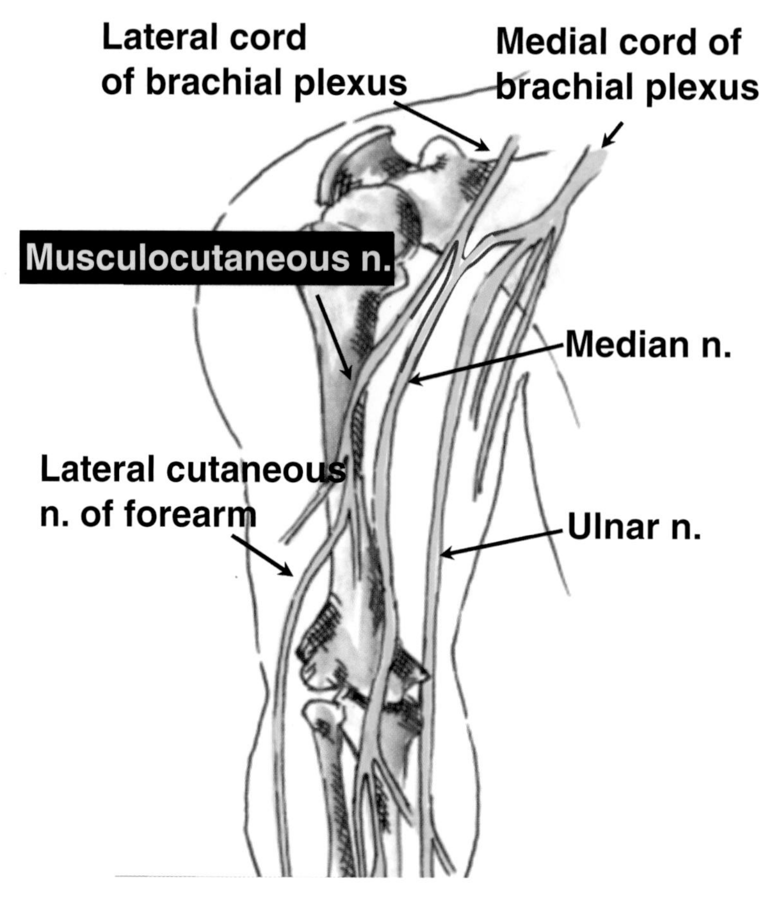

Figure 10.20. Peripheral nerve paths in the upper arm. The musculocutaneous nerve leaves the plexus at the coracoid process and continues as the lateral cutaneous nerve of the forearm.

10.4.2. Patient Positioning and Surface Anatomy

10.4.2.1. Patient Positioning

The patient's elbow is flexed, arm supinated, and shoulder abducted as in a similar position for axillary brachial plexus block. The hand and forearm should be loosely placed to allow elbow flexion during nerve stimulation.

10.4.2.2. Surface Anatomy (Figure 10.21)

- Proximal
  - Superiorly, the deltopectoral groove between pectoralis major insertion and anterior fibers of the deltoid muscle
  - Inferiorly, the axilla
- Distal
  - Laterally, the belly of biceps brachii muscle
  - Midline, the coracobrachialis muscle
  - The brachial artery pulse may be felt between biceps and coracobrachialis muscle bellies
  - Medially, the triceps muscle

10.4.3. Sonographic Imaging and Needle Insertion Technique

Prepare the needle insertion site and skin surface with an antiseptic solution. Prepare the ultrasound probe surface by applying a sterile adhesive dressing to it prior to needling as discussed earlier (see Chapters 3 and 4).

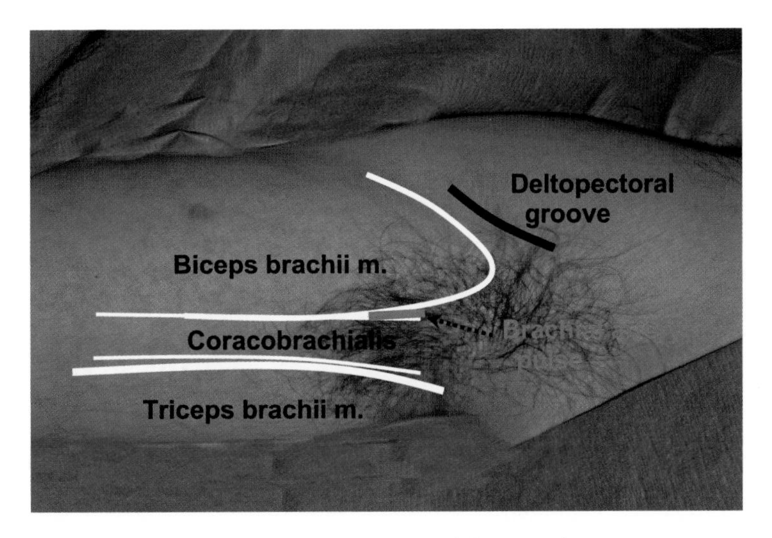

Figure 10.21. Surface anatomy for block of the musculocutaneous nerve.

10.4.3.1. *Scanning Technique*

- At a similar location to a distally located axillary block (i.e., 4–5 cm distal to the axillary crease at the brachial artery pulse location), in short axis to the humerus with a 10- to 15-MHz linear probe [Figure 10.22(A)].
  - The biceps and coracobrachialis muscles are seen on the lateral aspect (biceps most superficial) and the triceps is seen on the medial side, deeper than the biceps.
  - The musculocutaneous nerve is commonly located in the hyperechoic plane between biceps and coracobrachialis muscles; it may appear round/oval or triangular, or sometimes even linear.
- With the probe in this short-axis plane, all the peripheral nerves may be visible once the bright humeral shaft is located and placed along the lateral edge of the screen and the anechoic axillary artery is positioned in the middle of the screen.
- The depth of penetration for this nerve within the coracobrachialis is usually 2 to 3 cm.
- Placing the musculocutaneous nerve in the center field and rotating the probe to view the nerve in the long-axis plane may locate it as a tubular structure sandwiched within the hyperechoic connective tissue within or between the fascicular appearing muscles.
- Scanning distally along the medial aspect of the humerus, the musculocutaneous nerve becomes embedded within the coracobrachialis muscle [Figure 10.22(B)] and eventually leaves the coracobrachialis to lie between the two (short and long) heads of the biceps brachii muscle.

10.4.3.2. *Sonographic Appearance*

- At a proximal location similar to that used in axillary blocks [Figure 10.22(A)]:
  - The musculocutaneous nerve appears fairly hyperechoic, oval in shape and close to the well-demarcated humeral shaft.
  - The biceps and triceps brachii muscles appear heterogenous, hypoechoic, with few hyperechoic punctate areas, and lie in opposition to each other while bordering the neurovascular region; the coracobrachialis may be localized deep to the biceps where it sandwiches the musculocutaneous nerve.
  - The axillary artery and vein are positioned superficial and medial to the nerve (vein medial to artery).
  - The median and radial nerves lie superficial and deep to the axillary artery (respectively) and the ulnar nerve lies most superficial and medial.

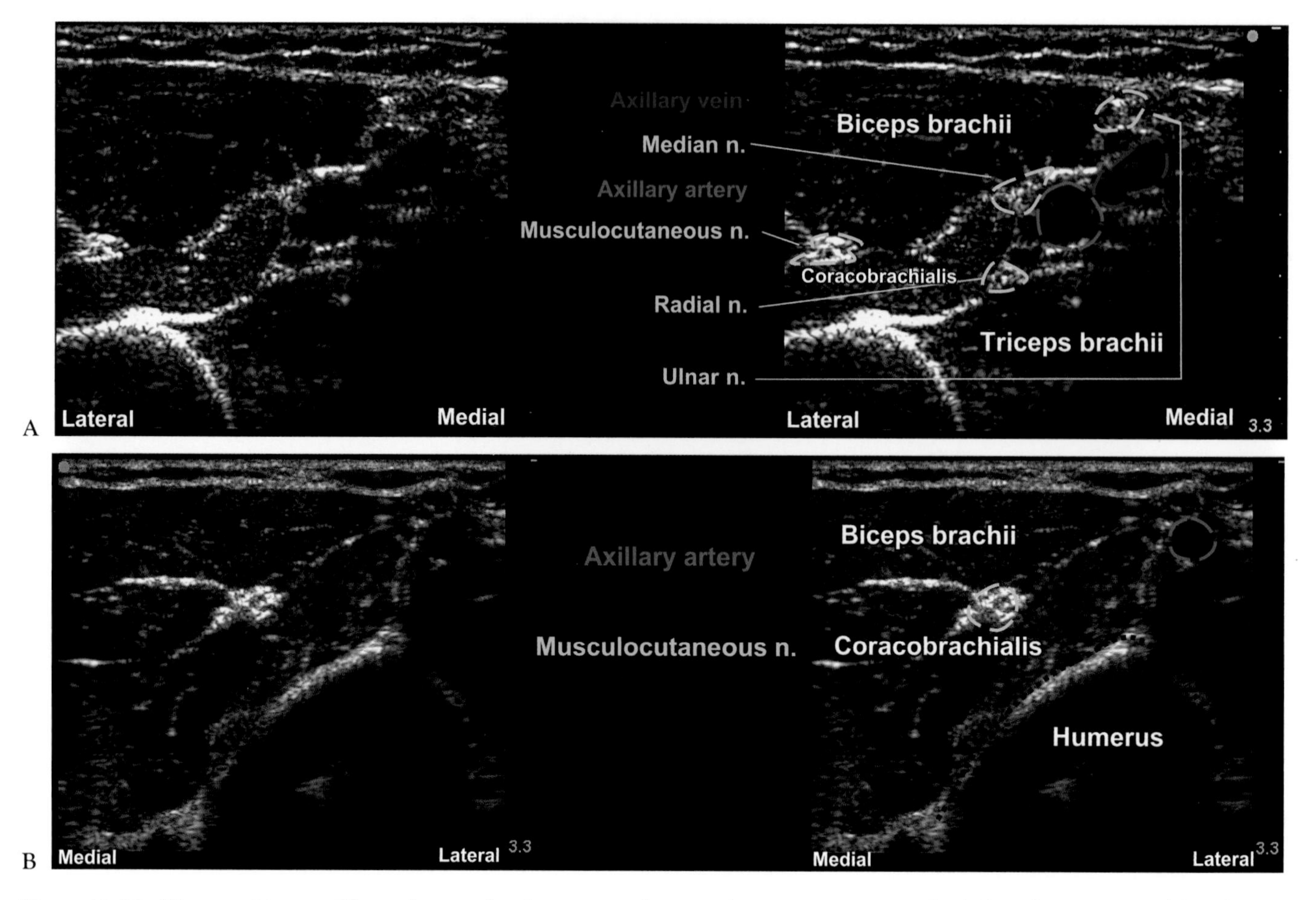

Figure 10.22. Ultrasound images. The probe was placed to capture the musculocutaneous nerve in the (A) axillary region and (B) the midhumeral region within the coracobrachialis muscle.

- More distally in a midhumeral location, deep within the coracobrachialis muscle, the nerve appears as an oval-to-round moderately echoic nodule surrounded by the bright [Figure 10.22(B)] fascial plane within the coracobrachialis (separating the two fused parts).
- A few centimeters distally the nerve may again be seen between all the muscles, with the coracobrachialis medial, the short head of biceps central and superficial, and the long head of biceps lateral; here the nerve may appear triangular and hyperechoic compared to the dark musculature.

10.4.3.3. *Needle Insertion Technique*

- Use a 3.5- to 5-cm insulated needle if using nerve stimulation.
- Both approaches (IP and OOP) can be used for this block.
- OOP technique includes (Figure 10.23):
  - Adjusting the ultrasound image to have the nerve located in the middle of the screen.
  - Inserting the needle approximately 1 to 2 cm distal to the transversely placed probe at a 30° to 45° angle.
- IP needling in an anterior (biceps) to posterior (triceps) direction will allow good visibility of the needle trajectory (Figure 10.24).

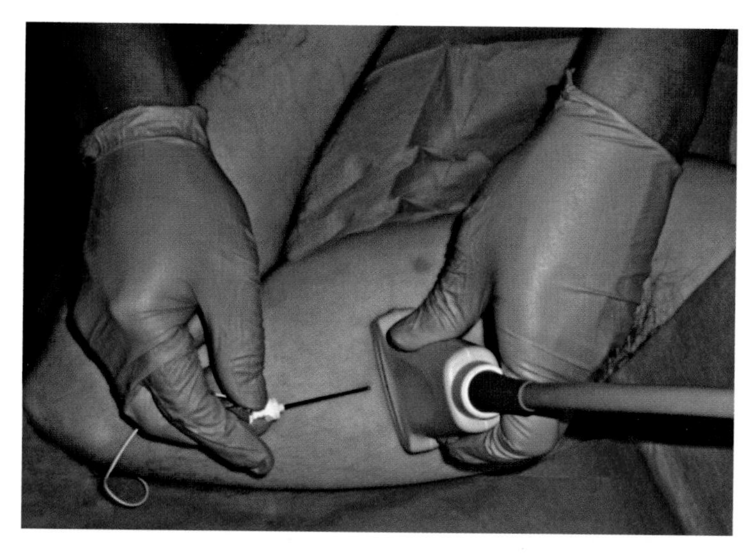

Figure 10.23. Needling technique using a linear probe and an out-of-plane (OOP) needle alignment.

10.4.4. Nerve Stimulation

- The correct nerve stimulation response for musculocutaneous nerve blockade at the midhumeral location is elbow flexion.
- Blood withdrawal into the tubing suggests axillary artery or vein puncture and the needle should be reinserted after pressure treatment; contact with the humerus indicates that the needle is too deep.

10.4.5. Local Anesthetic Application

- Performing a test dose with D5W is recommended prior to local anesthetic application to visualize the spread and confirm nerve localization (see Chapter 4 sidebar).
- Aim to spread approximately 5 mL (perhaps more if for surgical anesthesia rather than rescue analgesia) of local anesthetic around the nerve in a circular fashion in order to avoid needle contact with the nerve but obtain a complete block.
- The local anesthetic will appear similar to what it does in other blocks, with the injectate appearing as an expansion of hypoechogenicity surrounding the nerve; as it expands it may separate the nerve from the muscle tissue (Figure 10.24).

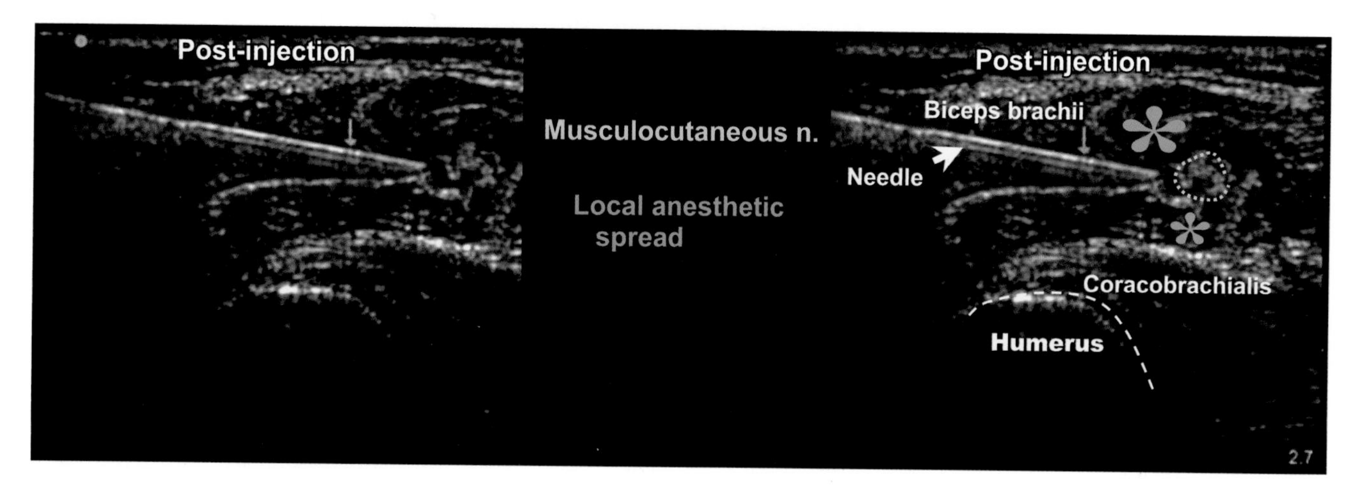

Figure 10.24. Local anesthetic application using in-plane (IP) needling technique from the anterior to posterior arm. The needle is clearly seen with this IP approach.

10.5. Ulnar Nerve

Ulnar nerve block at the midforearm may be used for rescue analgesia or blockade of the fifth digit for surgery. Blockade at this site is less likely to cause neuritis or neuropraxia than blockade at the cubital tunnel behind the medial epicondyle. The ulnar nerve in the midforearm is commonly located lying just medial to the pulsatile ulnar artery.

10.5.1. Clinical Anatomy

The origin of the nerve can be reviewed in Figure 10.2 and Table 10.1 as well as in Chapter 5.

- The ulnar nerve originates from C8 and T1 roots; in the forearm it innervates muscles that produce flexion of the ring (fourth) and little (fifth) fingers and ulnar deviation of wrist.
- The ulnar nerve is the continuation of the medial cord from the anterior division of lower trunk.
- Initially the nerve courses between the axillary artery and vein and then along the medial aspect of the brachial artery to the midpoint of the humerus before passing posteriorly and following the anterior surface of the medial head of the triceps.
- It then passes behind the medial epicondyle of the humerus (in the condylar groove), divides between the humeral and ulnar heads of the flexor carpi ulnaris and lies on the medial aspect of the elbow joint.
- During its descent through the forearm (Figure 10.14), the nerve courses anteriorly, coming to lie deep to the flexor carpi ulnaris and flexor digitorum superficialis (Figure 10.25), to approach the ulnar artery near the midline of the forearm at its midpoint (Figure 10.26); the nerve and artery lie directly anterior to the ulna at the junction of the lower third and upper two thirds of the forearm.
- At the wrist it crosses superficial to the flexor retinaculum immediately lateral to the pisiform bone in its own compartment (Guyon's canal) and divides into superficial and deep branches; the ulnar artery lies anterolateral to the nerve at the wrist.

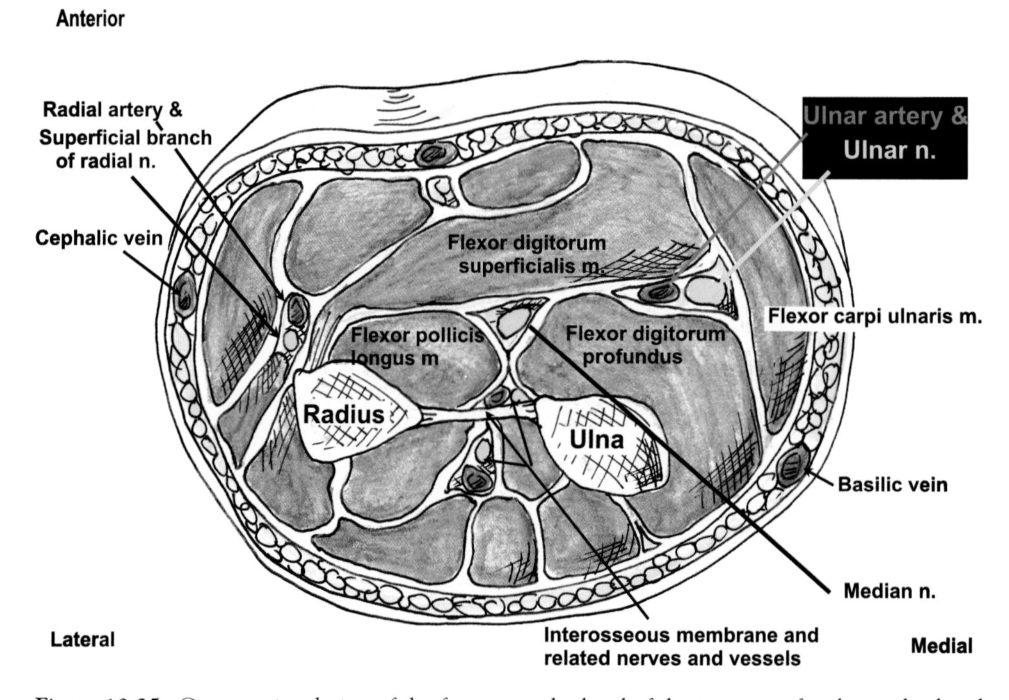

Figure 10.25. Cross-sectional view of the forearm at the level of the junction of its lower third and its upper two-thirds.

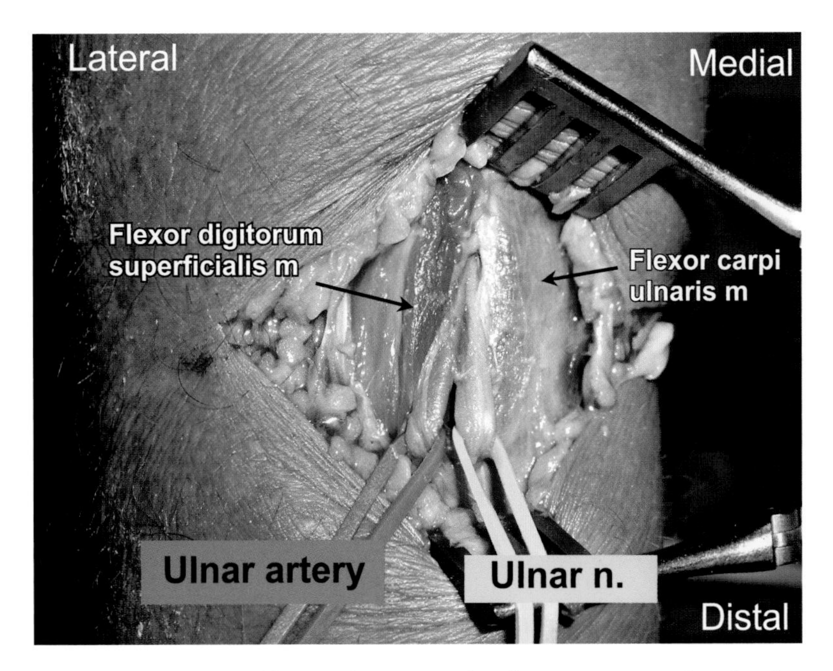

Figure 10.26. Dissection at midforearm location as the ulnar nerve approaches the ulnar artery.

- The nerve supplies all the intrinsic muscles of the hand except those supplied by the median nerve (i.e., all the interossei, the medial two lumbricals, the hypothenar muscles, the adductor pollicis, and the deep head of flexor pollicis brevis).
- Through its innervation of the interossei and medial two lumbricals, the nerve causes flexion of the metacarpophalangeal joints and extension of the interphalangeal joints of digits four and five.
- Dorsal and palmar cutaneous branches of the nerve branch 5 to 10 cm proximal to the wrist and generally supply the medial half of the fourth and all of the fifth digit (there may be some variation in overlap with the cutaneous branches of the median supplying the lateral three and a half digits).

10.5.2. Patient Positioning and Surface Anatomy

10.5.2.1. *Patient Positioning*

The patient's arm is flexed at the elbow with the shoulder externally rotated and forearm supinated. The forearm can rest on an arm board with an additional pillow under the wrist.

10.5.2.2. *Surface Anatomy* (Figure 10.27)

- Ulna
  - Palpate the bone at the junction of the middle and lower thirds of the forearm.
- Ulnar artery pulse
  - This will be difficult to palpate in many individuals.

10.5.3. Sonographic Imaging and Needle Insertion Technique

The ulnar nerve is depicted within the forearm using MRI in Figure 10.28, which can be used for reference with the ultrasound image [Figure 10.29(A,B)].

A linear or curved array probe may be used and a small footprint (25 mm; e.g., a "hockey stick" probe) will be helpful for easy manipulation on the forearm and for good alignment of the needle using IP technique. The linear probes are often used as they provide good needle tracking during IP approaches.

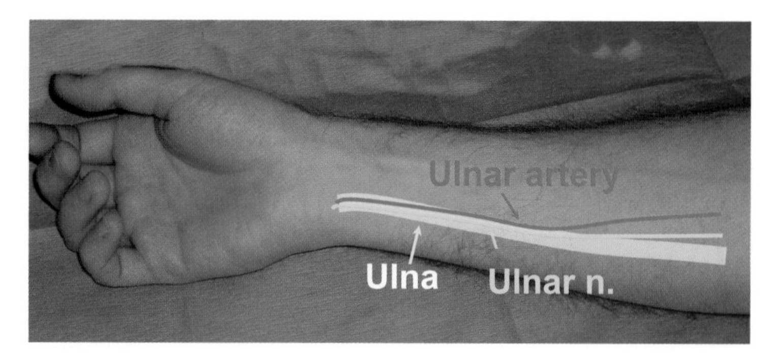

Figure 10.27. Surface anatomy for the ulnar nerve block in the midforearm.

Prepare the needle insertion site and skin surface with an antiseptic solution. Prepare the ultrasound probe surface by applying a sterile adhesive dressing to it prior to needling as discussed earlier (see Chapters 3 and 4).

10.5.3.1. *Scanning Technique*

- A high-frequency (10–15 MHz) linear probe is often used for this block.
- Place the probe transversely just above the midforearm level to view the ulnar nerve in short axis as it approaches the ulnar artery.
- Place the probe above the ulna and belly of the flexor carpi ulnaris, on the anterior surface of the arm, rather than medially to contact the bone.
- Scan downwards slowly until the pulsatile artery and nerve are viewed adjacent to each other [Figure 10.29(A); Doppler may be very valuable here].
- Confirm the identity of the nerve by dynamically scanning proximally [Figure 10.29(B)] and distally to confirm that it is separate from the artery proximally and converges to join the artery at the midforearm.

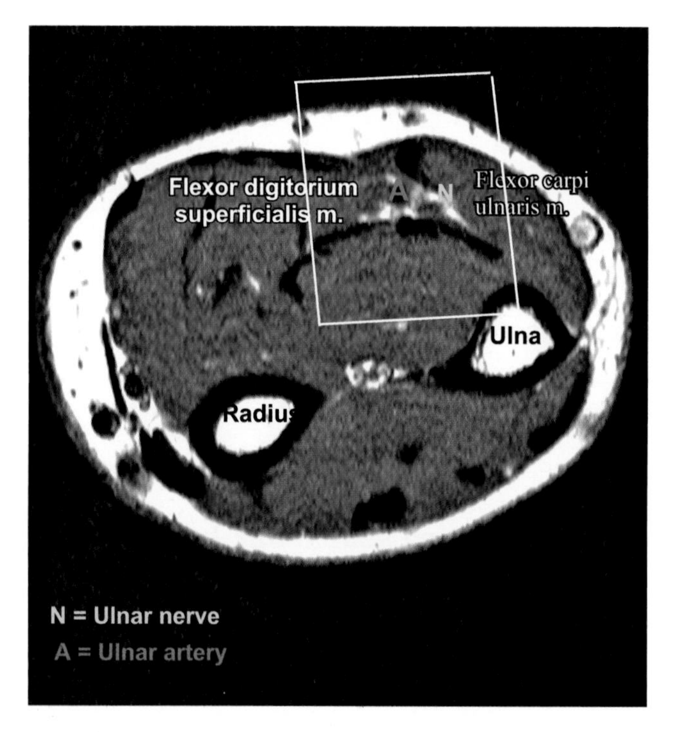

Figure 10.28. MRI image from a scan at the midforearm block location.

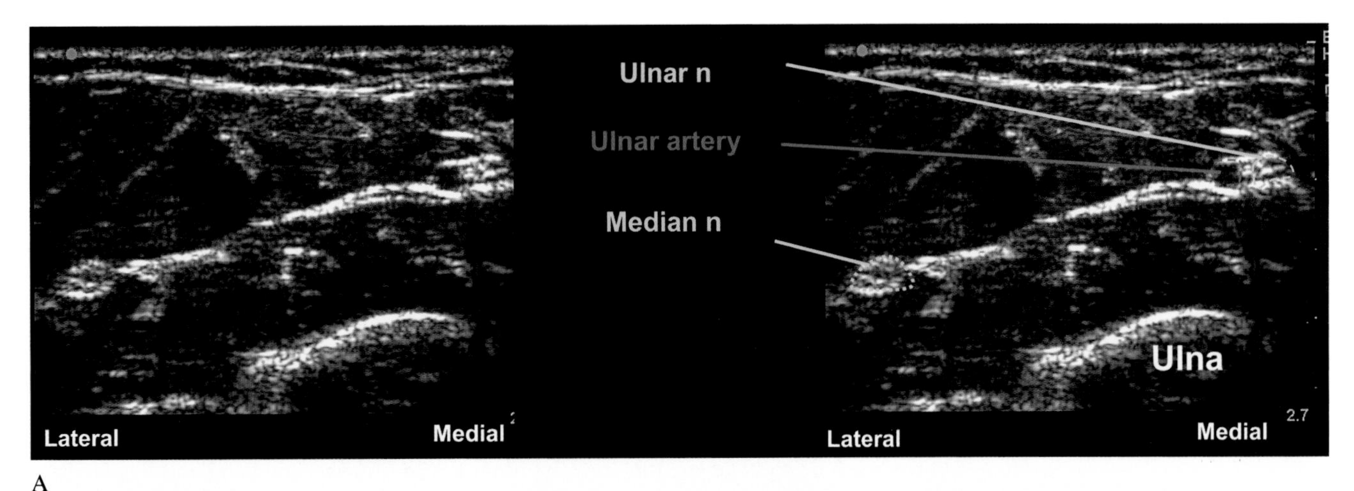

A

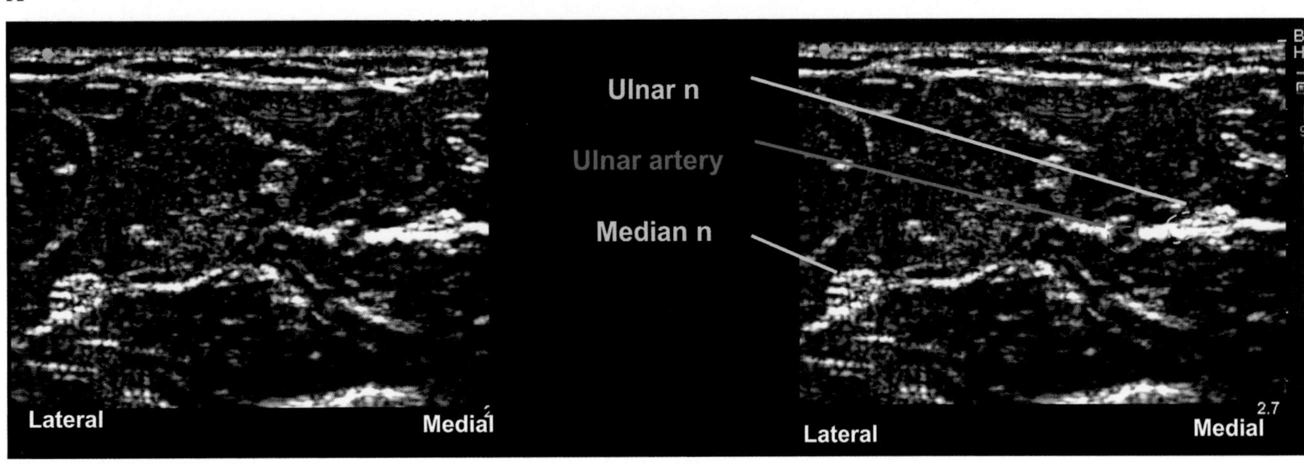

B

Figure 10.29. Ultrasound image of the ulnar nerve in the forearm medial to the ulnar artery: (A) the ulnar nerve and artery close together; (B) scanning proximally, the ulnar nerve and artery diverge from each other.

- Move the image of the nerve to the most lateral edge of the screen for good visibility of the needle shaft during IP advancement.
- At the level of the wrist the ulnar nerve may be hard to distinguish from the adjacent tendons.

> **Clinical Pearl**
>
> The ulnar nerve can be localized and blocked just proximal to the wrist (see Figure 3.10) in a similar manner to that which Chan (2006) suggests for the median nerve (see section 10.3).

10.5.3.2. *Sonographic Appearance*

- The nerve in short axis is viewed as a honeycomb oval-shaped structure, including hypoechoic fascicular structures surrounded significantly by hyperechoic tissue (Figure 10.29).
- The adjacent ulnar artery appears anechoic and roughly similar in size to the nerve and lateral to it.

- Proximal to the point where the nerve and artery are immediately adjacent [Figure 10.29(A)], the nerve can be traced to the point where the artery travels more laterally [Figure 10.29(B)].
- If able to demarcate the muscles they are located as follows: the flexor carpi ulnaris is superficial below the skin and subcutaneous layers; the flexor digitorum superficialis is superolateral to the nerve and artery; the flexor digitorum profundus is medial and deep to the nerve and artery (Figure 10.25).
- The nerve may be seen in long axis as a hyperechoic tubular structure.
- If seen, the deep hyperechoic ulna will have a bony shadow underneath.
- The median nerve may be seen at the lateral edge of the image and appears similar to the ulnar nerve in size and shape (Figure 10.29).

10.5.3.3. *Needle Insertion Technique*

- On the medial aspect of the forearm, the ulnar nerve is fairly superficial and lies medial to the ulnar artery, therefore a short (2–3 cm) needle can be used in a medial to lateral direction to reduce the risk of vascular puncture.
- With the probe placed transversely to the nerve:
  - An IP technique can be used effectively to allow good visualization of the needle shaft and tip.
    - Using a small footprint linear probe ("hockey stick"; Figure 10.30) is suitable for this block technique.
  - An OOP technique:
    - A small footprint or even L38 (Figure 10.31; SonoSite, Inc., Bothell, WA, USA) probe can be used for this approach.
    - Using a walk down needling approach (see Chapter 4) may allow better visualization of the needle tip in relation to the nerve and reduce potential nerve injury or vascular puncture.

10.5.4. Nerve Stimulation

- The correct nerve stimulation response for ulnar nerve blockade at this location is flexion of the ring (fouth) and little (fifth) fingers and ulnar deviation of the wrist.

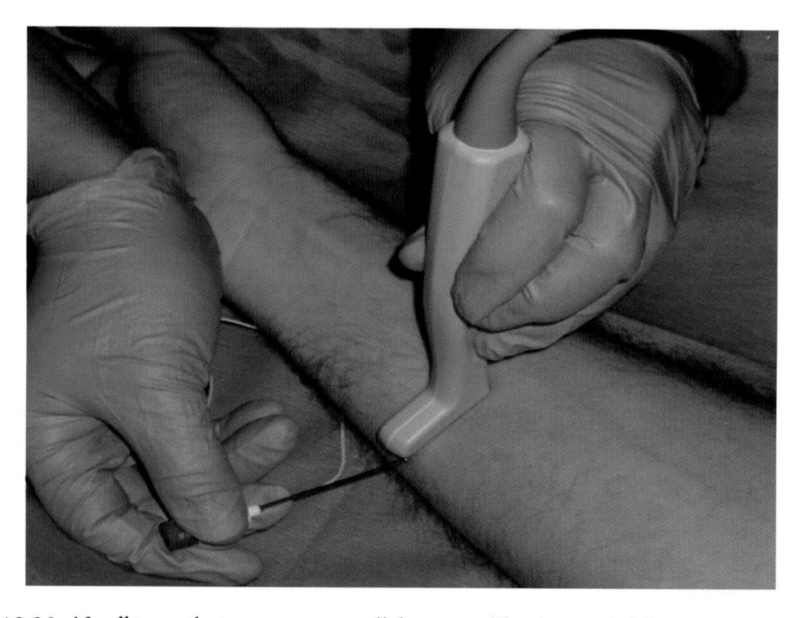

Figure 10.30. Needling technique using a small footprint ("hockey stick") linear probe with an in-plane (IP) needle alignment.

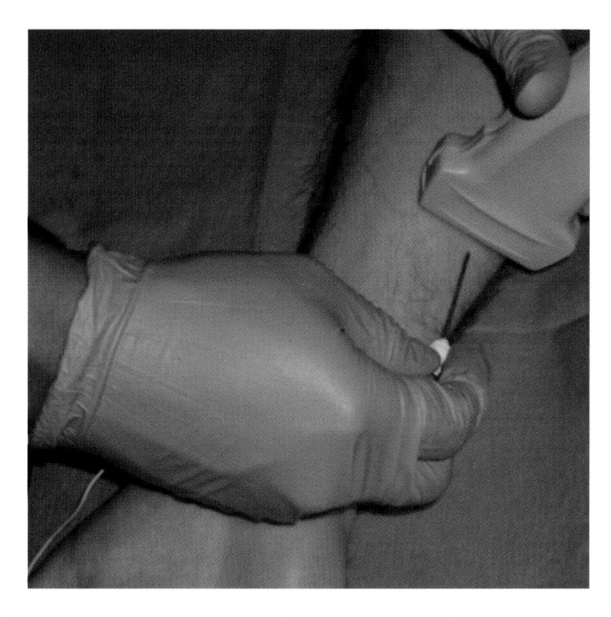

Figure 10.31. Needling technique using a linear probe with an out-of-plane (OOP) needle alignment.

- Blood withdrawal into the tubing suggests ulnar artery puncture and the needle should be reinserted after pressure treatment; contact with the ulna indicates that the needle is too deep.

10.5.5. Local Anesthetic Application

- Performing a test dose with D5W is recommended prior to local anesthetic application to visualize the spread and confirm nerve localization (see Chapter 4 sidebar).
- Aim to spread approximately 5 mL of local anesthetic around the nerve in a circular fashion in order to avoid nerve contact but to obtain a complete block.
- The local anesthetic injection will appear similar to what it does in other blocks, with the injectate appearing as an expansion of hypoechogenicity surrounding the nerve, which may separate the nerve from the artery (Figure 10.32).

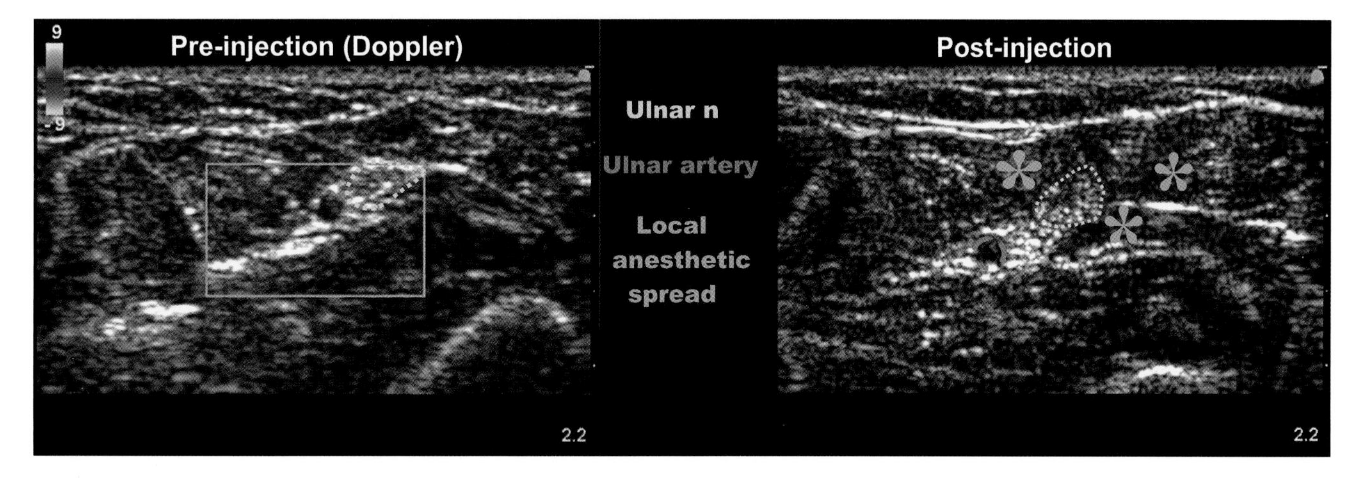

Figure 10.32. Local anesthetic application in the midforearm using an OOP approach with the needle between the ulnar nerve and artery.

Suggested Reading and References

Chan VWS. The use of ultrasound for peripheral nerve blocks. In: Boezaart AP, ed. Anesthesia and orthopaedic surgery. New York: McGraw-Hill; 2006; pp. 283–290.

Fornage BD. Peripheral nerves of the extremities: imaging with US. Radiology 1988;167:179–182.

Gray AT, Schafhalter-Zoppoth I. Ultrasound guidance for ulnar nerve block in the forearm. Reg Anesth Pain Med 2003;28:335–339.

Loewy J. Sonography of the median, ulnar and radial nerves. Can Assoc Radiol J 2002;53:33–38.

Retzl G, Kapral S, Greher M, Mauritz W. Ultrasonographic findings of the axillary part of the brachial plexus. 2001;92:1271–1275.

Schafhalyter-Zoppoth I, Gray AT. The musculocutaneous nerve: ultrasonic appearance for peripheral nerve block. Reg Anesth Pain Med 2005;30:385–390.

Silvestri E, Martinoli C, Derchi LE, Bertolotto M, Chiaramondia M, Rosenberg I. Echotexture of peripheral nerves: correlation between US and histologic findings and criteria to differentiate tendons. Radiology 1995;197:291–296.

11 Clinical Anatomy for Lower Limb Blocks

Ban C.H. Tsui

This chapter provides an overview of the lumbar and sacral plexuses and the distribution of the spinal nerves arising from these nerve plexuses to skin, muscles, and bones (i.e., dermatomes, myotomes, and osteotomes, respectively). The anatomy of individual terminal nerves is described in greater detail in the respective chapters on nerve blockade.

11.1. Origin of Spinal Nerves

The spinal nerves are part of the peripheral nervous system along with the cranial and autonomic nerves and their ganglia. There are 31 pairs of spinal nerves of the peripheral nervous system that arise segmentally from five regions of the spinal cord. There are 8 cervical (C1–C8), 12 thoracic (T1–T12), 5 lumbar (L1–L5), 5 sacral (S1–S5), and 1 coccygeal spinal nerves. These spinal nerves are formed from the union of the ventral (anterior) and dorsal (posterior) spinal nerve roots, which in turn are formed from the fusion of several smaller rootlets (Figure 11.1). A typical spinal nerve contains both sensory and motor fibers from the dorsal and ventral nerve roots, respectively. In addition, all spinal nerves contain sympathetic fibers that supply blood vessels, smooth muscle, and glands in the skin. Soon

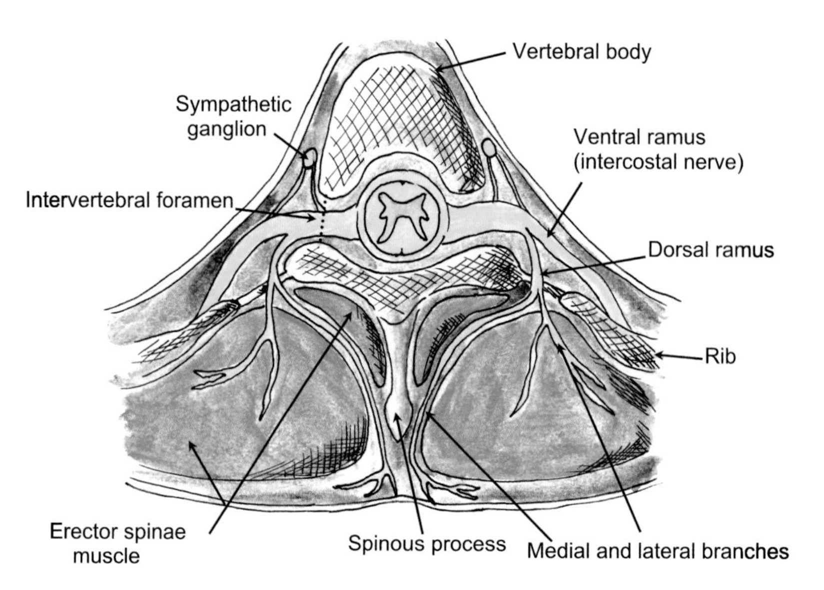

Figure 11.1. Spinal nerve anatomy at the thoracic spine.

after exiting the intervertebral (spinal) foramina, each of the spinal nerves divides into a larger ventral and smaller dorsal ramus. The ventral rami swing around laterally and anteriorly and supply the muscles, subcutaneous tissues (superficial fascia) and skin of the neck, extremities, and trunk laterally and anteriorly, while the dorsal rami course posteriorly and supply the paravertebral muscles, subcutaneous tissues, and skin close to the midline on the back.

11.2. Lumbar and Sacral Plexuses

The lumbar and sacral plexuses and their peripheral nerves are depicted in Figure 11.2. The individual peripheral nerves arising from these plexuses are described in greater detail in subsequent chapters.

11.2.1. Formation and Branches of the Lumbar Plexus

- The lumbar plexus (Figures 11.2 and 11.3) is formed by the union of the anterior primary rami of L1 to L3 and part of L4; 50% of the population also receive a small twig from T12 (termed *prefixed*) or an L5 extension (termed *postfixed*).
- The plexus supplies the skin and muscles of the lower part of the anterior abdominal wall (including the external genitalia) and the skin and muscles of the anterior and medial compartments of the thigh.
- The plexus assembles within the psoas major muscle, anterior to the transverse processes of the lumbar vertebrae.
- L1 bifurcates into two parts: upper (iliohypogastric and ilio-inguinal nerves) and lower (joins with L2 branch to form the genitofemoral nerve). L3, with portions of L2 and L4, divides into anterior and posterior divisions.
  - Anterior division: forms the obturator (L2–L4) and accessory obturator (L3, L4; when present) nerves.
    - The obturator nerve enters the pelvic cavity proper at the pelvic brim, passing behind the common iliac vessels and lateral to the internal iliac vessels; it then traverses the pelvic cavity along the pelvic side wall toward the obturator canal, through which it enters the upper part of the medial aspect of the thigh (Figure 11.4).

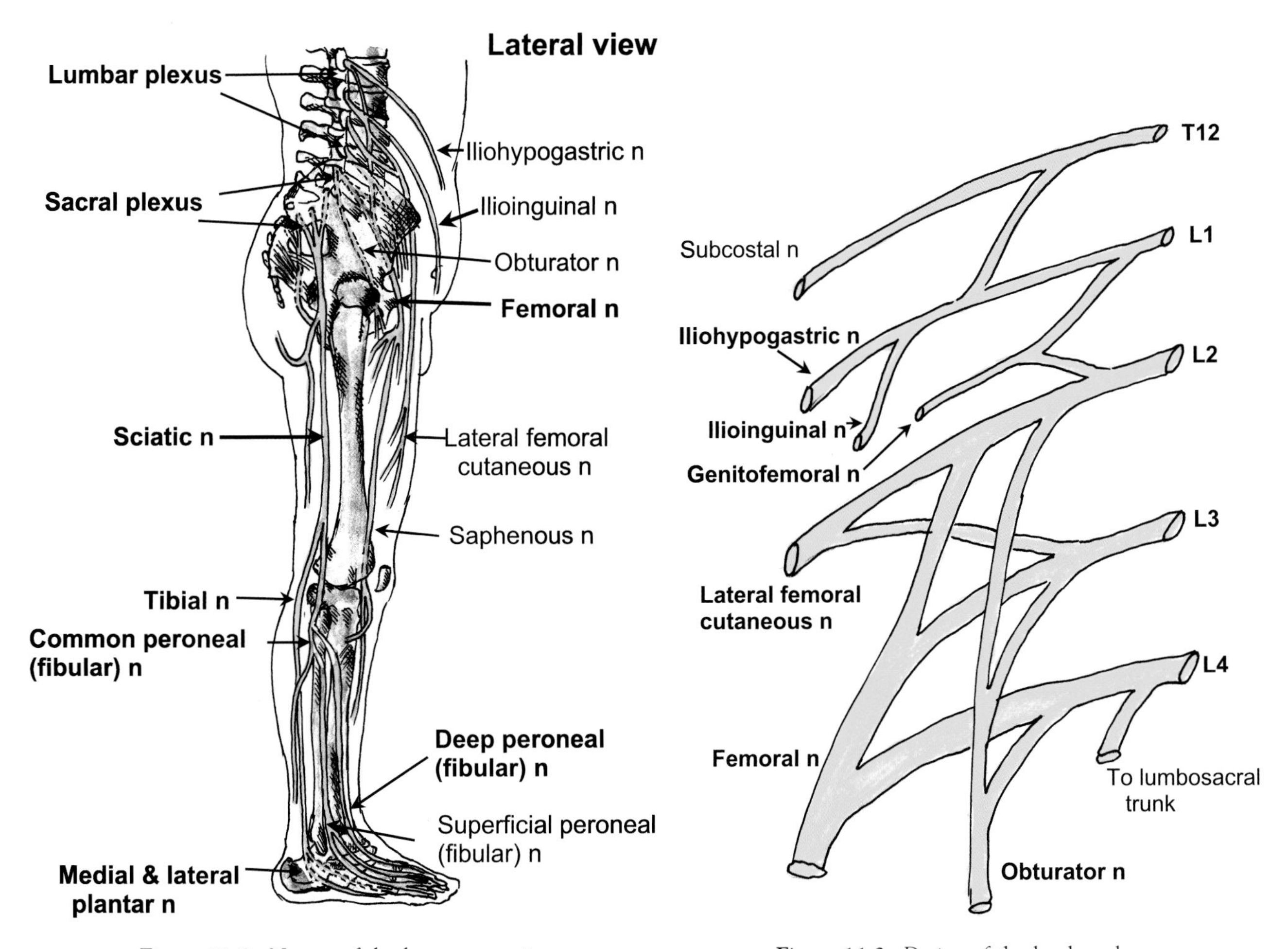

Figure 11.2. Nerves of the lower extremity.

Figure 11.3. Design of the lumbar plexus.

  - Posterior division: Forms the lateral (femoral) cutaneous nerve of the thigh (L2–L3) and the femoral nerve (L2–L4; Figure 11.4).
    - The lateral cutaneous nerve of the thigh (lateral femoral cutaneous nerve) passes obliquely from the lateral border of the psoas major muscle over the iliacus muscle, to enter the thigh just medial to the anterior superior iliac spine and deep to the inguinal ligament.
    - The femoral nerve emerges from the lateral aspect of the lower part of the psoas major muscle and courses inferiorly to enter the thigh under the inguinal ligament; just beyond the femoral triangle it branches into anterior and posterior branches (divisions).
- Additional muscular branches to:
  - Psoas major
  - Psoas minor
  - Iliacus
  - Quadratus lumborum
- In anatomical relation to the psoas major muscle, the obturator (L2–L4) and accessory obturator nerves emerge from its medial border; the genitofemoral (L1, L2) pierces the muscle to lie on its anterior surface; all others emerge from its lateral border.

11.2.2. Formation and Relations of the Sacral Plexus

- At the medial border of the psoas major muscle, the lumbosacral trunk is formed by the union of a branch of L4 and the anterior ramus of L5 (Figures 11.3 and 11.5).

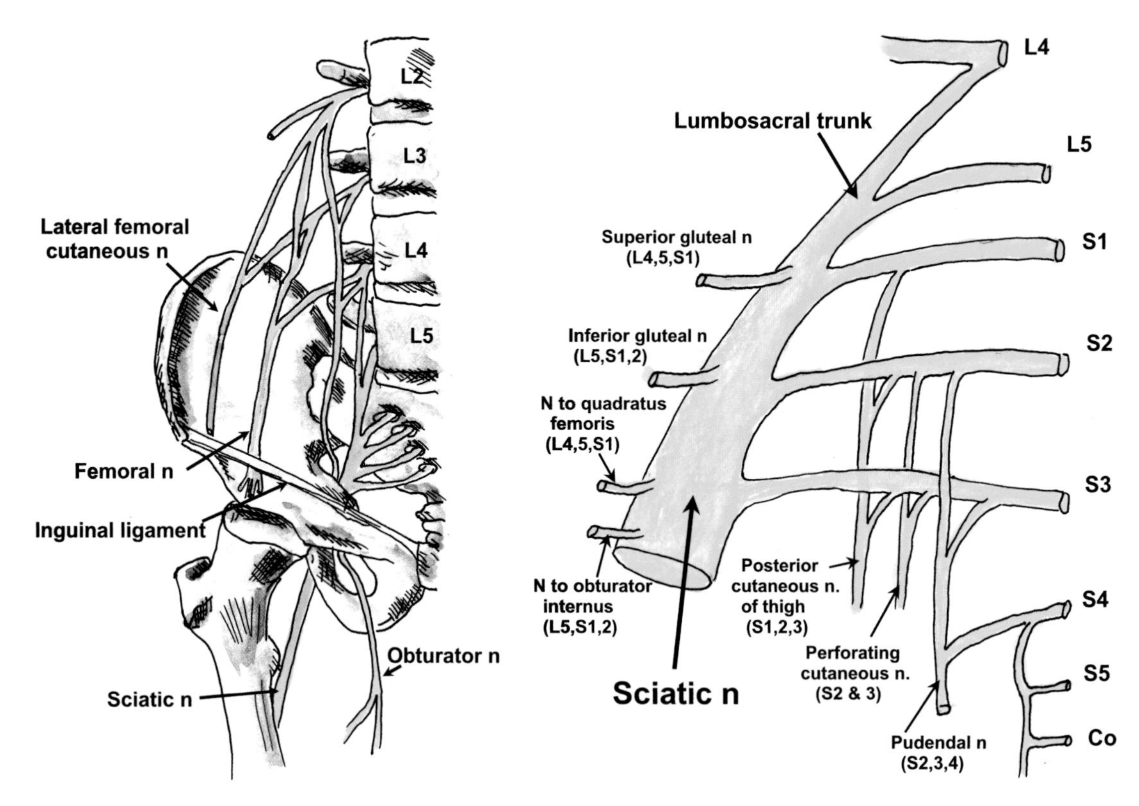

Figure 11.4. Lumbar and sacral plexuses within the skeleton.

Figure 11.5. Design of the sacral plexus.

- After passing over the pelvic brim, the lumbosacral trunk crosses in front of the sacroiliac joint and joins with the ventral ramus of S1.
- After exiting through the anterior sacral foramina, the anterior primary rami of S1 to S4 join the lumbosacral trunk to form the sacral plexus (Figure 11.5).
- The nerves of the plexus converge towards the greater sciatic foramen anterior to the piriformis muscle on the posterior pelvic wall.
- The main terminal nerves are the sciatic nerve (continuation of the plexus) and the pudendal nerves (terminal branches); several other small branches are given off, including
  - Muscular collateral branches
    - Inferior (L5, S1, S2) and superior (L4, L5, S1) gluteal nerves, and nerves to quadratus femoris (L4, L5, S1), piriformis (S1, S2), obturator internus (L5, S1, S2), levator ani (S4), coccygeus (S4), and external anal sphincter (S4) muscles
  - Cutaneous collateral branches
    - Posterior cutaneous nerve of the thigh (S1–S3) and perforating cutaneous nerve (S2, S3)
  - Visceral (parasympathetic) collateral branches
    - Pelvic splanchnic nerves (S2, S3, S4)
- Anatomical relationships to vessels:
  - The superior gluteal vessels pass between the lumbosacral trunk (L4, L5) and S1, or between S1 and S2 roots.
  - The inferior gluteal vessels pass between either roots S1 and S2 or S2 and S3 (gluteal vessels follow the course of the sacral nerves in the anterior plane).
  - The internal pudendal vessels pass from the greater to the lesser sciatic foramina, superficial to the sacrospinous ligament but deep to the sacrotuberous ligament, between the sciatic and pudendal nerves.

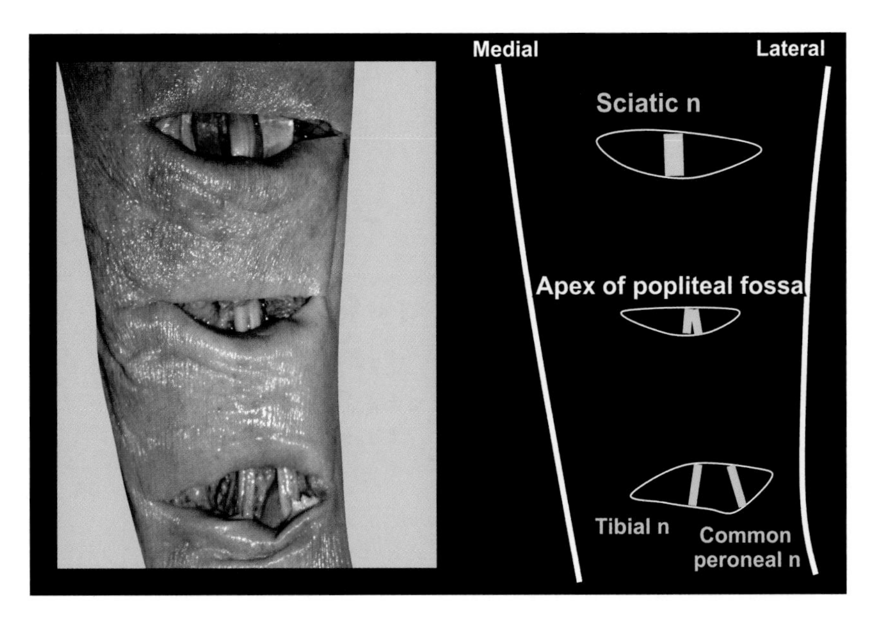

Figure 11.6. Sciatic nerve bifurcation in the posterior thigh.

- The sciatic nerve splits in the posterior thigh into tibial (medial) and common peroneal, or fibular, (lateral) nerves, although in about 10% of cases these nerves are separate right from the origin of the plexus. Figure 11.6 shows a dissected cadaver with the bifurcation of the sciatic into the tibial and common peroneal (fibular) nerves.

11.3. Distribution of Spinal Nerves in the Lower Extremity

Although it is generally more useful to consider musculoskeletal regions (i.e., hip, knee, etc.) for anesthesia procedures, a sound knowledge of the complex arrangement of spinal nerves and their segmentation patterns in the lower extremity will be beneficial for a true appreciation of the applications of regional blocks in this area.

11.3.1. Dermatomes

Within each spinal nerve (except C1, which does not have a sensory component), the fibers from the dorsal root of the spinal cord supply a specific area or band of skin. This band of skin is referred to as a *dermatome*. The C5 to T1 and L1 to S2 spinal nerves supply the skin of the upper extremity and the lower extremity, respectively. There is considerable overlap between contiguous dermatomes, with individual dermatomes extending beyond the boundaries of the adjacent dermatome. The dermatomes are generally arranged as consecutive horizontal bands on the surface of the axial skeleton, and more or less vertical bands on the extremities (Figures 11.7 and 11.8). Dermatomes are important particularly for peripheral nerve blockade, and specific cutaneous areas can be targeted based on the dermatomal pattern produced through the terminal nerves in that part of the body (Figures 11.9 and 11.10).

11.3.1.1. Segmental Sensory Innervation (Dermatomes) of the Lower Limb

- L1: Pelvic region (anterior) and upper medial thigh
- L2: Upper and lateral aspects of thigh
- L3: Lower anterior medial aspect of thigh and knee

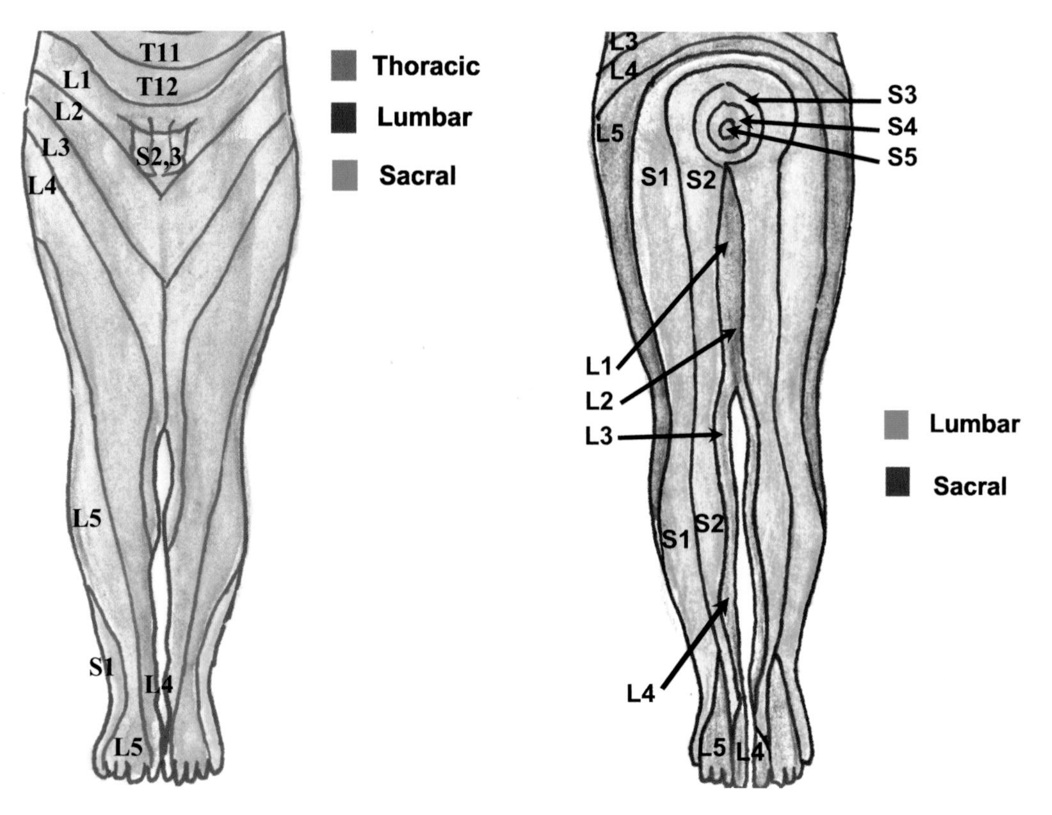

Figure 11.7. Dermatomes of the lower extremity, anterior view.

Figure 11.8. Dermatomes of the lower extremity, posterior view.

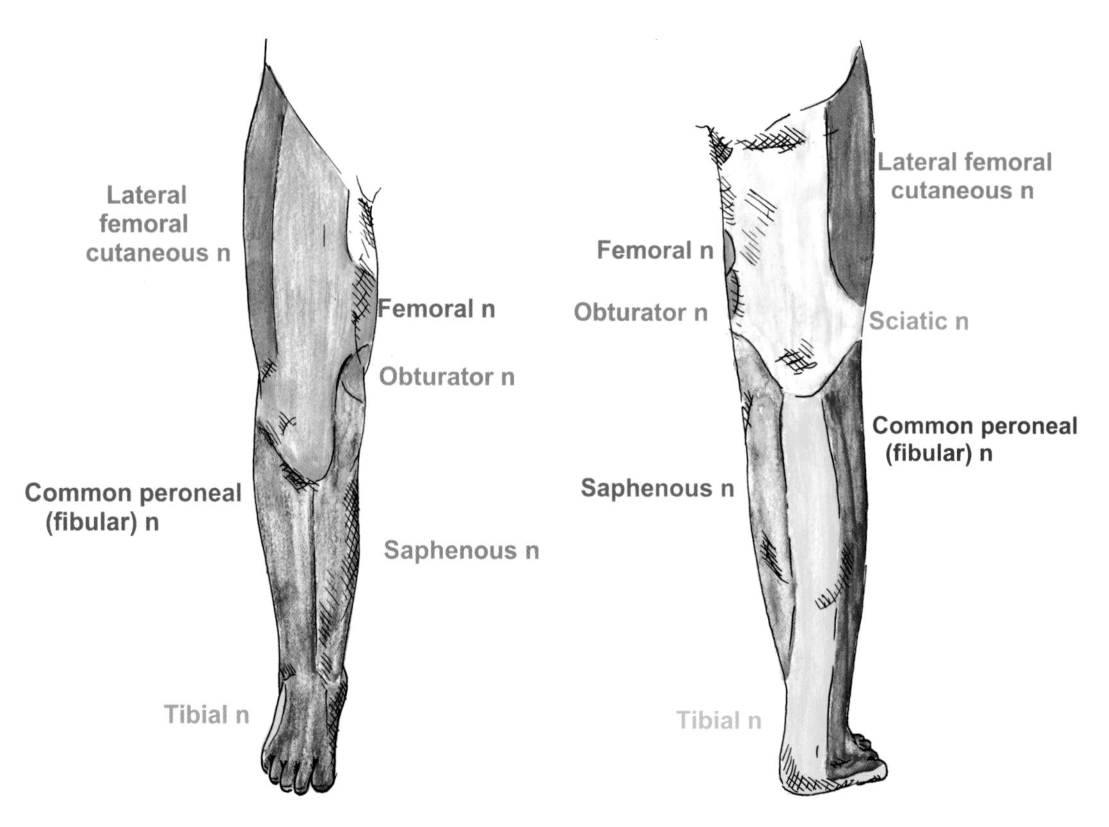

Figure 11.9. Cutaneous distribution of the peripheral nerves in the lower extremity, anterior view.

Figure 11.10. Cutaneous distribution of the peripheral nerves in the lower extremity, posterior view.

- L4: Anteromedial aspect of leg and medial ankle
- L5: Anterolateral aspect of leg, medial aspect of foot, upper surface of first to third toes
- S1: Lateral side of foot and sole
- S2: Posterior surface of thigh and leg
- S3 and S4: Gluteal and perianal (posterior pelvic) region

11.3.2. Myotomes

The ventral roots of the spinal cord contribute to the motor innervation of skeletal muscle by providing motor nerve fibers to the spinal nerves. A *myotome* is a group of skeletal muscle that is supplied segmentally by the ventral roots of a particular spinal nerve. Movements of the extremities and trunk that are created by these myotomes can thus be classified segmentally (see below). In general, segmental innervation of the muscles is fairly well differentiated. For clinical practice, it is important to understand that there is also a specific distribution of innervation to skeletal muscles that is derived from the terminal nerves (Figures 11.11 and 11.12). Tables 11.1 and 11.2 summarize the origin of each terminal motor nerve and its related movements; the segmental innervation of the lower extremity is depicted indirectly, through the origin of the terminal nerves. This table will be repeated in subsequent chapters to describe motor response associated with nerve stimulation.

11.3.2.1. Segmental Motor Responses Associated with Nerve Stimulation

- L2 and L3: Flexion, adduction, and medial rotation of hip
- L3 and L4: Extension of knee
- L4: Foot inversion

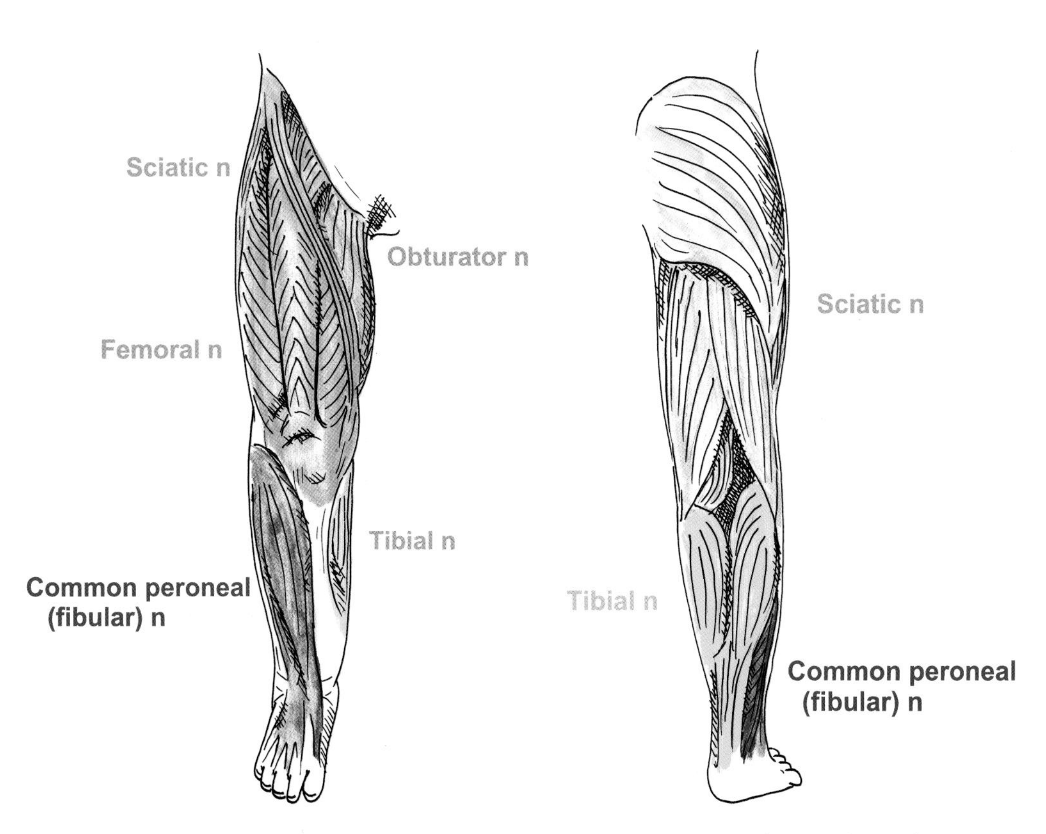

Figure 11.11. Distribution of muscular innervation by the terminal nerves of the lower extremity, anterior view.

Figure 11.12. Distribution of muscular innervation by the terminal nerves of the lower extremity, posterior view.

Table 11.1. Lumbar plexus terminal motor nerves: origin and motor responses associated with nerve stimulation.

Movement	Nerve	Plexus division	Root
Adduction and flexion of thigh	Obturator	Anterior	L2, 3, 4
Patellar twitch and knee extension	Femoral (main nerve and its posterior branch)	Posterior	L2, 3, 4
Thigh adduction only (pectineus m.)	Femoral (anterior branch below inguinal ligament)	Posterior	L2, 3, 4

- L4 and L5: Dorsiflexion of foot
- L5 and S1: Extension, abduction, and lateral rotation of hip and flexion of knee
- L5 and S1: Foot eversion
- S1 and S2: Plantar flexion of foot

11.3.2.2. *Muscular Distribution of Spinal Segments*

- L2: Psoas major, iliacus, gracilis, sartorius
- L3: Adductor longus and brevis, rectus femoris
- L4: Vastus lateralis and medialis, adductor magnus, tibialis anterior
- L5: Tibialis anterior, extensor digitorum longus, extensor hallucis longus, peroneus (fibularis) tertius, extensor digitorum brevis, tibialis posterior, flexor digitorum longus, semimembranosus, semitendinosus, short head biceps femoris, tensor fasciae latae, gluteus medius and minimus
- S1: Peroneus (fibularis) longus and brevis, medial and lateral gastrocnemius, soleus, biceps femoris, gluteus maximus, piriformis
- S2: Abductor hallucis, abductor digiti minimi (quinti), interossei
- S2 to S4: External anal sphincter
- S4: Bulbospongiosus (bulbocavernosus)

11.3.3. Osteotomes

Osteotomes refer to specific regions of the bones throughout the extremities that are innervated by the terminal nerves (rather than by spinal segment as with dermatomes; Figures 11.13 and 11.14). The innervation of bones can be significantly different from that of the

Table 11.2. Sciatic plexus branches and terminal motor nerves: origin and motor responses associated with nerve stimulation.

Movement	Nerve	Root
Anal sphincter	Pudendal	S2, S3, S4
Gluteal twitch/thigh abduction (gluteus minimus and medius)	Superior gluteal	L4, L5, S1
Gluteal twitch/thigh extension (gluteus maximus)	Inferior gluteal	L5, S1, S2
Knee flexion and ankle plantar flexion	Tibial (above and below sciatic bifurcation)	L4, L5, S1, S2, S3
Ankle dorsiflexion	Common peroneal (fibular)	L4, L5, S1, S2
Ankle and toe extension	Deep peroneal (fibular)	L5, S1
Foot eversion (peroneus longus and brevis)	Superficial peroneal (fibular)	L5, S1
First toe abduction	Medial plantar	S1, S2
Fifth toe abduction	Lateral plantar	S1, S2, S3

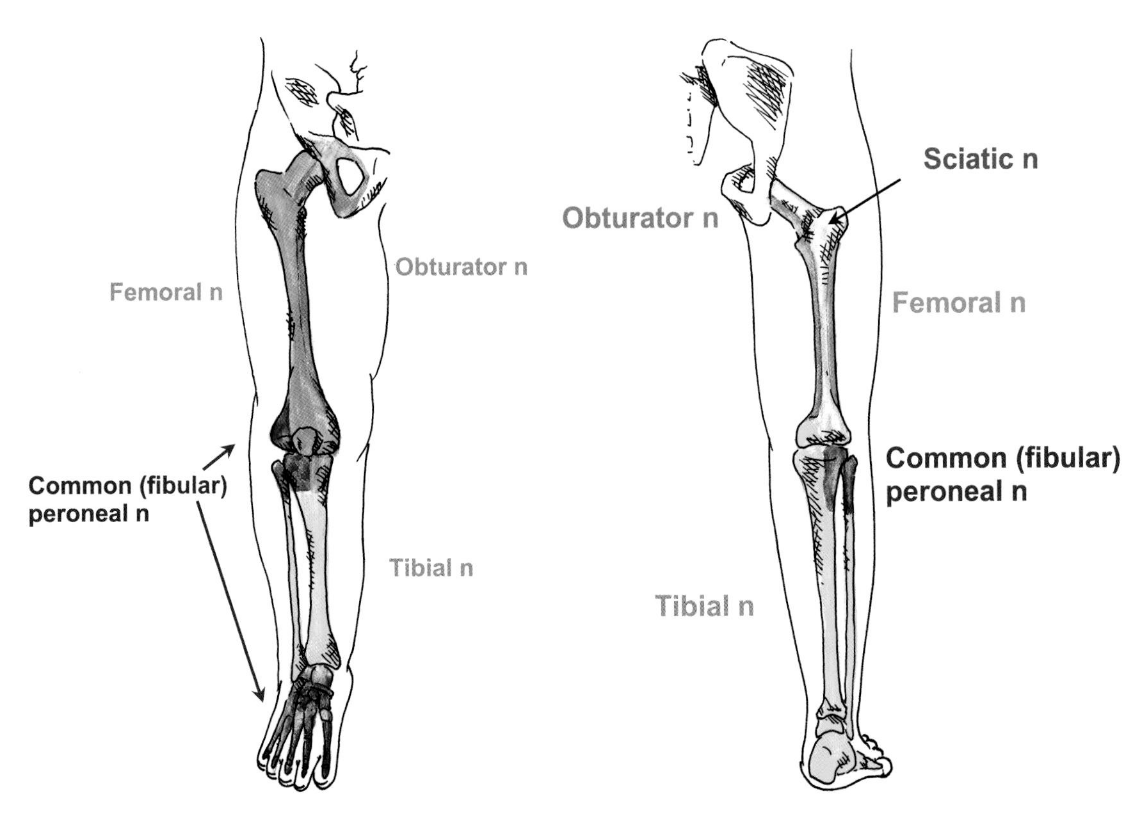

Figure 11.13. Osteotomes of the lower extremity, anterior view.

Figure 11.14. Osteotomes of the lower extremity, posterior view.

muscles and skin. A good knowledge of joint innervation is important for orthopedic surgery as well as other surgical specialties and neurology. Table 11.3 outlines the innervation of the lower extremity joints and the associated motor responses associated with nerve stimulation during nerve block procedures.

Table 11.3. Lower extremity joint innervation and motor responses associated with nerve stimulation.

Joint	Nerve	Root(s)	Motor response
Hip			
Anterior	Femoral (nerve to rectus femoris)	L2–L4	Patellar twitch (thigh adduction if posterior division only)
	Obturator (anterior division)	L2–L4	Thigh adduction
Posterior	Sciatic (nerve to quadratus femoris)	L4, L5, S1	Gluteal twitch (quadratus femoris)
Knee			
Anterior	Femoral (articular branches)	L2–L4	Patellar twitch
	Tibial (articular branches)	L4, L5, S1–S3	Knee and ankle flexion
	Common peroneal (fibular)	L4, L5, S1, S2	Ankle dorsiflexion
Posterior	Obturator	L2–L4	Thigh adduction
	Common peroneal (fibular)	L4, L5, S1–S2	Ankle dorsiflexion
	Tibial	L4, L5, S1–S3	Knee and ankle flexion
Ankle			
	Deep peroneal	L5, S1	Ankle and toes extension
	Superficial peroneal	L5, S1	Foot eversion
	Posterior tibial	L5, S1, S2	Ankle dorsiflexion
	Saphenous	L3, L4	None

Suggested Reading and References

Awad IT, Duggan EM. Posterior lumbar plexus block: anatomy, approaches and techniques. Reg Anesth Pain Med 2005;30:143–149.
Bo WJ, Meschan I, Krueger WA. Basic atlas of cross-sectional anatomy: a clinical approach. Philadelphia: Saunders; 1980.
Ellis H, Feldman S, Harrop-Griffiths W, eds. Anatomy for anaesthesiologists, 8th ed. Boston: Blackwell; 2004.
Lee B. Atlas of surgical and sectional anatomy. Stamford, CT: Appleton-Century-Crofts; 1983.
Netter FH. Atlas of human anatomy. Summit, NJ: CIBA-GEIGY Corporation; 1989.

12 Lumbar Plexus/Psoas Compartment Block

Ban C.H. Tsui

Despite the recent popularity of lumbar plexus blockade, the value of ultrasound guidance for this block is still limited and it is important to recognize the complexity of this block and the associated risks. Potential complications include an increased risk of causing retroperitoneal hematoma (even with correct injection), injury to retroperitoneal structures, systemic toxicity from injection into deep muscle tissue, and unintentional epidural or intrathecal local anesthetic spread. This block has the advantage of blocking the entire lumbar plexus (Figure 12.1) and therefore provides anesthesia/analgesia of the anterolateral and medial thigh, the knee, and the cutaneous distribution of the saphenous nerve below the knee (i.e., femoral nerve, obturator nerve, and the lateral cutaneous nerve of the thigh). It is often combined with a sciatic nerve block to provide complete surgical anesthesia to the entire lower extremity. Although this block has been used for inguinal hernia repair in children, it is generally not indicated for adults because the iliohypogastric, ilioinguinal, and genitofemoral (L1–L2) nerves may not be adequately blocked with the common lumbar plexus injection site at the more caudal L3–L5 level.

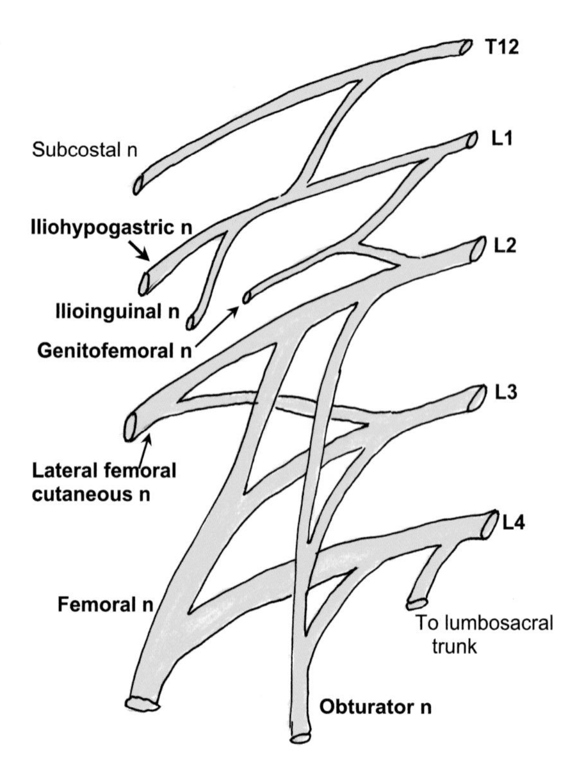

Figure 12.1. Design of the lumbar plexus.

12.1. Clinical Anatomy

12.1.1. Lumbar Plexus Within the Psoas Compartment

- The first lumbar nerve emerges between the first and second lumbar vertebrae; the last between the fifth lumbar vertebrae and the base of the sacrum (body of first sacral vertebra).
- The lumbar spinal nerves (ventral rami) lie within the substance of the psoas major muscle immediately after exiting the intervertebral foramina and divide into divisions anterior to the lumbar transverse processes (Figure 12.2). Major branches of the plexus (Figure 12.3) include the iliohypogastric, ilioinguinal, genitofemoral, lateral femoral cutaneous, femoral and obturator nerves (accessory obturator when present).
- The nerve roots, although technically within a single-massed psoas major muscle, can be accessed clinically in a space or compartment bordered medially by the psoas major muscle fiber insertions (onto the bodies of the lumbar vertebrae), posteriorly by the lumbar transverse processes, and anteriorly by the fascia iliaca (Figure 12.4).
- Iliohypogastric (L1) and ilioinguinal (L1) nerves indicated for inguinal hernia repair (Figures 12.1 through 12.4):
  - The iliohypogastric nerve penetrates the transverse abdominis muscle just above the iliac crest, supplies it, and divides into anterior and lateral cutaneous branches.
    - The anterior branch pierces and supplies the internal oblique muscle just 2 cm medial to the anterior superior iliac spine; it then courses deep to the external oblique muscle and superior to the inguinal canal and pierces the external oblique aponeurosis about 2 to 3 cm above the superficial inguinal ring, terminating subcutaneously in the skin of the suprapubic region.
    - The lateral branch supplies the posterolateral portion of the gluteal skin after piercing both the oblique muscles.
  - The ilioinguinal nerve pierces and supplies the internal oblique muscle and then enters the inguinal canal, in which it traverses outside the spermatic cord, to emerge through the superficial (external) inguinal ring (the external oblique aponeurosis) where it

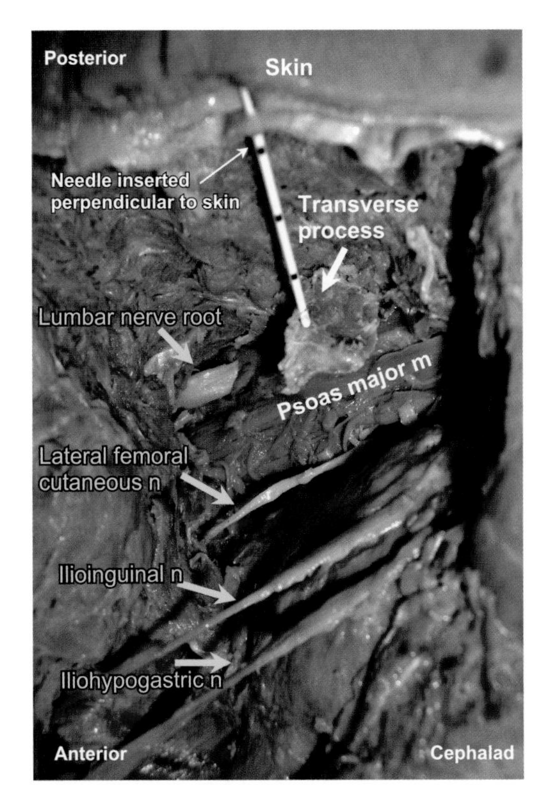

Figure 12.2. Transverse dissection at the lumbar spine showing the nerves of the lumbar plexus coursing anterior to the transverse processes and within the psoas major muscle.

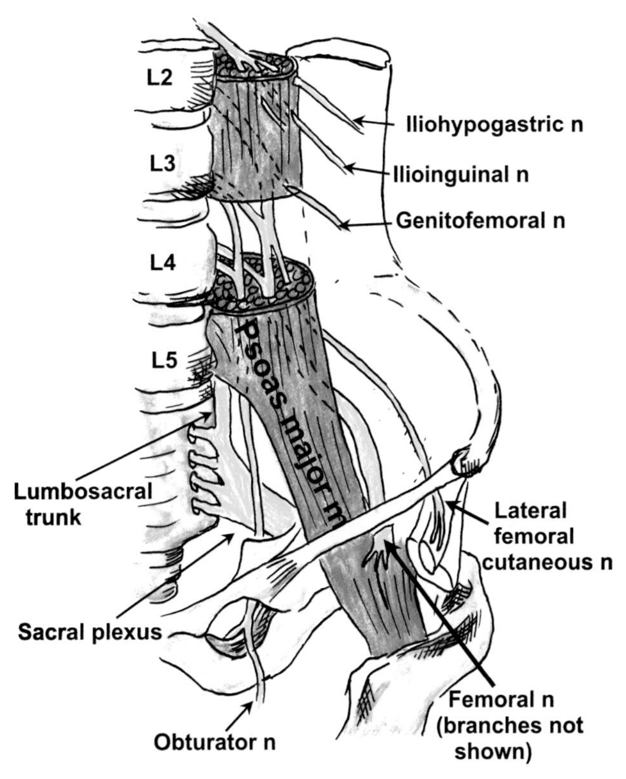

Figure 12.3. Major branches of the lumbar plexus.

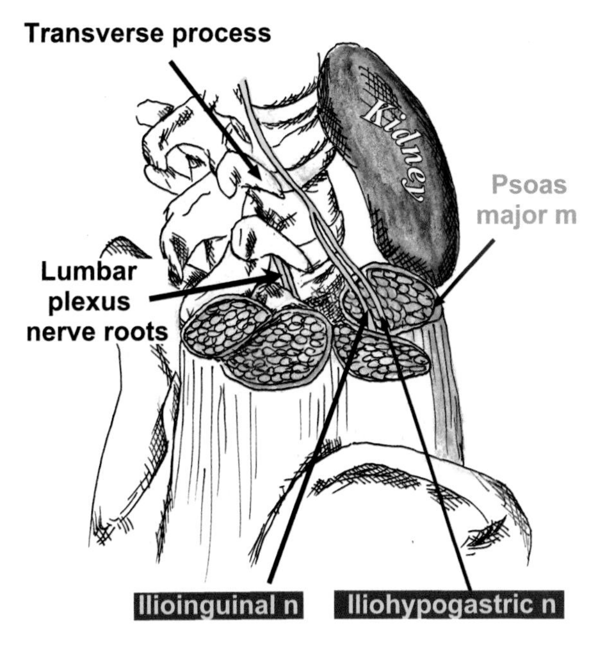

Figure 12.4. Psoas major muscle compartment.

provides cutaneous innervation to the skin of the scrotum (or labium majus) and adjacent thigh.

12.1.2. Terminal Nerves of Lumbar Plexus

- Genitofemoral nerve (L1, L2; Figure 12.1): at the lower border of L3, the genitofemoral nerve pierces then lies anterior to the psoas major muscle; it then descends subperitoneally and behind the ureter and divides into two branches (genital and femoral), at a variable distance above the inguinal ligament:
  - Genital branch: Crosses the external iliac artery and traverses the inguinal canal within the spermatic cord. In females it accompanies the round ligament of the uterus.
    - The nerve supplies the cremaster muscle; skin over the scrotum, and adjacent thigh (females, skin over anterior part of labium majus and mons pubis).
  - Femoral branch: Descends lateral to the external iliac artery, passes under the inguinal ligament, enters the femoral sheath lateral to the femoral artery, pierces the anterior layer of the femoral sheath and fascia lata.
    - It innervates the skin immediately below the crease of the groin anterior to the upper part of the femoral triangle.
- Lateral cutaneous nerve of thigh (a.k.a., lateral femoral cutaneous nerve; L2, L3; Figures 12.1 and 12.2): This nerve passes obliquely from the lateral border of the psoas major muscle over the iliacus to enter the thigh below or through the inguinal ligament, variably medial to the anterior superior iliac spine. On the right side of the body, the nerve passes posterolateral to the cecum and on the left it traverses behind the lower part of the descending colon. The nerve lies on top of the sartorius muscle before dividing into anterior (supplies skin over the anterolateral aspect of the thigh) and posterior (supplies skin on the lateral aspect of the thigh from the greater trochanter to the midthigh) branches.
  - Occasionally, this nerve is a branch of the femoral nerve rather than its own nerve.
- Femoral nerve (L2–L4; Figures 12.1 and 12.3): The femoral nerve is the largest nerve of this plexus, supplying muscles and skin on the anterior aspect of the thigh (its saphenous branch supplies the skin on the medial aspect of the leg below the knee and the skin on the medial aspect of the foot); it descends through the psoas major muscle and emerges low at its lateral border, coursing inferiorly between the iliacus and psoas major muscles to enter the thigh under the inguinal ligament; just beyond the femoral triangle, it branches into anterior and posterior branches (divisions).
  - Anterior branch (division): Gives muscular branches to pectineus and sartorius and cutaneous branches (intermediate and medial cutaneous nerves of thigh) to the skin on the anterior aspect of the thigh.
  - Posterior branch (division): Sends muscular branches to the quadriceps femoris muscle and gives rise to the saphenous nerve, its largest cutaneous branch. The saphenous nerve follows the femoral artery, lying lateral to it within the adductor (Hunter's, subsartorial) canal and then crossing it anteriorly to lie medial to the artery. Distal to the canal it leaves the artery to lie superficial at the medial aspect of the knee; the nerve then continues inferiorly (subcutaneously) with the long (great) saphenous vein along the medial aspect of the leg down to the tibial aspect of the ankle; it provides articular branches to the hip and knee joints.
- Obturator nerve (L2–L4; Figures 12.1 and 12.3): The obturator nerve emerges from the medial border of the psoas major muscle at the pelvic brim to pass behind the common iliac vessels and lateral to the internal iliac vessels; it then courses inferiorly and anteriorly along the lateral wall of the pelvic cavity on the obturator internus muscle toward the obturator canal, through which it enters the upper part of the medial aspect of the

Table 12.1. Target terminal nerves for lumbar plexus block: origin and motor responses associated with nerve stimulation.

Movement	Nerve	Plexus division	Root
Adduction and flexion of thigh	Obturator	Anterior	L2, 3, 4
Patellar twitch and knee extension	Femoral (main nerve and its posterior branch)	Posterior	L2, 3, 4
Thigh adduction only (pectineus m.)	Femoral (anterior branch below inguinal ligament)	Posterior	L2, 3, 4

thigh above and anterior to the obturator vessels. It divides into its anterior and posterior branches near the obturator foramen.
- Anterior branch: Passes into the thigh anterior to the obturator externus, descends in front of the adductor brevis, behind the pectineus and adductor longus muscle, with its terminal cutaneous branches emerging as it courses alongside the femoral artery. Behind the pectineus muscle it supplies the adductor longus, gracilis, adductor brevis (usually), and pectineus (often) muscles. Its cutaneous branches supply the skin on the medial aspect of the thigh.
- Posterior branch: Pierces the obturator externus muscle anteriorly and supplies it, then passes behind the adductor brevis muscle (sometimes supplies it) to descend on the anterior aspect of the adductor magnus muscle (medial to the anterior branch) which it supplies; it then traverses the adductor canal with the femoral artery and vein to enter the popliteal fossa, where it terminates as an articular branch to the back of the knee joint capsule (oblique popliteal ligament).

- Accessory obturator nerve (L3, L4): This nerve is present in about 30% of individuals; it descends along the medial border of the psoas major muscle, crosses the superior pubic ramus behind the pectineus muscle, supplies it, and gives articular branches to the hip joint.

Table 12.1 depicts the target nerves of the lumbar plexus block that contain motor fibers. This table shows the origin of the nerves originating from the lumbar plexus as well as the muscle movements associated with nerve stimulation.

12.2. Patient Positioning and Surface Anatomy

12.2.1. Patient Positioning [Figure 12.5(A,B)]

The patient lies in the semiprone position with the operative side up and with both hips flexed. The gluteal crease is not a reliable landmark in this dependant position.

12.2.2. Surface Anatomy

- Horizontal line
  - A line drawn through the uppermost aspects (peaks) of the iliac crests (corresponding to approximately L4 spinous process)
- Vertical line
  - A line perpendicular to the horizontal line and crossing through the ipsilateral posterior superior iliac spines (PSIS)

The traditional puncture site is the intersection of these two lines, although ultrasound imaging may identify a slightly different location.

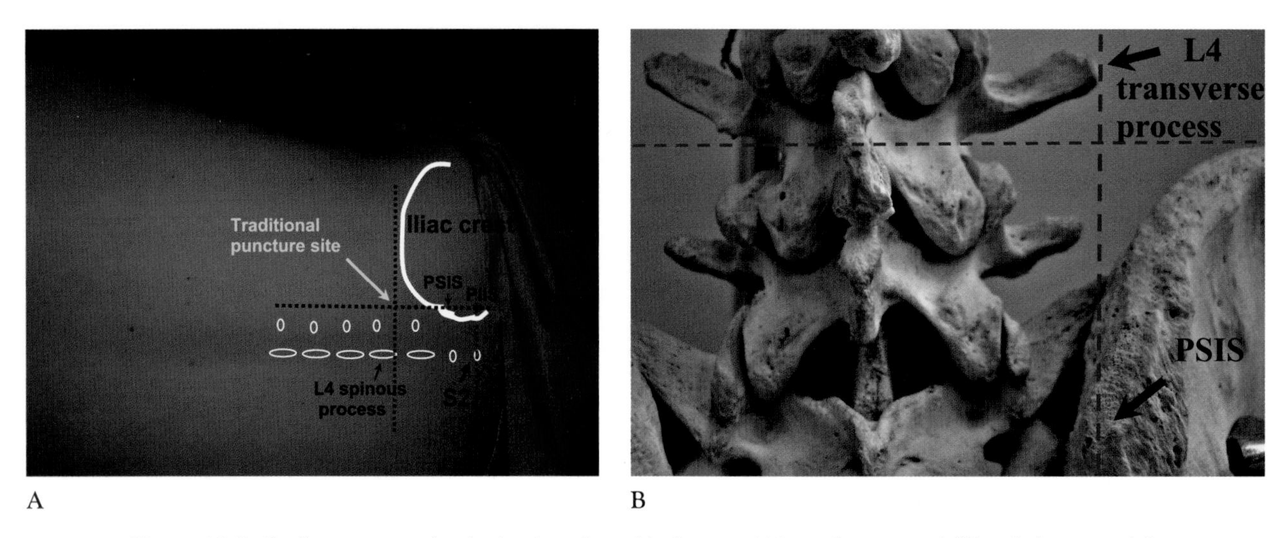

A B

Figure 12.5. Surface anatomy for the lumbar plexus block using (A) a volunteer and (B) a skeleton model.

12.3. Sonographic Imaging and Needle Insertion Technique

This discussion on ultrasound scanning, sonographic appearance, and needling technique for the lumbar plexus is quite similar to that for lumbar paravertebral blockade. Generally speaking, ultrasound scanning for lumbar paravertebral blockade is similar to that described for the thoracic paravertebral block (described in Chapter 19) although rib visualization only applies in the thoracic region.

Because the lumbar plexus is difficult to capture with both magnetic resonance imaging [MRI; Figures 12.6 and 12.7(A,B,C)] and ultrasound imaging, the primary role of the

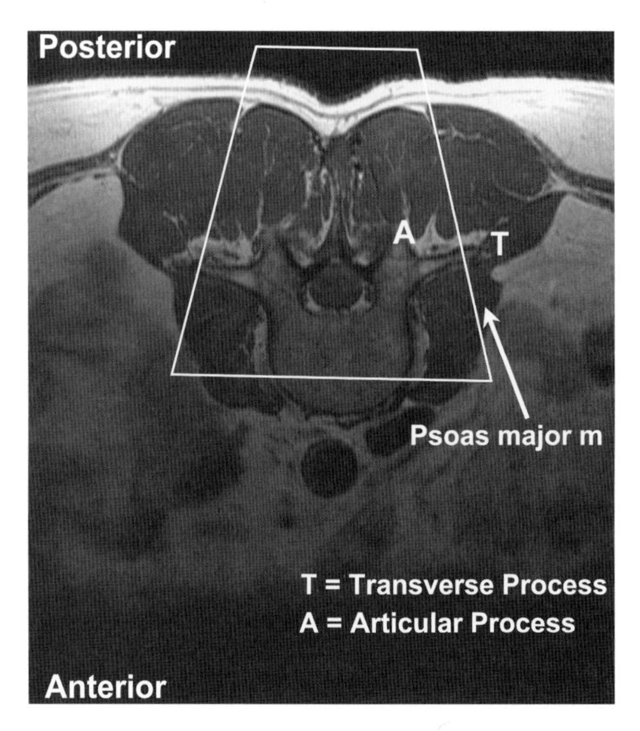

Figure 12.6. MRI image of a transverse section at L4.

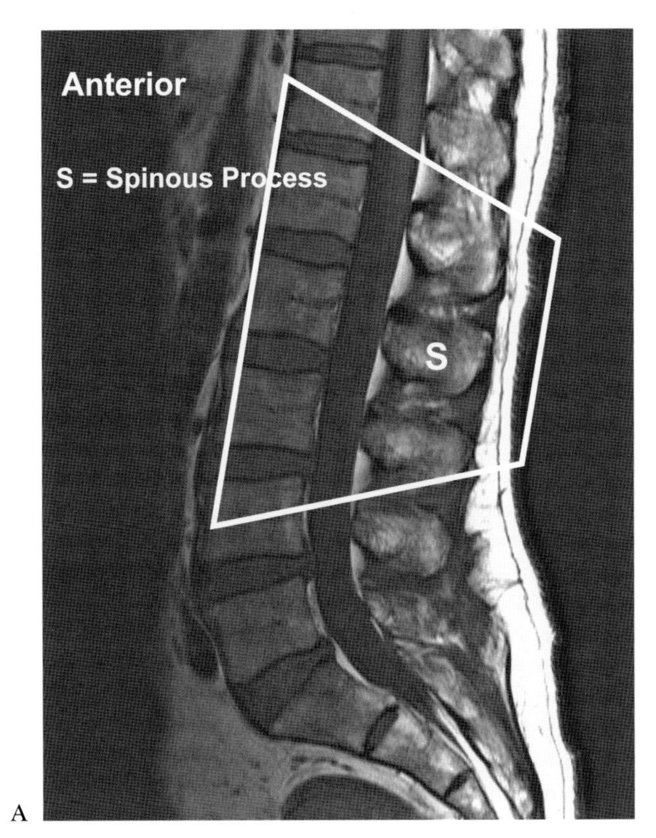

A

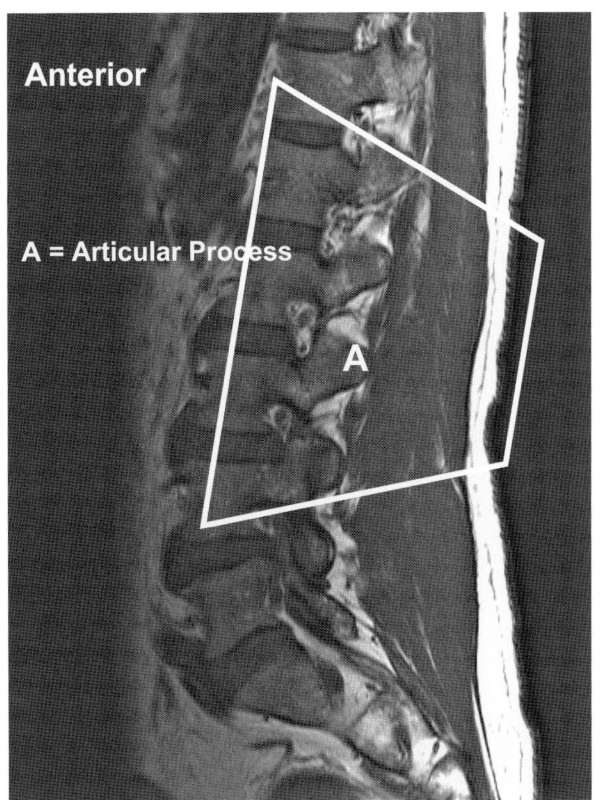

B

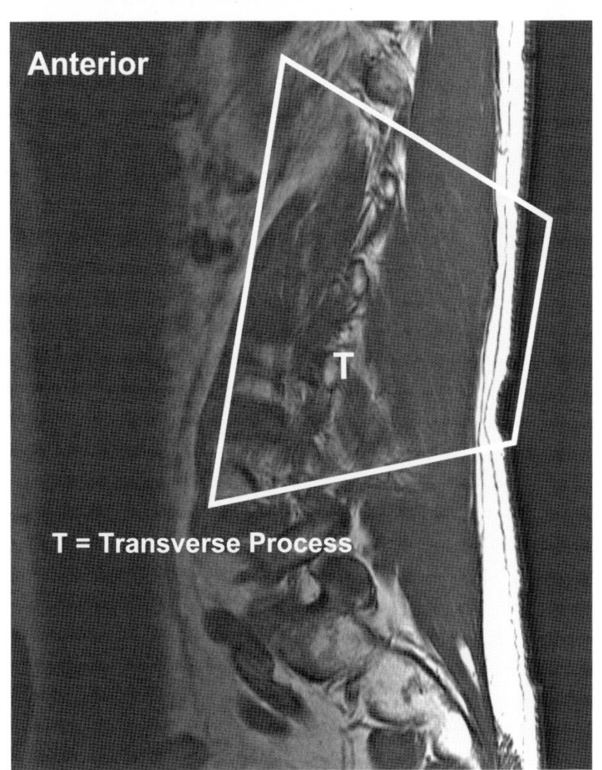

C

Figure 12.7. MRI images of longitudinal sections showing the (A) spinous, (B) articular, and (C) transverse processes.

transverse and longitudinal ultrasound scans (Figures 12.8, 12.9, 12.10, and 12.11) is to identify and locate bony landmarks (e.g., transverse, articular, and spinous processes).

Prepare the needle insertion site and skin surface with an antiseptic solution. Prepare the ultrasound probe surface by applying a sterile adhesive dressing to it prior to needling as discussed earlier (see Chapters 3 and 4).

12.3.1. Scanning Technique

There is limited information on lumbar plexus sonoanatomy. Kirchmair and colleagues described ultrasound techniques to localize the lumbar plexus and adjacent transverse processes, the erector spinae, psoas major and quadratus lumborum muscles, as well as articular processes mainly in the pediatric population. Ultrasound imaging of the lumbar plexus in adults, in the experience of the authors of this text, is difficult.

Traditionally, the approach for the lumbar plexus block has been at the L4 to L5 level to avoid renal hematoma or other complications at the level of the kidney (L2–L3; Figure 12.4). Ultrasound visualization of the kidneys and vascular structures [Figure 12.12(A,B)] may allow needle insertion at a more cephalad level (L1–L4) to provide more consistent blockade of the ilioinguinal and iliohypogastric nerves.

The mean skin to lumbar plexus depth at the level of L4 is 8.4 cm in adult men and 7.1 cm in adult women, based on computed tomography assessment. There is a positive correlation between body mass index and skin-to-plexus distance. The distance between the posterior edges of the transverse processes of the lumbar vertebrae and the lumbar plexus is about 1.8 cm.

The primary use of ultrasound for lumbar plexus block will be for locating anatomical landmarks of the block and measuring their distance from the skin and any other structures (e.g., the kidney if using a cephalad approach). See Section 12.3.3 for more details.

- Place a 5- to 7-MHz curved array probe in the transverse plane at the midline and at the L4 spinous process location (Figure 12.13) and identify the spinous, articular, and transverse processes of the lumbar vertebrae.
- In this view (if the field is large enough) the iliac crest peak may be visible laterally, but this location is too lateral for the block site as complications (e.g., retroperitoneal injection) may not be avoided.
- Other important structures, such as the kidney (inferior edge at L2) and its related vessels, should be carefully observed to assist with proper positioning of the probe (Figure 12.12). For instance, clear visibility of the kidney indicates that the probe is placed too cephalad and thus should be adjusted caudally.
- The position of the transverse processes can be verified by turning the probe to the longitudinal (sagittal) plane adjacent to the spinous processes of L4 and L5.
- Move the longitudinally aligned probe laterally from the midline to view along the transverse processes (Figures 12.11 and 12.14).
- Identify the point at which the transverse process is just visible (indicating its tip); this marks the ideal block location.
- In the longitudinal scan image, the L2 to L4 spinal nerves are located deep (anterior) and just lateral to the visible landmarks of the transverse processes. However, not only is it difficult to see the deeply positioned spinal nerves with the low resolution of the curved probe, but it is also difficult to track the needle at this depth.

Clinical Pearls

- In most situations, ultrasound is primarily useful for marking the location and depth of the transverse processes, rather than actually guiding the needle.
- This is an advanced ultrasound-guided block technique to be performed by experienced clinicians.

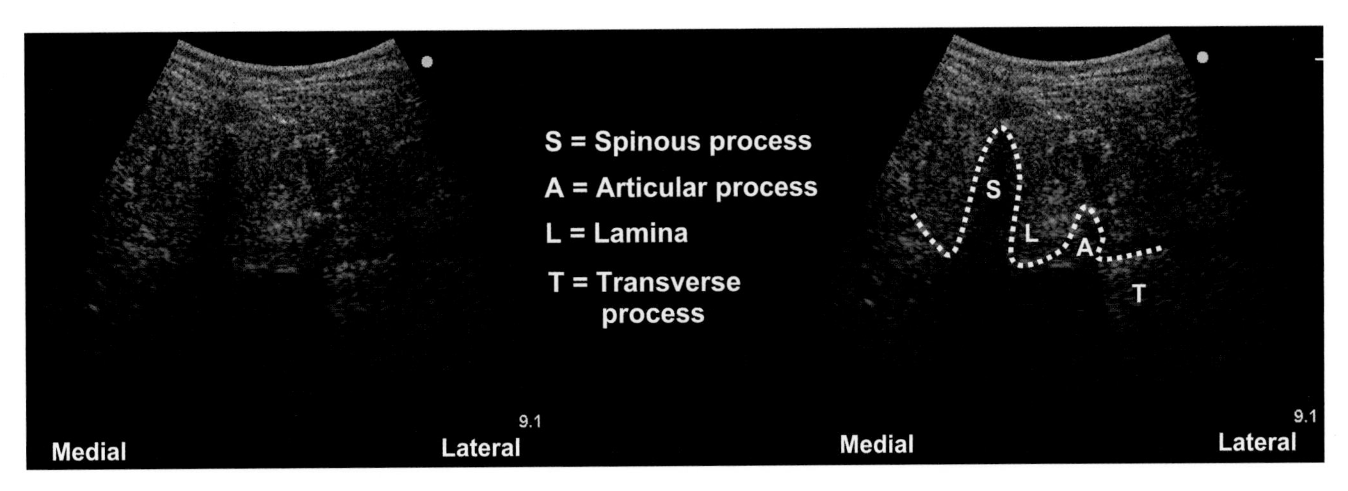

Figure 12.8. Ultrasound image of a transverse axis view at the lumbar spine (L4–L5).

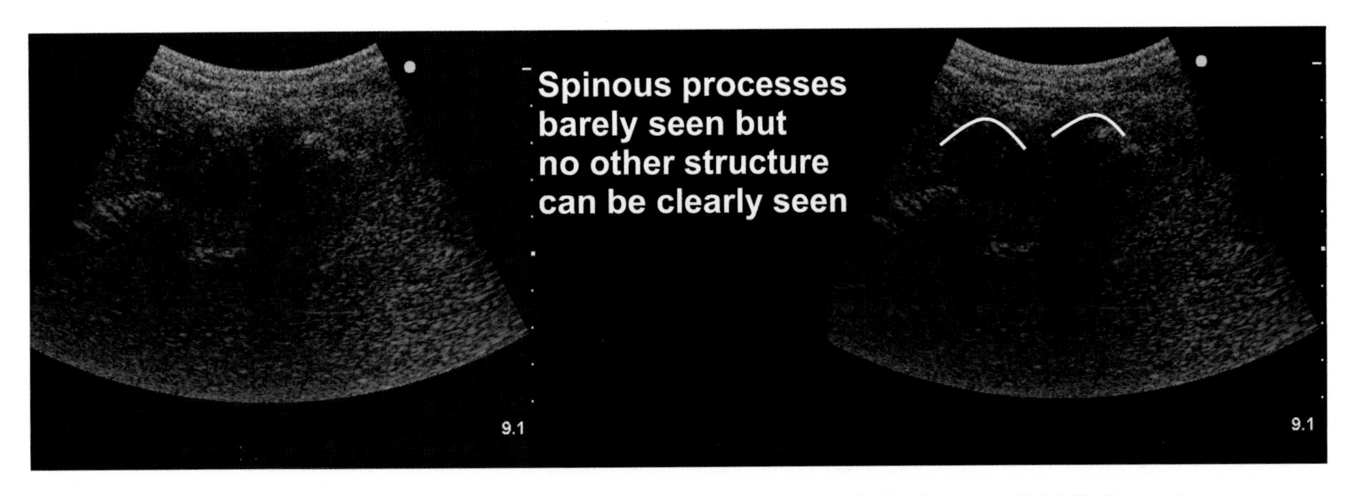

Figure 12.9. Ultrasound image of a longitudinal axis view of the spinous processes at the lumbar spine (L4–L5). Bony spinous process reflected most of ultrasound such that no clear structure can be seen.

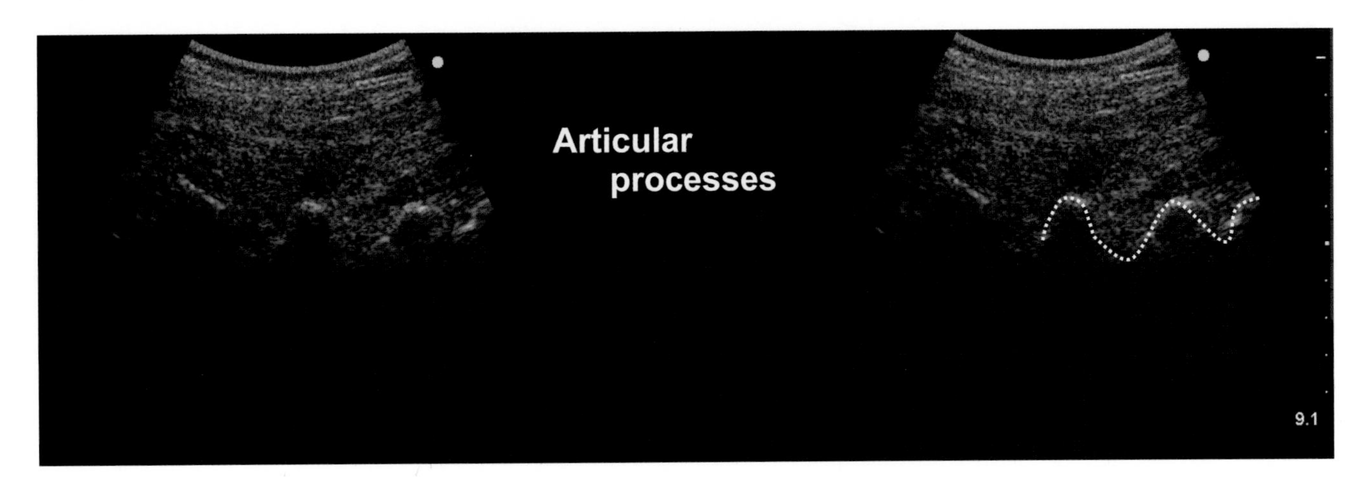

Figure 12.10. Ultrasound image of a longitudinal axis view of the articular processes in the lumbar spine (L4–L5).

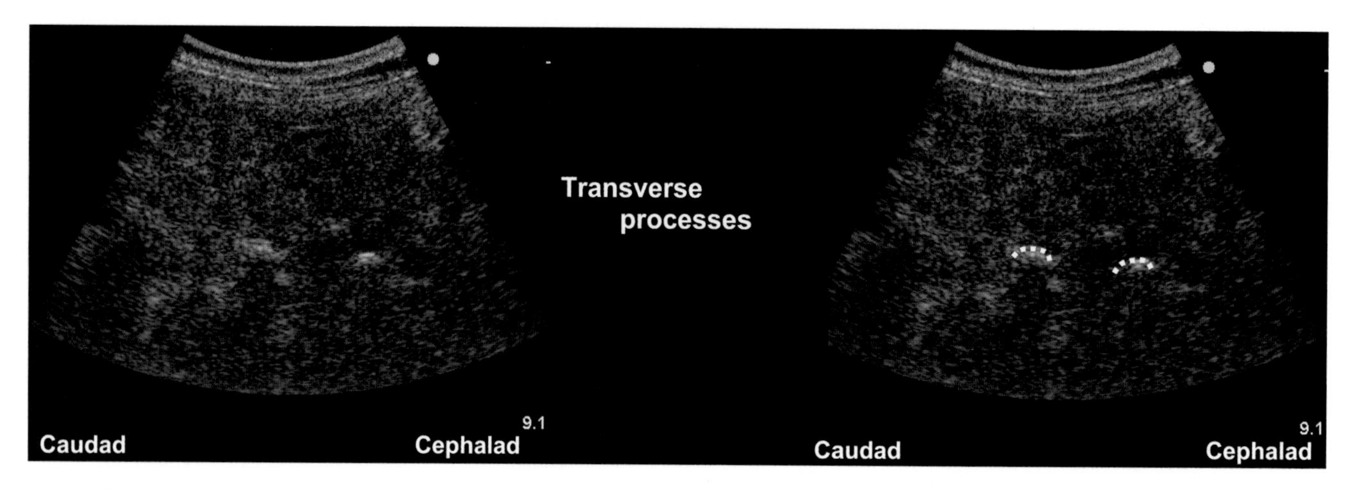

Figure 12.11. Ultrasound image of a longitudinal axis view at the transverse processes in the lumbar spine (L4–L5).

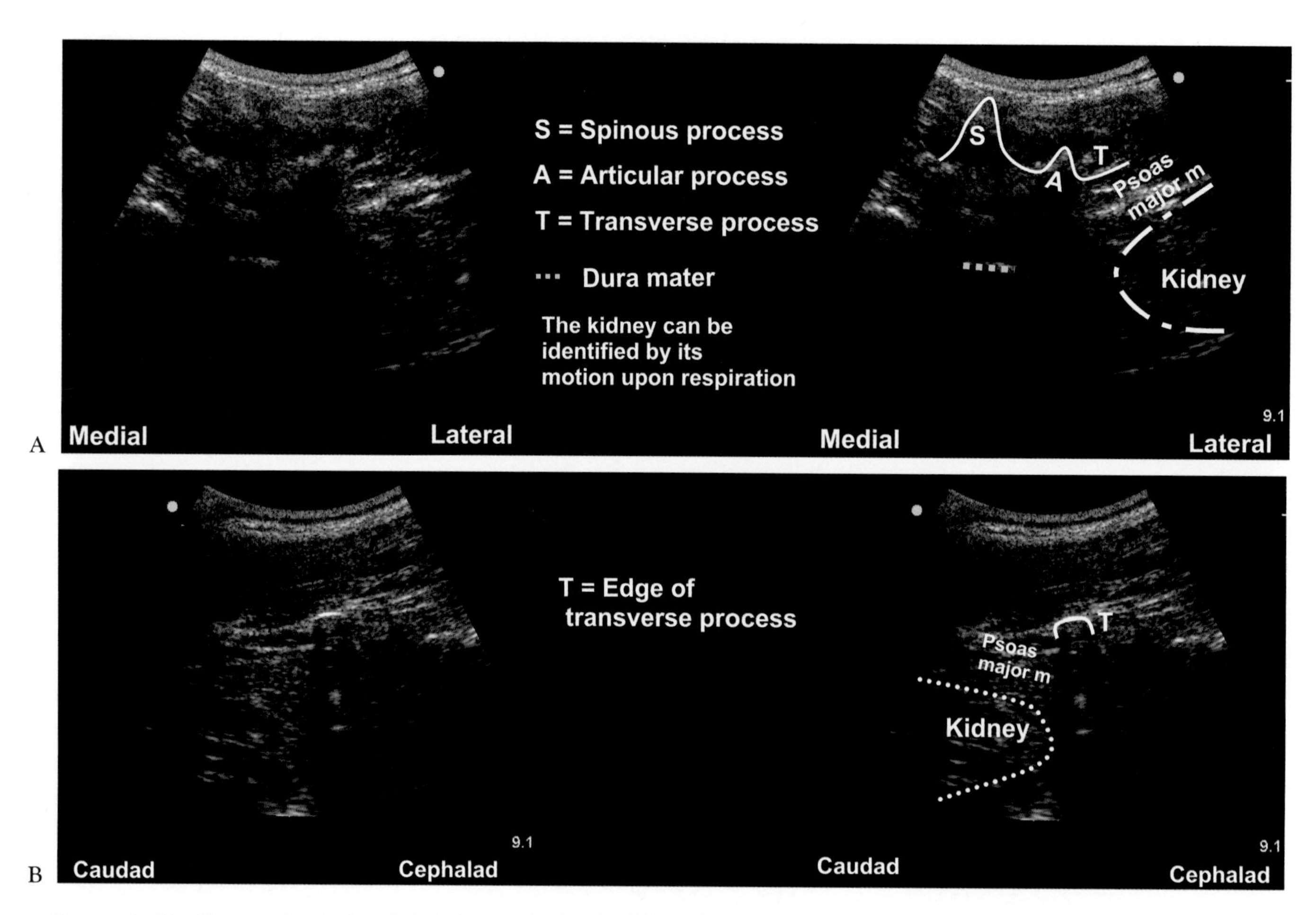

Figure 12.12. Ultrasound visibility of the kidney at the level of L1 in (A) transverse section and (B) longitudinal section using a curved array probe. In these still images, it can be difficult to clearly see the kidney. However, it can be easily recognized in real time as it moves with respiration.

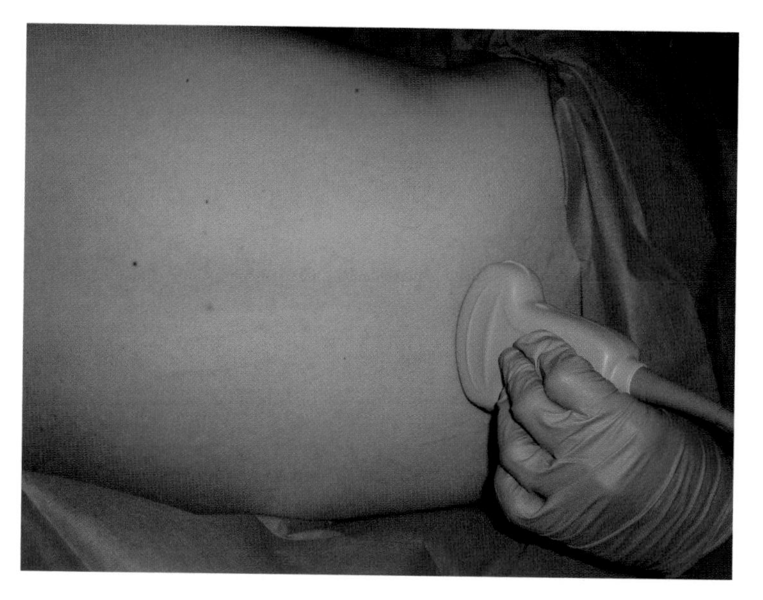

Figure 12.13. Scanning at L4 to L5 in the transverse (short-axis) plane with a curved array probe.

- A technique described by Kirchmair and colleagues from cadaveric and pediatric studies:
  - A curved array, 5- to 8-MHz transducer, is used to capture a longitudinal paravertebral sonogram at the relevant lumbar vertebral levels (L3–L5) by viewing from the cephalad portion of the sacrum and counting the transverse processes in a cranial direction.
  - Next, capture the transverse sonogram to view the psoas major, quadratus lumborum, and erector spinae muscles and use these for landmarks to identify the plexus within the psoas major muscle.
  - Alternate between transverse and longitudinal viewing to delineate the plexus.
  - These authors suggest that a linear array transducer can also be used.

12.3.2. Sonographic Appearance (5–8 MHz, Curved Array Probe)

- The deep location of this block precludes visibility of the lumbar plexus. Indeed, the transverse processes (which are the primary landmarks) are often very vaguely delineated.

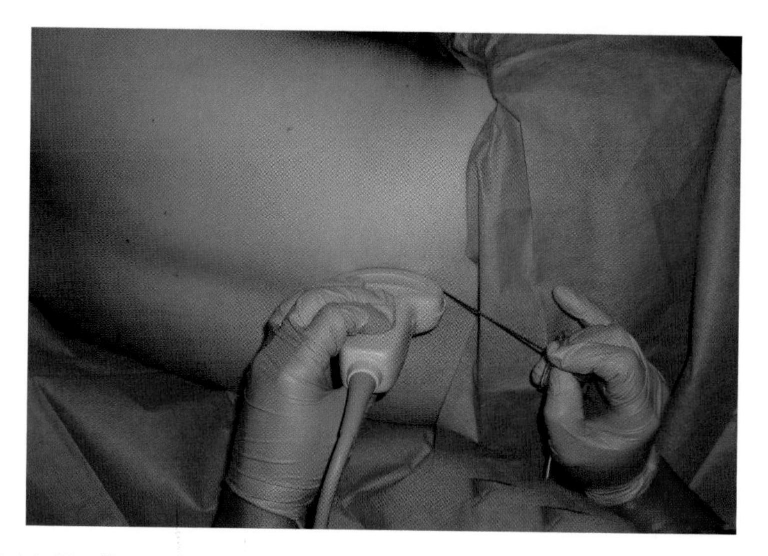

Figure 12.14. Needling technique using a curved array probe in a longitudinal plane and in-plane (IP) needle alignment.

Therefore, it is important to switch between transverse and longitudinal scanning between the spinous processes and the tip of the transverse processes to survey the area.

- Transverse/short-axis scan (between L3 and 4 transverse processes; Figure 12.8):
  - A "starry night" appearance of the muscles is evident, with hyperechoic divisions representing septae; the quadratus lumborum and erector spinae muscles are superficial with the quadratus lumborum muscle deep and lateral to the erector spinae (these muscles may not be clearly evident).
  - The articular and transverse processes are located deep to the erector spinae but superficial to the psoas major muscles.
  - The spinous processes appear hypoechoic (likely due to dorsal shadowing effect) and extend superficially.
  - The vertebral body/disk, if identified, is at the deepest aspect of the image and will be dark due to considerable shadowing from the surrounding bony structures.
  - The psoas major muscle lies superficial and lateral to the vertebral body; it lies deep to and at the intersection of the other muscles (quadratus lumborum and erector spinae).
  - Plexus fascicles or fascicle groups lie adjacent to both the psoas major muscle and the vertebral body, theoretically with hypoechoic dots surrounded by relatively bright tissue resembling connective tissue (the plexus will not likely be seen).
- Longitudinal/long-axis scan (3–4 cm parallel to spinous processes, between L3 and L5):
  - A striated-appearing erector spinae muscle layer lies most superficial with the psoas major muscle appearing rounded and between the lumbar transverse processes.
  - The transverse processes are located deep to the erector spinae muscles at roughly equal spacing, and appear slightly tubular with bright reflections and adjacent dark (hypoechoic) bony shadowing (Figure 12.11).
  - Medial to the transverse processes, a circular largely hypoechoic vertebral body may be seen deep to a more echoic articular process (Figure 12.10), both interspersed between the psoas major musculature; the spinous processes can be captured and appear short and broad in long-axis view (Figure 12.9).
  - If seen, the plexus is reported to appear with hypoechoic parallel bands bordered by hyperechoic striations, embedded within the posterior one third of the psoas major muscle and between the lumbar transverse processes.

12.3.3. Needle Insertion Technique

- Both in-plane (IP) and out-of-plane (OOP) techniques can be used (see Chapter 4). However, we have found that ultrasound imaging is most useful for surveying the region and identifying the location and depth of important bony and muscular anatomical landmarks before performing this block. This is *supported* or *offline* scanning that is often used before performing ultrasound-guided epidurals (preprocedurally; see the ultrasound section in Chapter 18). Using *real-time*, or *online*, scanning to track and control the needle trajectory within the deep muscle layers is difficult (Figures 12.14 and 12.15).
- Supported, or offline, technique using ultrasound imaging for identifying the landmarks:
  - As stated in the above sections, it is critical to use both transverse and longitudinal scanning during offline scanning to provide double confirmation of the structures' identities and location.
  - Refer to Section 12.3.1 to locate the ideal block site at the tips of the transverse processes (Figure 12.11).
    - Needling at more cephalad levels is possible, however, it is important to visualize the kidney (Figure 12.12) and the operator should have adequate experience.
  - Mark the lateral edge of the transverse process and record the skin-to-transverse process distance.
  - After assessing the region and identifying landmarks with ultrasound, perform the needling.

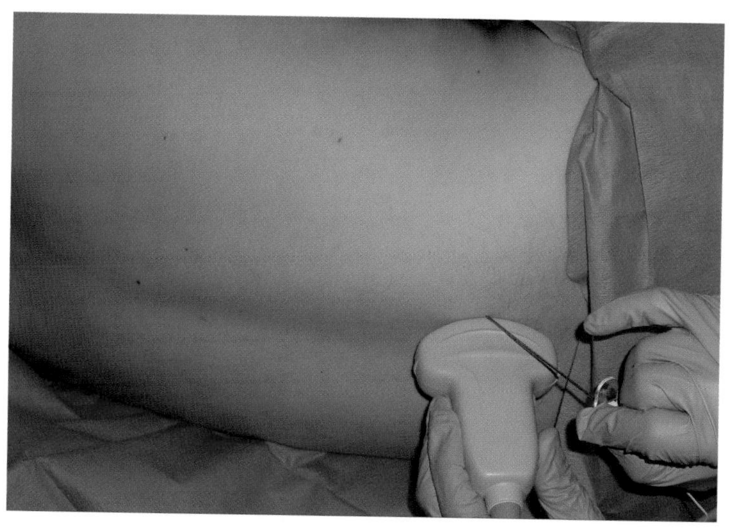

Figure 12.15. Needling technique with a curved probe in longitudinal axis with out-of-plane (OOP) needle alignment. This needling technique bears a higher risk than others.

- Use a puncture site as determined by ultrasound (usually about 4 cm lateral to the midline) and insert the needle perpendicular to the skin (without any significant medial or lateral angle) to reach the transverse process. In an average adult use a 100-mm, 20-ga insulated needle.
- After needle contact with the transverse process, redirect the needle in a caudal direction in order to advance the needle until a "pop" is felt or to the point indicated by nerve stimulation; this caudal direction is used to avoid inadvertent kidney puncture.
  - Occasionally a distinct "pop" will be felt 2 to 3 cm deep to the transverse processes when entering the psoas major muscle compartment.
  - The total needle insertion depth is usually between 7 to 9 cm beneath the skin.

- In thin individuals, both IP and OOP real-time, or online needling under ultrasound guidance may be possible as the shorter distance to many of the anatomical structures may allow needle visibility with the lower resolution probe. The needle may be seen as it is first inserted towards the transverse process and then walked off the bone and into the psoas muscle compartment. However, it can be very difficult to track the needle and the ultrasound probe may ultimately be a source of distraction without benefit during needling.
  - Theoretically, an OOP needle alignment with a longitudinally placed probe (Figure 12.15), or an IP alignment with a transversely placed probe (not shown) may have a high risk potential as the needle can easily be angled either too medially (i.e., toward the nerve roots or spinal cord) or laterally (i.e., toward the abdominal cavity or even pleura if too cephalad) as it is difficult to track the needle tip.
  - It is therefore advised to use an IP alignment to a longitudinally placed probe (Figure 12.14) or an OOP alignment for the transversely placed probe (not shown).
  - This author prefers to use ultrasound as an offline support tool to locate and mark the landmarks prior to block procedure.

12.4. Nerve Stimulation

Table 12.2 shows the expected motor response associated with nerve stimulation during lumbar plexus block. We recommend combining nerve stimulation with ultrasound imaging for this block because the nerve roots/plexus are difficult to visualize.

Table 12.2. Responses and recommended needle adjustments for use with nerve stimulation during lumbar plexus blocks.

Correct Response from Nerve Stimulation
Quadriceps muscle twitch (palpable or visual) at 0.5 to 1.0 mA intensity

Other Common Responses and Necessary Needle Adjustment

- Muscle twitches from electrical stimulation
  - Paraspinal (local twitch from direct stimulation)
    - *Explanation*: Needle tip too superficial
    - *Needle Adjustment*: Advance needle tip
  - Hamstring (roots of sciatic nerve)
    - *Explanation*: Needle inserted too caudally
    - *Needle Adjustment*: Withdraw completely and reinsert 3 to 5 cm cranially
  - Thigh flexion (quite deep 7+cm, psoas major muscle stimulation)
    - *Explanation*: Needle tip too deep (close to peritoneal cavity)
    - *Needle Adjustment*: Withdraw needle and follow protocol
- Bone contact
  - Transverse Process (4–6 cm deep)
    - *Explanation*: Close placement; angle slightly off
    - *Needle Adjustment*: Withdraw to subcutaneous tissue and reinsert with an angle 5° more cranial or caudal
- No response despite deep placement
  - Past transverse process and lumbar plexus
    - *Explanation*: Needle tip too deep
    - *Needle Adjustment:* Withdraw completely and reinsert

12.5. Local Anesthetic Application

The hypoechoic spread of local anesthetic may be traced on the sonographic screen to the posterior portion of the psoas major muscle, but it is often difficult to see any spread of the local anesthetic.

Suggested Reading and References

Awad IT, Duggan EM. Posterior lumbar plexus block: anatomy, approaches, and techniques. Reg Anesth Pain Med 2005;30:143–149.

Capdevila X, Macaire P, Dadure C, et al. Continuous psoas compartment block for postoperative analgesia after total hip arthroplasty: new landmarks, technical guidelines, and clinical evaluation. Anesth Analg 2002;94:1606–1613.

Johr M. The right thing in the right place: lumbar plexus block in children [comment on Kirchmair et al., 2004]. Anesthesiology 2005;102:865.

Kirchmair L, Tanja E, Jorg W, Bernhard M, Kapral S, Mitterschiffthaler G. A study of the paravertebral anatomy for ultrasound-guided posterior lumbar plexus block. Anesth Analg 2001; 93:477–481.

Kirchmair L, Entner T, Kapral S, Mitterschiffhaler G. Ultrasound guidance for the psoas compartment block: an imaging study. Anesth Analg 2002;94:706–710.

Kirchmair L, Enna B, Mitterschiffthaler G, et al. Lumbar plexus in children. A sonographic study and its relevance to pediatric regional anesthesia. Anesthesiology 2004;101:445–450.

13

Femoral Block

Ban C.H. Tsui

Blockade of the femoral nerve is indicated for surgical anesthesia and postoperative analgesia in the anterior thigh and knee as well as quadriceps tendon repair. Motor response to nerve stimulation is ipsilateral quadriceps contraction (*patellar twitch*). Combined with a sciatic nerve block, complete anesthesia below the midthigh can be achieved. Prior to the 1990s, an anterior lumbar block approach (a.k.a., femoral 3-in-1 approach), first described by Winnie and colleagues in 1973, was performed based on the assumption that local anesthetic injection into the femoral nerve sheath would initiate spread of the solution proximally to anesthetize the obturator and lateral femoral cutaneous nerves as well. Later reports of failures with this approach, however, have led to the femoral block being considered as an individual nerve block, and advocated the posterior lumbar block approach for accessing the whole lumbar plexus (including a modified Winnie approach called *psoas compartment block*). At present, there is limited published methodology, and no experiential recommendations from this author regarding the use of ultrasound guidance for the obturator nerve block; therefore this approach will not be discussed in this text.

13.1. Clinical Anatomy

- The femoral nerve (L2–L4) is the largest branch of the lumbar plexus (Figure 13.1).
- It descends through the psoas major muscle, exiting the muscle at its lower lateral border, before coursing between the psoas major and iliacus muscles, deep to the fascia iliaca (iliopectineal fascia), towards the inguinal ligament (the inguinal ligament is the lower

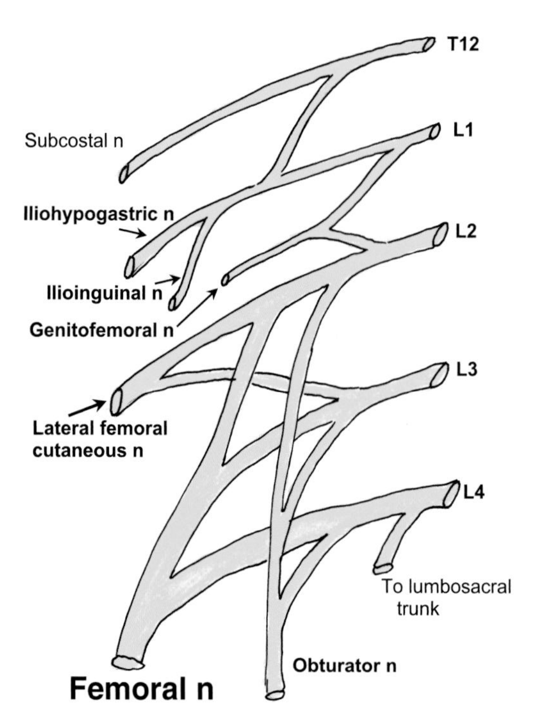

Figure 13.1. Schematic diagram of the lumbar plexus.

in-turned border of the external oblique aponeurosis extending between the pubic tubercle medially and anterior superior iliac spine laterally).

- At the inguinal ligament and just distal to it, the nerve lies slightly deeper (0.5–1 cm) and lateral (approximately 1.5 cm) to the femoral artery; the vein is medial to the artery (VAN is the mnemonic for the anatomical relationship, starting medially; Figures 13.2 and 13.3).

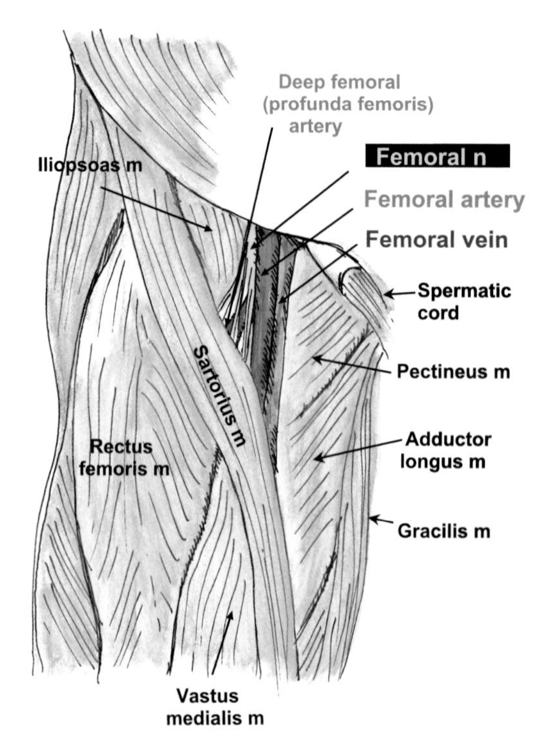

Figure 13.2. Relationship between the femoral nerve, artery, and vein beyond the inguinal ligament.

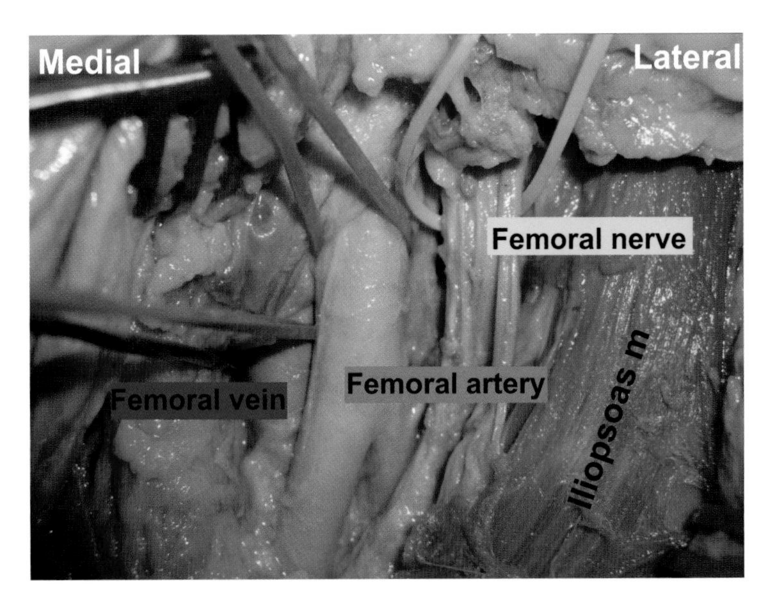

Figure 13.3. Dissection of the anterior thigh below the femoral (inguinal) crease.

- At the femoral (inguinal) crease (a few centimeters caudad to the inguinal ligament) the nerve lies underneath the fascia iliaca (iliopectineal fascia), deep to the fascia lata (Figure 13.4), and is separated from the femoral artery (pulse is superficial and palpable here) and vein by the iliopectineal (Cooper's) ligament and often a portion of the psoas major muscle.

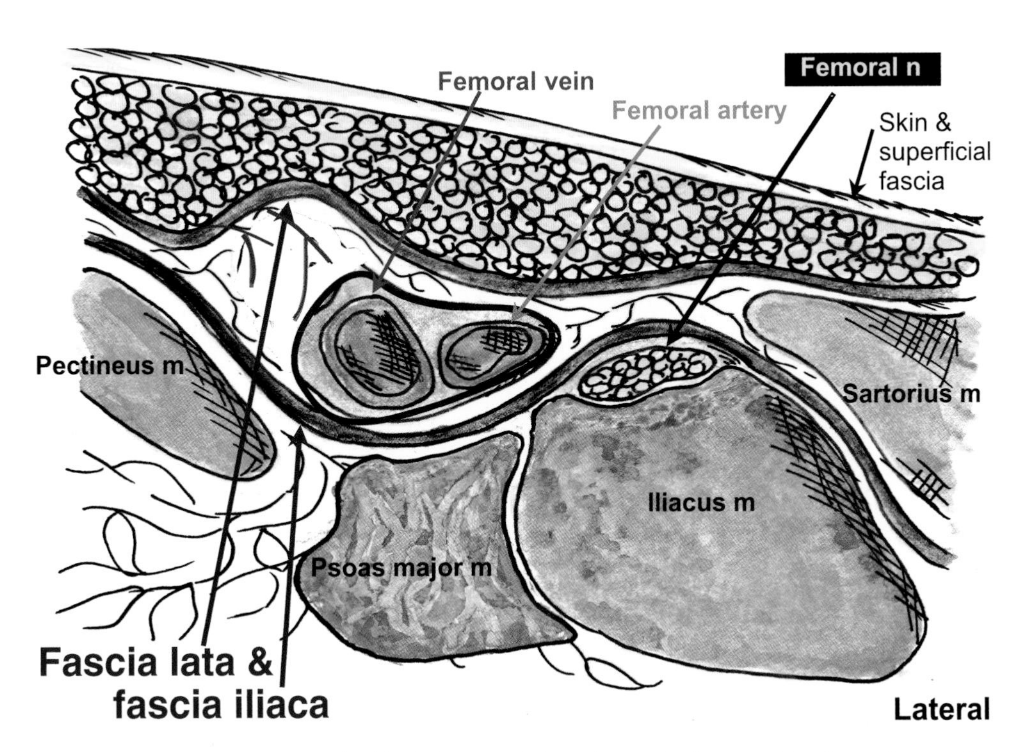

Figure 13.4. Cross-section at the block location below the inguinal crease. The femoral nerve lies deep to the fascia lata and fascia iliaca (iliopectineal fascia) and is separated from the artery and vein(s).

Table 13.1. Target terminal motor nerves of the femoral nerve block.

Movement	Nerve	Plexus division	Root
Patellar twitch and knee extension	Femoral (main nerve and its posterior branch)	Posterior	L2, 3, 4
Thigh adduction only (pectineus m.)	Femoral (anterior branch below inguinal ligament)	Posterior	L2, 3, 4

- The nerve divides into anterior and posterior branches in the proximal thigh; branches to the sartorius muscle arise just inferior to the inguinal ligament and leave the femoral nerve proximal to the main block location site. A response to stimulation of this muscle often indicates the needle is too superficial and medial to the main femoral nerve block site (the femoral nerve block requires injection deep to fascia iliaca).
- There are variations to this branching pattern with the femoral nerve branching more proximally in many cases.
- In the proximal thigh, the femoral artery gives rise to the profunda femoris (deep femoral) artery from its lateral aspect. This is a useful landmark because if ultrasound scanning fails to locate the nerve immediately lateral to the femoral artery at the block location, the profunda femoris artery can be traced proximally to locate the femoral nerve before it divides.
- The saphenous nerve is the terminal branch of the femoral nerve and it innervates the skin over the medial aspect of the leg and foot.

Table 13.1 summarizes the origin of the femoral nerve (including divisions) and the associated movement with nerve stimulation.

13.2. Patient Positioning and Surface Anatomy

13.2.1. Patient Positioning

The patient lies supine with the legs extended and the thighs externally rotated approximately 15°. If ultrasound imaging is not utilized, a pillow is placed under the patient's hip to facilitate palpation of the femoral pulse and accentuate other pertinent landmarks for ease of palpation.

13.2.2. Surface Anatomy (Figure 13.5)

- Inguinal ligament
  - Medial attachment to the pubic tubercle (2–3 cm from midline on upper pubis border), lateral to the anterior superior iliac spine.
- Femoral/inguinal crease
  - Natural oblique skin fold parallel and 3 to 6 cm distal to the ligament; the femoral artery is most superficial here.
- Femoral artery pulse
  - Lies at the midinguinal point, at the junction between the medial third and lateral two thirds of the inguinal crease, although it is most superficial at the femoral crease.
  - Is approximately 1–1.5 cm medial to the nerve.
  - Although not palpable, the branching point of the femoral artery where the profunda (deep femoral) femoris artery arises is a good landmark for ultrasound guidance; this branching usually occurs 4 cm inferior to the inguinal crease in an average adult.

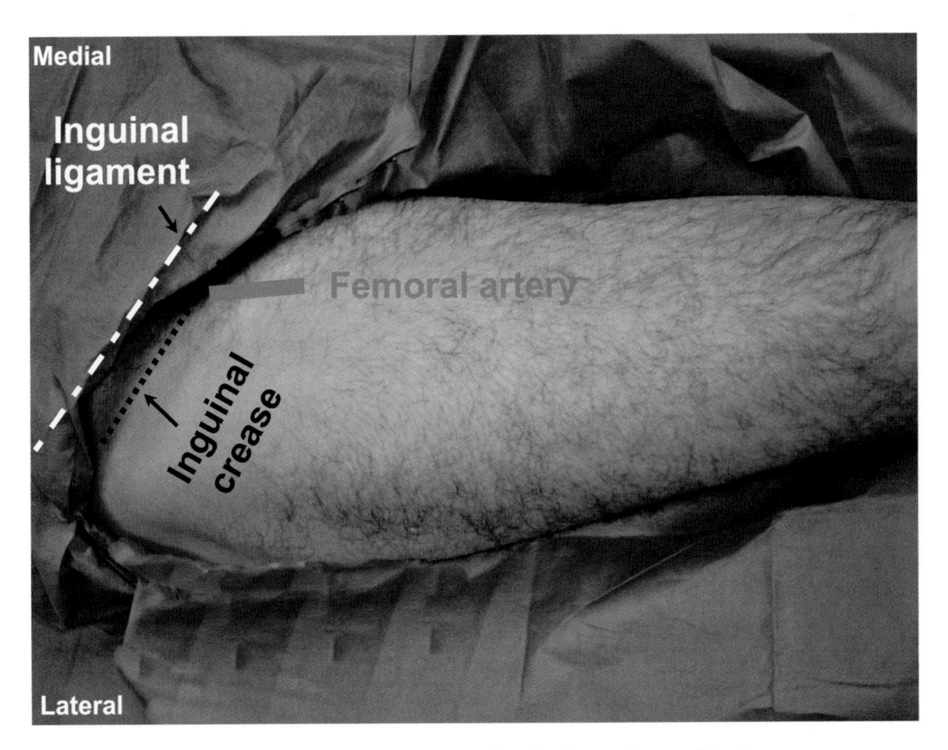

Figure 13.5. Surface anatomy for the femoral nerve block.

13.3. Sonographic Imaging and Needle Insertion Technique

The magnetic resonance imaging (MRI) scans [Figure 13.6(A,B)] show the femoral nerve at the block location (just distal to the inguinal ligament) and more distally at the point where the femoral artery gives off the profunda femoris (deep femoral) artery. The reader can refer to these images when studying the sonographic images captured at the same locations (Figures 13.7 and 13.8).

Prepare the needle insertion site and skin surface with an antiseptic solution. Prepare the ultrasound probe surface by applying a sterile adhesive dressing to it prior to needling as discussed earlier (see Chapters 3 and 4).

13.3.1. Scanning Technique

- A 10+MHz transducer can be used if the neurovascular structures are not located too deep (i.e., thin individuals) as this will show good distinction between the nerve (fascicular appearance) and the surrounding structures (vessels and muscles). A midrange 5- to 7.5-MHz linear transducer is recommended if the nerve and artery are deep (>4 cm).
- Position the probe transverse to the nerve axis in the proximal thigh approximately 2 to 3 cm inferior to the inguinal ligament and along the inguinal crease. The nerve should appear approximately 1 cm deeper than and 1.5 cm lateral to the femoral artery (color Doppler may be used to localize the femoral artery and vein; Figure 13.7).
- Depth of penetration is approximately 2 to 4 cm from the skin surface.
- The ideal block location should be proximal to significant branching of the femoral nerve. This branching occurs at approximately the same location to where the femoral artery gives rise to the profunda femoris (deep femoral) artery (about 4 cm below the crease) (see Nerve Localization sidebar).

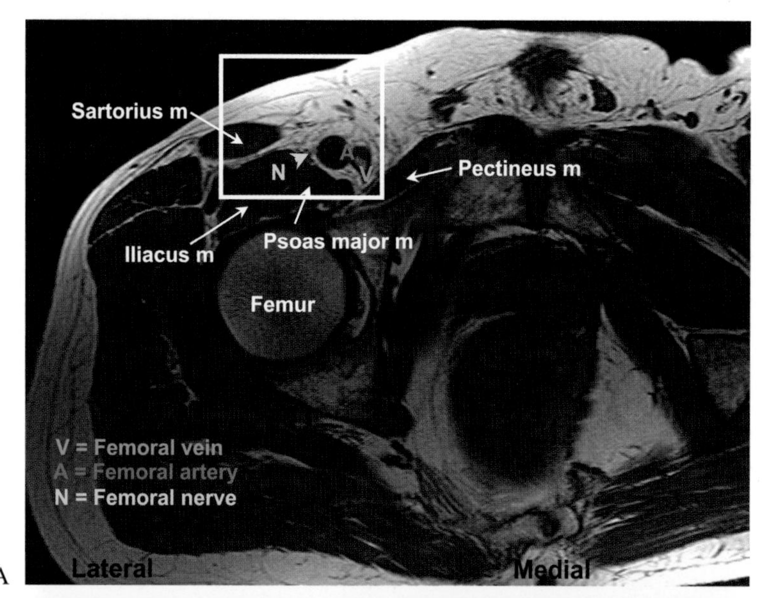

A

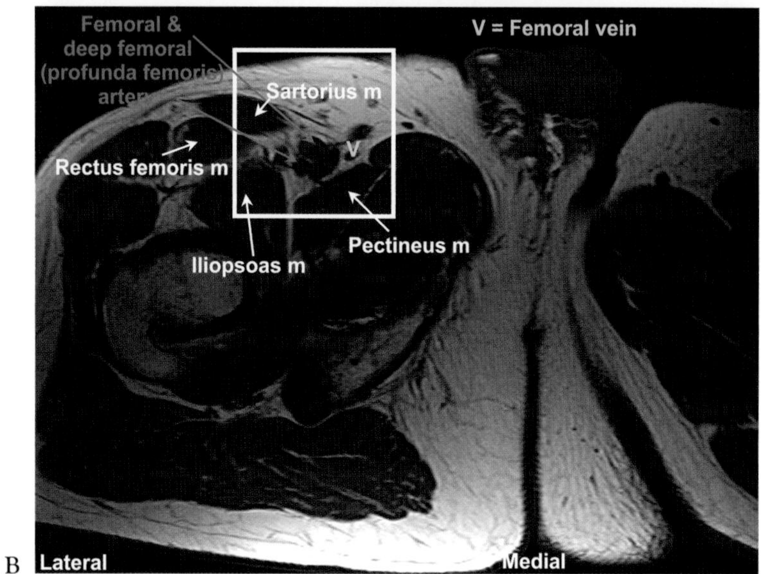

B

Figure 13.6. MRI images at (A) the block location and (B) approximately 4 cm distal at the profunda (deep) femoris branch point.

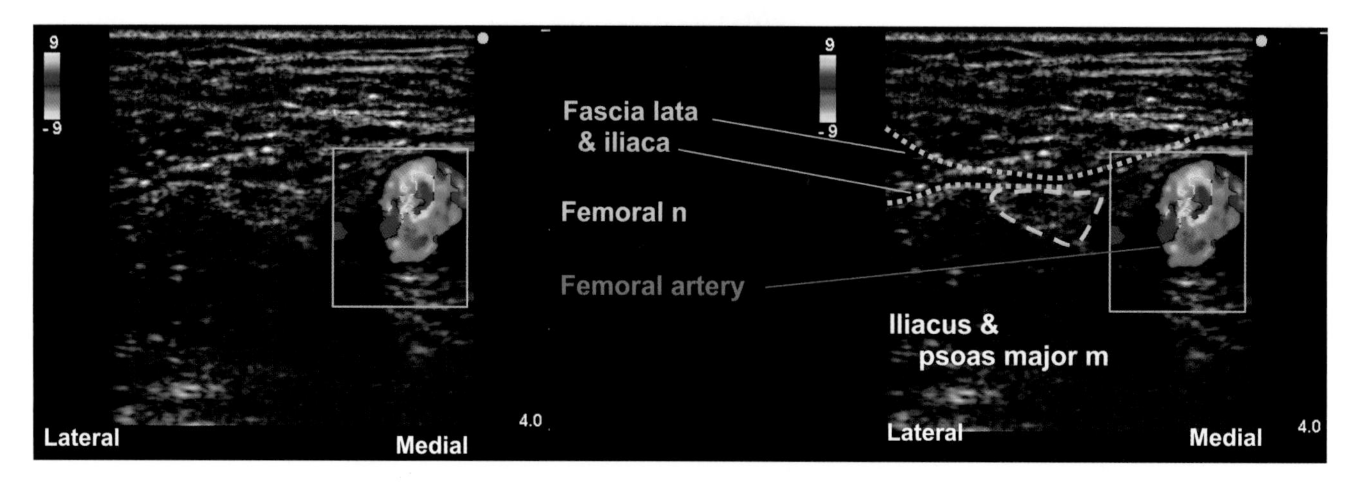

Figure 13.7. Ultrasound image using color Doppler at the block location with the oval–triangular nerve lateral to the illuminated pulsating artery and deep to the fascia iliaca.

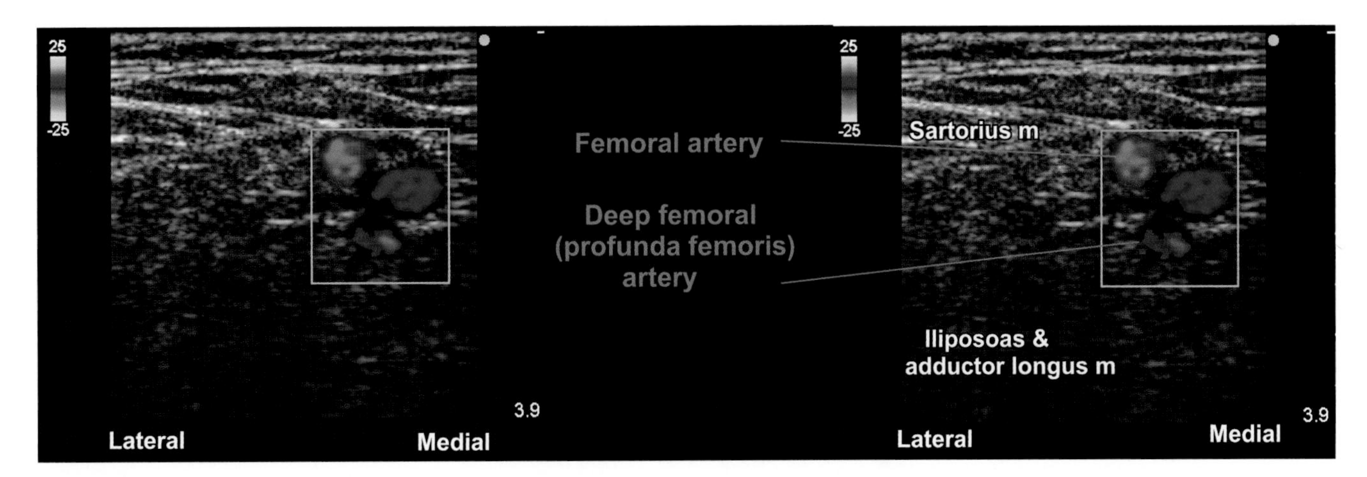

Figure 13.8. Ultrasound image from a scan distal to the block location where the profunda femoris (deep femoral) artery diverges from the femoral artery. This location can be suitable in some cases (e.g., obesity) for artery localization and subsequent tracing towards the femoral crease to the nerve.

Nerve Localization

Using the ultrasound probe, the femoral artery is first identified at a distance of about 1 cm from the inguinal crease and the nerve usually lies lateral to the artery. It is sometimes difficult to determine the exact location of the inguinal ligament and/or crease due to anatomical distortion or extreme obesity. In these cases, we recommend to use Doppler to identify the femoral artery and ensure that the block location is proximal to where the profunda femoris (deep femoral) artery branches off from the femoral artery (Figure 13.8). This arterial junction usually occurs 4 cm inferior to the inguinal crease in the average adult. By adopting this new technology and tracing back along the paths of these arteries, the optimal needle placement can be achieved.

13.3.2. Sonographic Appearance (10-MHz Linear Probe)

- Short-axis plane below inguinal crease (Figure 13.7):
  - The nerve lies about 1 cm lateral and deep to the large, circular, and anechoic femoral artery.
  - The fascia lata (most superficial) and iliaca (immediately above the nerve), may be seen superficial to the femoral nerve, and often appear bright and longitudinally angled (occasionally the fascia may be better identified after being highlighted from local anesthetic injection).
  - The femoral nerve often appears triangular in shape and of variable size, due to its irregular course; early division above the inguinal ligament can increase the transverse diameter of the nerve.

13.3.3. Needle Insertion Technique

- A 5- to 7-cm, 22-ga needle can be inserted in-plane (IP) or out-of-plane (OOP) to the transverse probe (see Chapter 4), at the location identified by ultrasound (approximately at the inguinal crease).

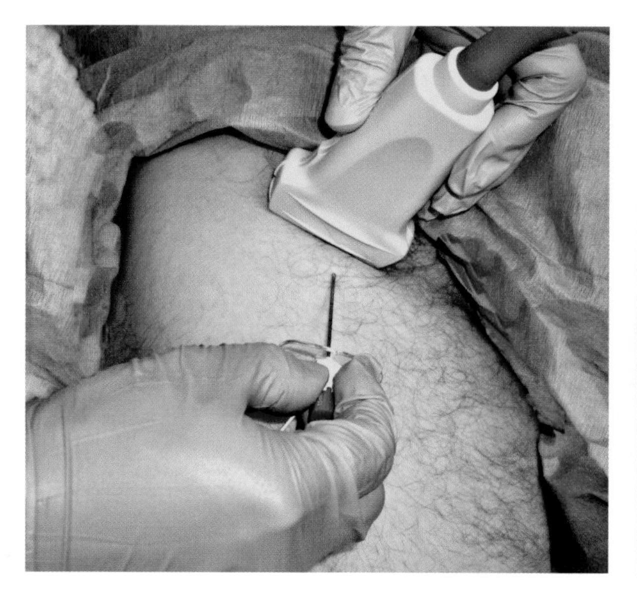

Figure 13.9. Needling technique using a linear probe and an out-of-plane (OOP) needle alignment.

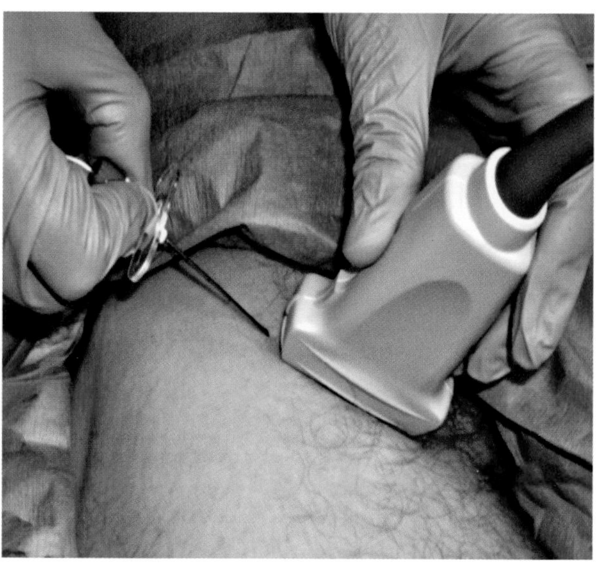

Figure 13.10. Needling technique using a linear probe and in-plane (IP) needle alignment in a lateral to medial direction.

Anisotropy

Imaging of the femoral nerve is highly sensitive to anisotropy, therefore, it is important to pay attention to the tilt angle of the transducer (Chapter 3). A 10° angle shift (caudal or cephalad) in the transducer has been shown to make the nerve isoechoic with the surrounding muscles. The best image obtained by using the correct transducer angle will brighten the nerve considerably compared to a very hypoechoic iliopsoas muscle immediately deep to the nerve.

- OOP approach (Figure 13.9):
  - Insert the needle 2 cm below the probe in an acute angle (30°–45°) to the skin.
  - An OOP walk down approach with incremental, stepwise angulation of the needle will provide immediate localization of the needle tip as a bright dot, with subsequent ease in following it to the required depth (see Chapter 4 for a detailed description of the technique).
- IP approach (Figure 13.10):
  - Insert the needle in a lateral to medial direction from the lateral edge of the probe.
  - This medially directed approach will help ensure the needle approaches the nerve first, rather than the artery or vein.
- Steeper angles and longer needles may be required in obese patients.
- Try to localize the needle tip within the fascial space surrounding the nerve.

13.4. Nerve Stimulation

Table 13.2 summarizes the optimal motor responses associated with nerve stimulation during the femoral nerve block and the recommended adjustments with other common responses. Ultrasound will likely reduce several common incorrect responses (e.g., contacting the femur) during nerve stimulation, although nerve stimulation is still recommended for most blocks at this time.

Table 13.2. Responses and recommended needle adjustments for use with nerve stimulation during femoral nerve block.

Correct Response from Nerve Stimulation

The most reliable response is a visible or palpable ipsilateral femoral muscle twitch (patella twitch) at 0.3 to 0.5 mA current, which indicates that one is stimulating the posterior division of the nerve. If twitches of the sartorius muscle occur, the needle may be outside the nerve sheath and one may be stimulating the proximal branch which supplies the sartorius muscle.

Other Common Responses and Necessary Needle Adjustment

- Muscle twitches from electrical stimulation
  - Iliopsoas or pectineus (direct stimulation of muscle)
    - *Explanation*: Too superior or deep needle tip placement
    - *Needle Adjustment*: Withdraw needle completely and reinsert
  - Sartorius (branches of sciatic nerve to sartorius)
    - *Explanation:* Needle tip too anteromedial to main femoral nerve trunk
    - *Needle Adjustment:* Redirect needle laterally and advance 1 to 3 mm deeper
- Bone contact
  - Hip or superior ramus of pubic bone
    - *Explanation*: Needle tip too deep
    - *Needle Adjustment*: Withdraw needle to subcutaneous tissue and reinsert
- No response
    - *Explanation*: Needle tip often too medial or lateral
    - *Needle Adjustment:* Withdraw completely and reinsert after checking landmarks
- Vascular puncture
  - Femoral artery or vein
    - *Explanation:* Needle tip too medial
    - *Needle Adjustment:* Withdraw needle completely and reinsert 1 cm lateral

13.5. Local Anesthetic Application

- Performing a test dose with dextrose 5% in water (D5W) is recommended prior to local anesthetic application to visualize the spread and confirm nerve localization (see Chapter 4 sidebar).
- Local anesthetic spread should occur within the fascial space surrounding the nerve (Figure 13.11).
- The solution may displace the nerve medially towards or laterally away from the artery.

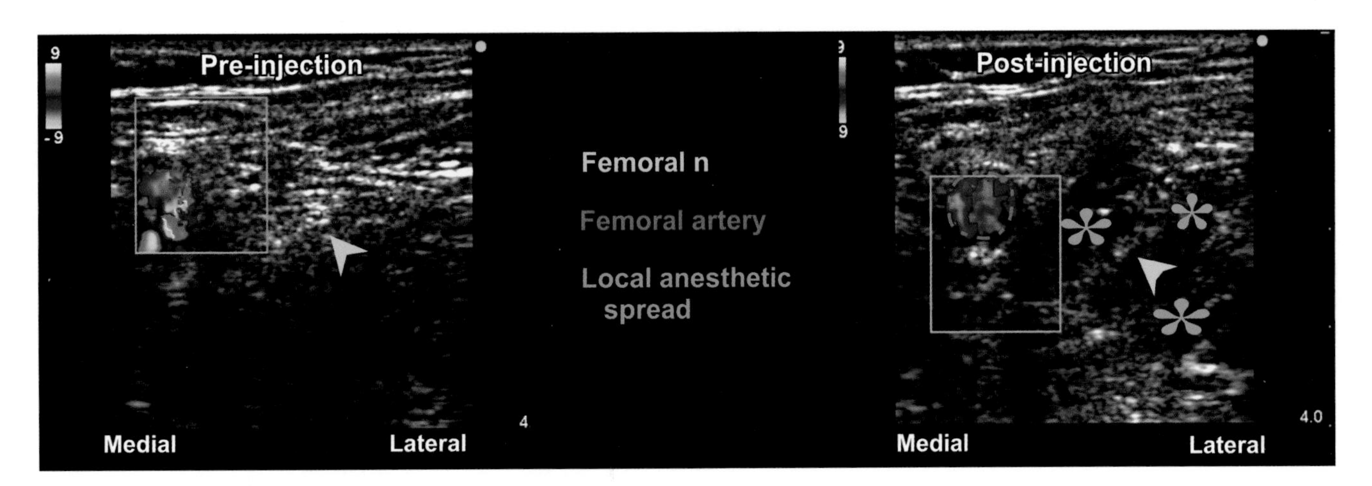

Figure 13.11. Local anesthetic application surrounding the femoral nerve.

Suggested Reading and References

Agur AM, Dalley AF. Grant's Atlas of Anatomy. 11 ed. Philadelphia: Lippincott Williams & Wilkiins, 2005.

Marhofer P, Schrogendorfer K, Wallner T, et al. Ultrasonographic guidance reduces the amount of local anesthetic for 3-in-1 blocks. Reg Anesth Pain Med 1998;23:584–588.

Schafhalter-Zoppoth I, Moriggl B. Aspects of femoral nerve block. Reg Anesth Pain Med 2006;31:92–93.

Sites BD, Beach M, Gallagher LD, et al. A single injection ultrasound-assisted femoral nerve block provides side effect-sparing analgesia when compared with intrathecal morphine in patients undergoing total knee arthroplasty. Anesth Analg 2004;99:1539–1543.

Soong J, Schafhalter-Zoppath I, Gray A. The importance of transducer angle to ultrasound visibility of the femoral nerve. Reg Anesth Pain Med 2005;30:505.

Winnie AP, Ramanurthy S, Durrani Z. The inguinal paravascular techniques of lumbar plexus anesthesia: the "3-in1 block." Anesth Analg 1973;52:989–996.

14

Sciatic and Popliteal Blocks

Ban C.H. Tsui

The large sciatic nerve lies deep within the gluteal region and may be difficult to locate blindly or with ultrasound. Of benefit during ultrasound-guided blockade of the sciatic nerve and its terminal branches (tibial and common peroneal nerves) are the numerous bony and vascular landmarks that can be used for ease of identification. Knowledge of anatomy is paramount with these blocks and the block location and approach will ultimately depend on the surgical requirement. The sciatic nerve is commonly blocked at the gluteal (Labat approach) or subgluteal region if anesthesia of the thigh and knee is required in addition to that of the lower leg. The sciatic nerve terminates by dividing into tibial and common peroneal (fibular) nerves, both contained within the common epineural sheath of the sciatic nerve. For procedures below the knee, the sciatic nerve is often blocked (posteriorly or laterally) in the popliteal fossa although it may be necessary to block both the tibial and common peroneal (fibular) nerves separately if the sciatic nerve has already divided (there are variable proximal and distal bifurcation points). Blockade of both tibial and common peroneal (fibular) nerves will target the entire leg below the knee except for the area of skin supplied exclusively by the saphenous nerve on the anteromedial leg and foot.

14.1. Clinical Anatomy

- Sciatic nerve (L4, L5, S1–S3)
  - The sciatic nerve is part of the sacral plexus (Figures 14.1 and 14.2); about 2 cm broad at its origin in the adult and a flattened oval in cross-section, the sciatic nerve is the broadest and largest peripheral nerve in the human body.
  - The nerve leaves the pelvis through the greater sciatic foramen below the piriformis (generally) and descends just medial to the midpoint of a line between the greater trochanter of the femur and the ischial tuberosity along the back of the thigh (Figures 14.3 and 14.4); it is accompanied medially by the posterior femoral cutaneous nerve and proximally by the inferior gluteal artery (not shown).

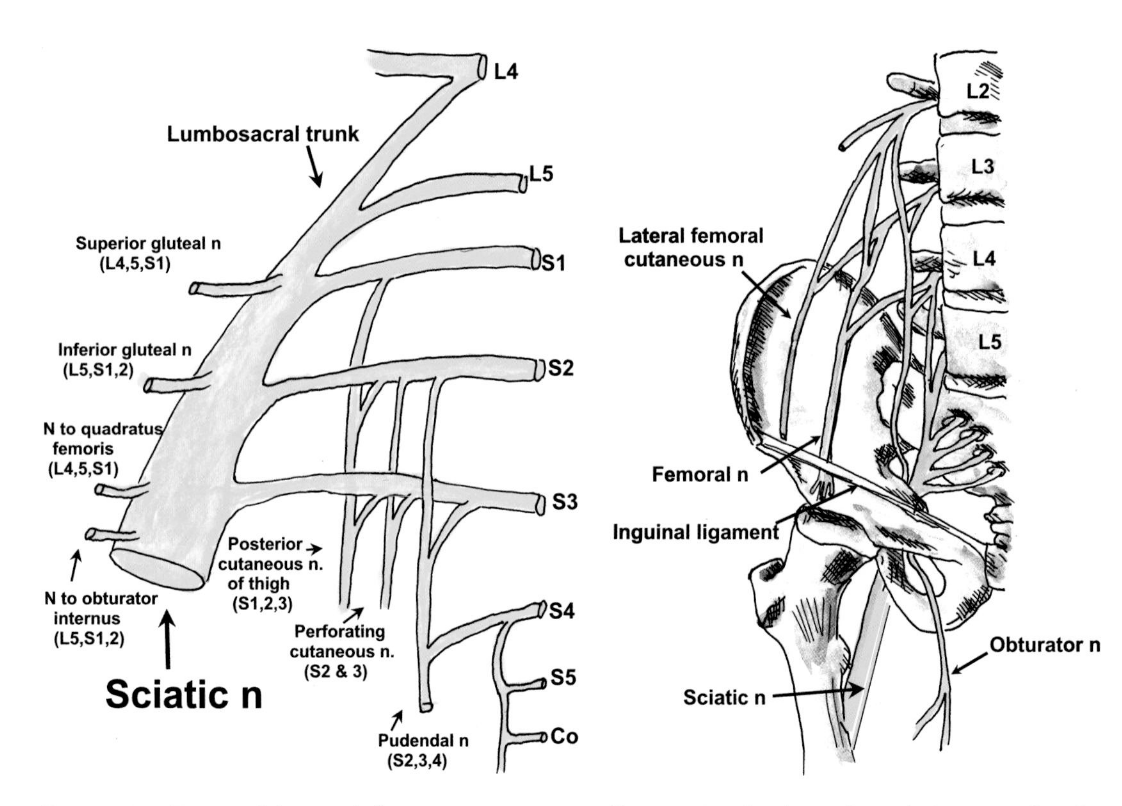

Figure 14.1. Design of the sacral plexus.

Figure 14.2. Lumbar and sacral plexuses within the skeleton.

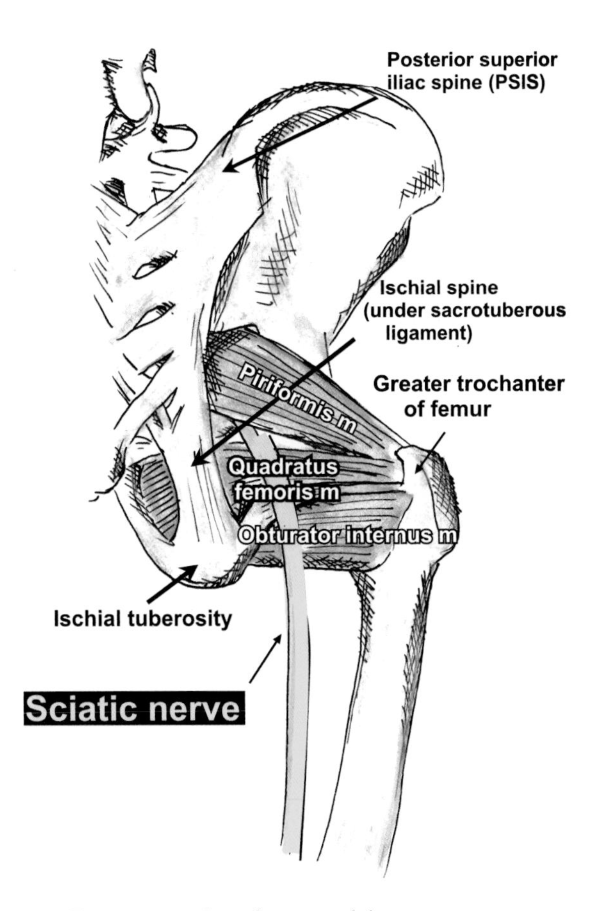

Figure 14.3. Initial course of the sciatic nerve.

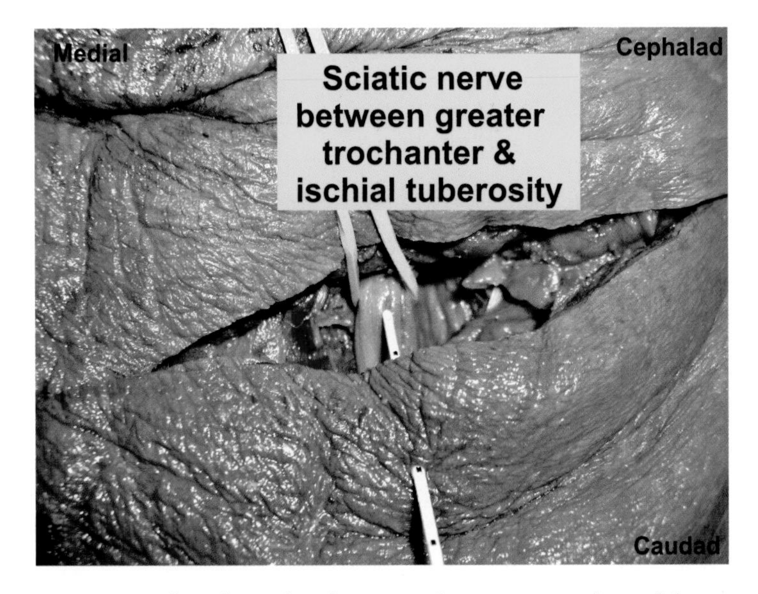

Figure 14.4. Dissection at the inferior gluteal region as the sciatic nerve descends between the greater trochanter of the femur and the ischial tuberosity.

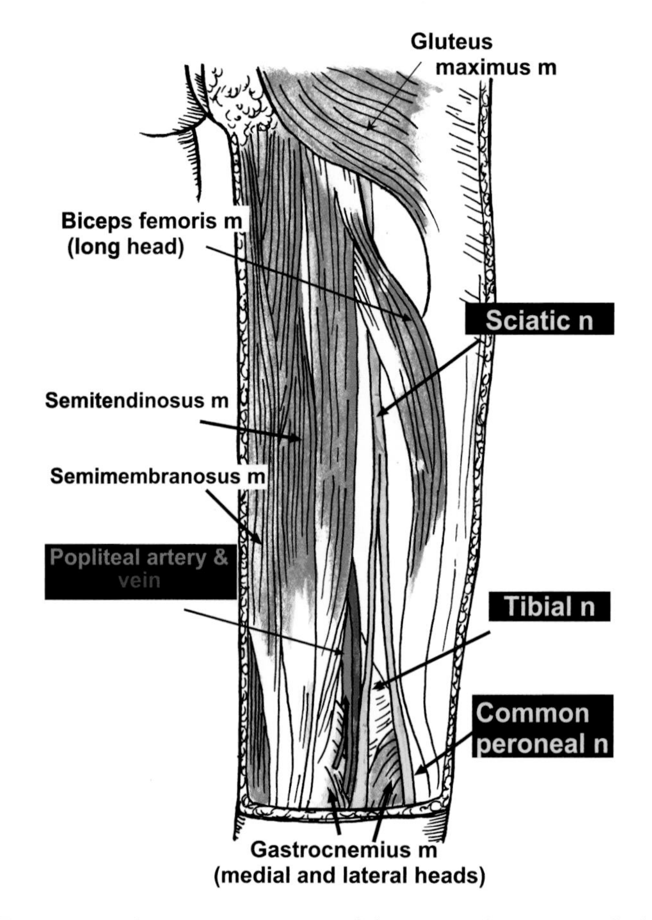

Figure 14.5. Sciatic nerve course and division in the posterior thigh.

- Proximally, the nerve lies deep to the gluteus maximus (Figures 14.5 and 14.6), resting first on the posterior ischial surface and then coursing inferiorly posterior to the obturator internus, gamelli, and quadratus femoris muscles to enter into the back of the thigh where it usually divides. Inferior to the lower border of the gluteus maximus the nerve

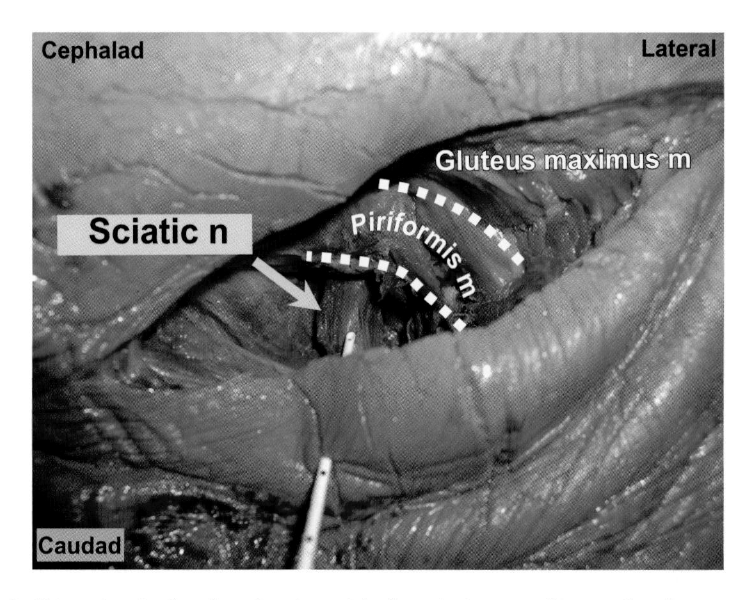

Figure 14.6. Dissection in the gluteal region with the sciatic nerve deep to the gluteus maximus and piriformis muscles.

is relatively superficial, after which it lies under cover of the long head of the biceps femoris muscle.
  - The nerve generally divides into the tibial nerve medially and the common peroneal (fibular) nerve laterally near the apex of the popliteal fossa (approximately two thirds of the way down the thigh; Figure 14.5); however, its division is variable and can occur at a more proximal location, anywhere between the piriformis muscle and the popliteal fossa, or occasionally at a more distal location.
  - The nerve has its own artery, the artery to the sciatic nerve or the arteria comitans (from the inferior gluteal artery), which lies on the posterior aspect of the nerve and is contained within the fibrous sheath surrounding the nerve.
  - Anteriorly, the nerve lies in front of the ischium on the adductor magnus muscle.
  - Branches of the sciatic nerve include:
    - Muscular to semitendinosus, semimembranosus, and biceps femoris muscles and the ischial (hamstring) part of the adductor magnus muscle (the adductor part is supplied by the obturator nerve).
    - Articular to the hip joint capsule.
    - Terminal: tibial and common peroneal (fibular) nerves.
- Tibial nerve (L4, L5, S1–S3)
  - The tibial nerve (Figure 14.5) is the larger of the two sciatic divisions. At its divergence from the common peroneal (fibular) nerve, generally near the apex of the popliteal fossa (Figure 14.7), it is covered medially by the semitendinosus and semimembranosus muscles, and laterally by the biceps femoris muscle; lower down near the base of the popliteal fossa it is covered by both heads of the gastrocnemius muscle.
  - Within the popliteal fossa the nerve becomes more superficial, courses lateral to the popliteal vessels becoming superficial to them at the knee, and crosses to the medial side of the popliteal artery near the base of the fossa.
  - Its surface projection is on a vertical line extending from the apex of the popliteal fossa to the level of the fibular neck and from there to a point halfway between the medial malleolus and the calcaneal (Achilles) tendon.
  - Branches in the popliteal fossa:
    - Muscular (from lateral aspect of the nerve) to popliteus, gastrocnemius, soleus, and plantaris muscles.
    - Cutaneous sural nerve descends along the lateral aspect of the leg, passes behind the lateral malleolus, and on to the lateral aspect of the foot.
    - Articular to the knee.

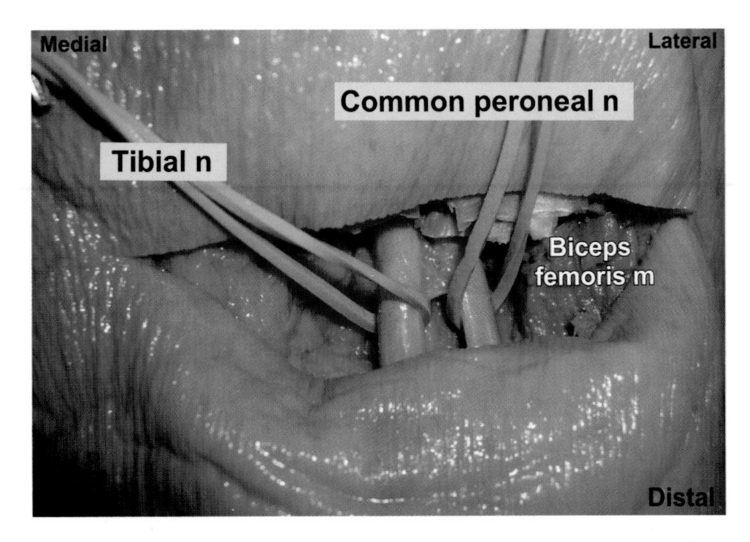

Figure 14.7. Dissection at the midthigh near the sciatic nerve bifurcation into tibial and common peroneal nerves.

- The nerve continues down the posterior compartment of the leg with the posterior tibial vessels deep to the soleus muscle and on the surface of the tibialis posterior, finally reaching the posterior surface of the tibial shaft (it may be called the posterior tibial nerve here), where it ends between the medial malleolus and the calcaneal tuberosity (heel) deep to the flexor retinaculum by dividing into its terminal branches.
- Branches in the calf and foot:
  - Muscular to tibialis posterior, flexor digitorum longus, flexor hallucis longus, and soleus muscles.
  - Cutaneous (medial calcaneal nerve) to medial side of the heel and sole.
  - Articular to ankle joint.
  - Terminal branches include medial and lateral plantar nerves.

- Common peroneal (fibular) nerve (L4, L5, S1, S2)
  - The common peroneal (fibular) nerve (Figure 14.5) is about half the size of the tibial nerve.
  - After splitting off from the sciatic nerve (tibial component), it descends obliquely along the lateral border of the popliteal fossa toward the fibular head, medial to the biceps femoris (Figure 14.7) and between its tendon and the lateral head of the gastrocnemius.
  - The nerve winds along the lateral aspect of the fibular neck deep to the peroneus (fibularis) longus muscle, where it is palpable (can be rolled against the bone) just before diving into the muscle; here it divides into its terminal branches, the deep and superficial peroneal (fibular) nerves (Figure 14.8).
  - Branches near the fibula:
    - Cutaneous: sural communicating nerve (joins sural nerve) and lateral cutaneous nerve of calf.
    - Articular to knee.
  - The deep peroneal (fibular) nerve descends on the anterior aspect of the interosseous membrane deep to the extensor digitorum longus, reaching the anterior tibial artery

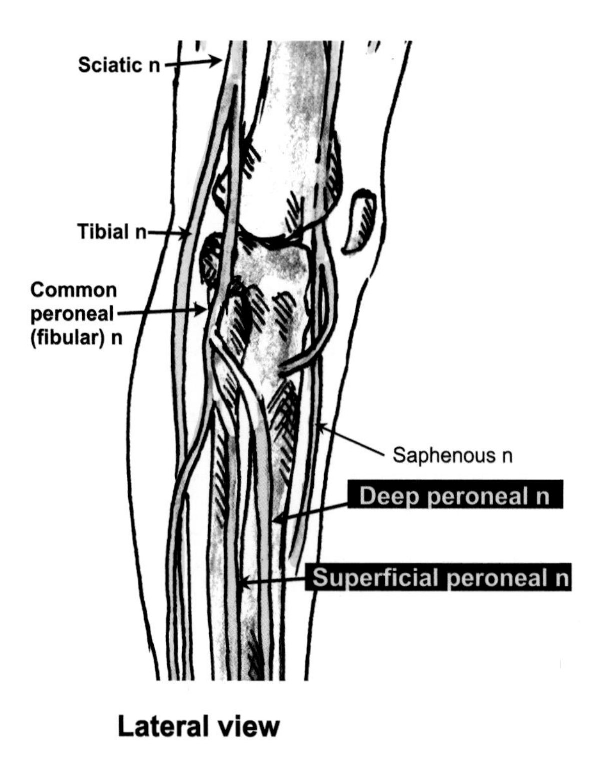

Figure 14.8. Lower extremity nerves entering the leg. The common peroneal nerve's terminal branches (deep and superficial peroneal nerves) enter the leg just distal to the fibular neck.

in the lower third of the leg; it then lies on the anterior aspect of the lower third of tibia with the anterior tibial artery, before crossing the ankle under the extensor retinaculum and terminating as medial (cutaneous) and lateral (motor) branches.
  - The deep peroneal (fibular) motor branches supply:
    - Muscles in the anterior compartment of the leg (tibialis anterior, extensor hallucis longus, extensor digitorum longus, peroneus (fibularis) tertius muscles).
    - The extensor digitorum brevis, the only muscle on the dorsum of the foot.
  - The deep peroneal (fibular) sensory branches supply:
    - The ankle joint capsule.
    - The web of skin between the first and second toes.
  - The superficial peroneal (fibular) nerve descends along the intermuscular septum between the peroneal (fibular) muscles and the extensor digitorum longus (anterior compartment) to pierce the deep fascia in the leg's distal third and become superficial, where it divides into medial and lateral branches which supply the skin on the dorsum of the foot and the toes.
  - The superficial peroneal (fibular) nerve supplies the peroneus (fibularis) longus, peroneus (fibularis) brevis, and the skin on the lateral aspect of the lower half of the leg and the dorsum of the foot.
- Popliteal fossa
  - This is the space at the back of the knee between the skin and the popliteal surface of the femur, and is bordered superolaterally by the biceps femoris muscle, superomedially by the semimembranosus and semitendinosus muscles, and inferiorly by both heads of the gastrocnemius muscle.
  - Its apex is proximal and base distal at the crease of the popliteal fossa (crease of knee joint).
  - The popliteal vessels and tibial and common peroneal (fibular) nerves are found in its anterolateral part.
  - The area surrounding the vessels and nerves is filled with dense connective adipose tissue; this is good for ultrasound identification due to its contrasting echogenicity.

Table 14.1 depicts the target motor nerves of the sacral plexus, many of which will be anesthetized by the sciatic blocks and some by the popliteal blocks. This table also summarizes the motor responses that can be used during nerve stimulation.

Table 14.1. Target nerves of the sciatic nerve blocks: origin and associated movement for use with nerve stimulation.

Movement	Nerve	Root
Anal sphincter	Pudendal	S2, 3, 4
Gluteal twitch / thigh abduction (gluteus minimus and medius)	Superior gluteal	L4, 5 & S1
Gluteal twitch / thigh extension (gluteus maximus)	Inferior gluteal	L5 & S1, 2
Knee flexion, foot inversion and ankle plantar flexion	Tibial (above and below sciatic bifurcation)	L4, 5, & S1, 2, 3
Ankle dorsiflexion	Common peroneal	L4, 5 & S1, 2
Ankle and toe extension	Deep peroneal	L5 & S1
Foot eversion (peroneus longus and brevis)	Superficial peroneal	L5 & S1
First toe abduction	Medial plantar (Tibial)	S1, 2
Fifth toe abduction	Lateral plantar (Tibial)	S1, 2, 3

Clinical Pearls

- Ultrasound imaging of the sciatic nerve is often more complex than for the brachial plexus or other peripheral nerves in the upper or lower extremity, because the nerve is located so deeply. It is often necessary to utilize probes of lower frequency resulting in images of lower resolution. Also, the steep angle of needle insertion often required makes it challenging to track the needle within the tissues.
- The nerve is often wide and flat, thus it can be difficult to recognize the nerve during transverse imaging.
- Scanning to obtain the long-axis (longitudinal) view of the sciatic nerve can be useful to further visualize the course of the nerve, the inserted catheter, and the spread of local anesthetic.
- Inserting the needle at some distance from the probe may reduce the angle and improve imaging of the needle.
- It is advisable to use an ultrasound machine with higher resolution (e.g., Phillips ATL HDI 5000, Philips Medical Systems, Bothell, WA, USA) if available, for obtaining reliable imaging.

Nerve Stimulation

In patients with significant peripheral neuropathy (e.g., from diabetes or renal failure), it may be necessary to use currents of up to 1.0 mA to stimulate the sciatic nerve. This is acceptable as long as the responses are clear and specific to the nerve.

14.2. Labat (Gluteal) Sciatic Nerve Block Approach

14.2.1. Patient Positioning and Surface Anatomy

14.2.1.1. Patient Positioning

Place the patient in the lateral or semiprone (Sim's) position, with the hip and knee flexed and the operative side uppermost.

14.2.1.2. Surface Anatomy [Figures 14.3, 14.9(A,B)]

- Oblique line
  - Joining the posterior superior iliac spine (PSIS) to the midpoint of the greater trochanter (on its medial aspect)
- Parahorizontal line
  - Joining the greater trochanter (at above location) to the sacral hiatus

A perpendicular line drawn at the midpoint of the oblique line and reaching the parahorizontal line is the traditional puncture site (this intersection should be approximately 5 cm caudad along the perpendicular line).

14.2.2. Sonographic Imaging and Needle Insertion Technique

An image of the sciatic nerve in the gluteal region as captured by magnetic resonance imaging (MRI; Figure 14.10) can be used as reference for the corresponding ultrasound image (Figure 14.11).

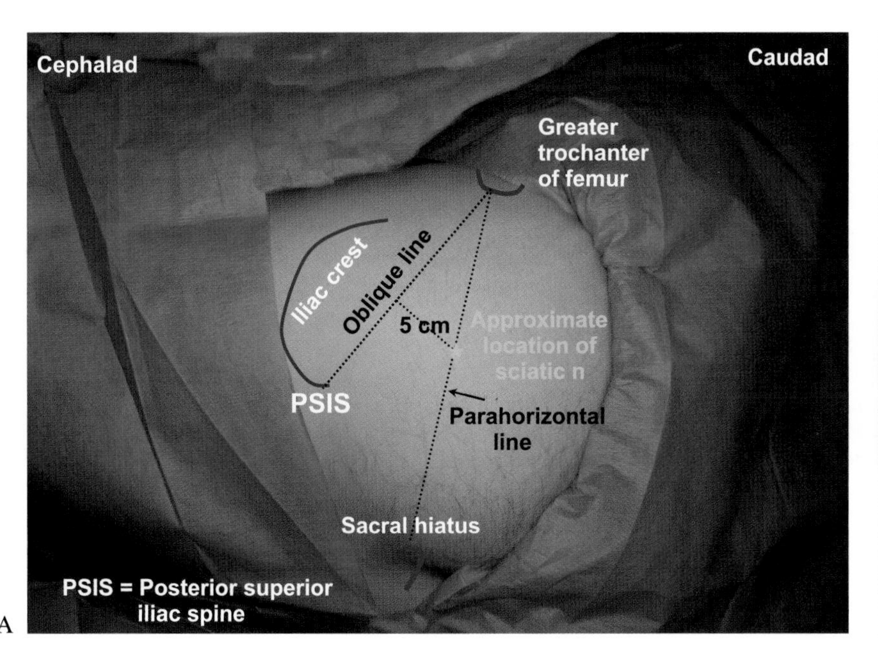

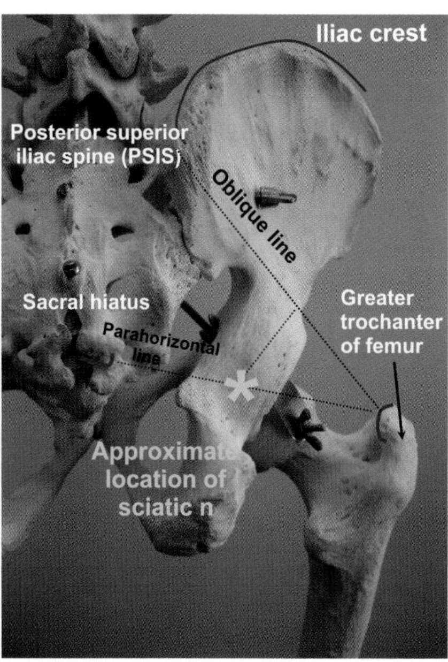

Figure 14.9. Surface anatomy for the Labat block using (A) a volunteer in the lateral decubitus position and (B) a skeleton model.

Prepare the needle insertion site and skin surface with an antiseptic solution. Prepare the ultrasound probe surface by applying a sterile adhesive dressing to it prior to needling as discussed earlier (see Chapters 3 and 4).

The nerve structures are most visible when the angle of incidence is approximately 90° to the ultrasound beam.

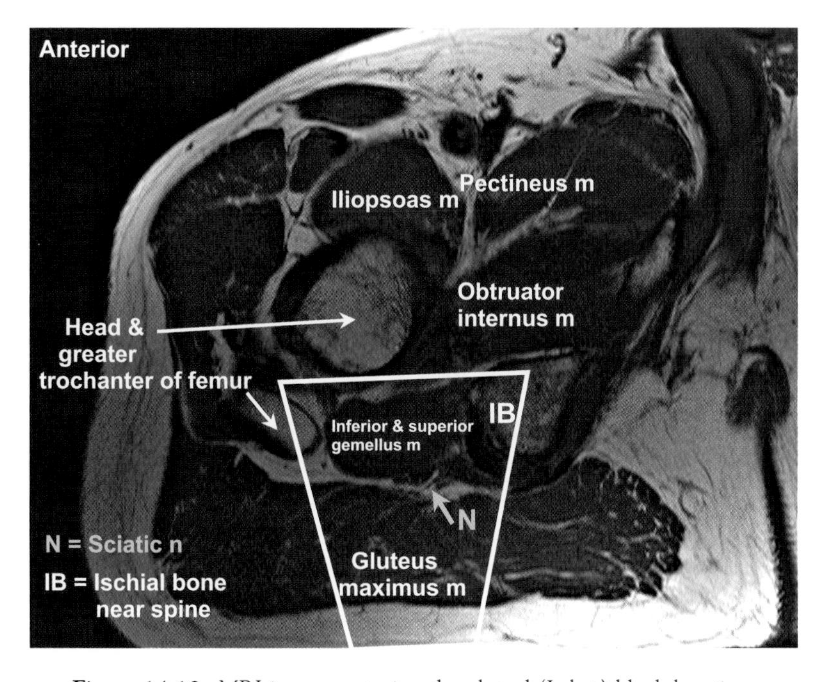

Figure 14.10. MRI image capturing the gluteal (Labat) block location.

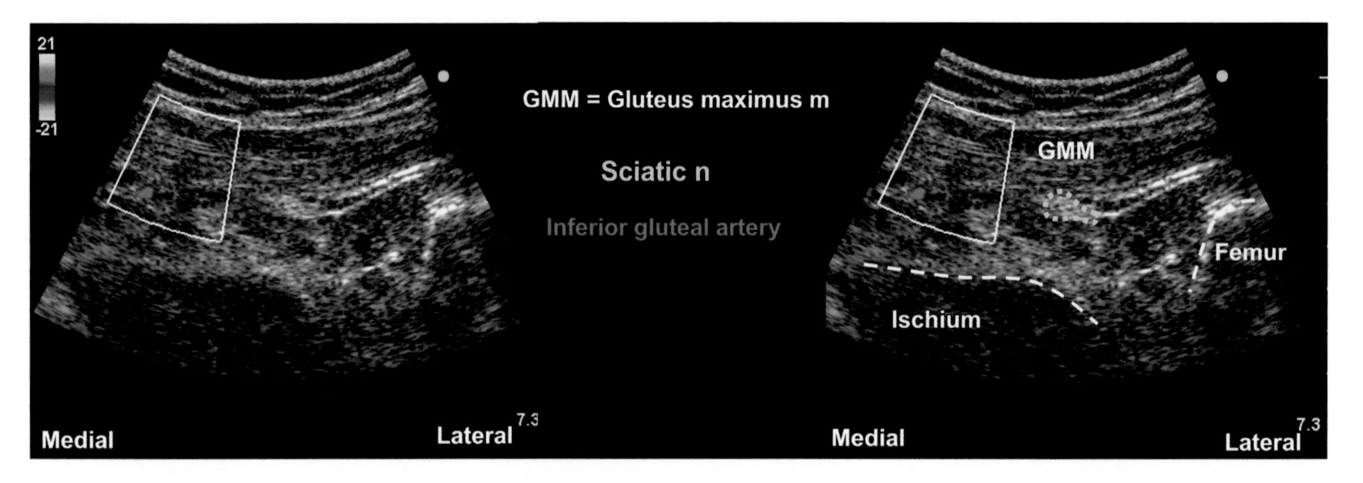

Figure 14.11. Ultrasound image of sciatic nerve in short-axis view using a curved probe at the gluteal block location.

14.2.2.1. *Scanning Technique*

- Use a curved, lower frequency 2- to 5-MHz probe for scanning the gluteal region.
- The depth of penetration is often more than 4 cm from the skin surface.
- First identify the bony structures that are adjacent to the sciatic nerve (e.g., the ischial bone).
- Move the probe cephalad and caudad in the gluteal region to examine the ischial bone (a hyperechoic line with bony shadowing underneath). Locate the widest portion of the ischial bone and the ischial spine medially.
- Use color Doppler to try to locate the inferior gluteal artery that is adjacent to the ischial spine that is medial to the sciatic nerve (Figure 14.11). The author has had occasional success producing a color Doppler effect with the particular angles of probe alignment required and the depth of the structures.
- Locate the bulky gluteus maximus muscle that is superficial and posterior to the sciatic nerve.
- Other vascular structures that may be noted immediately adjacent to the sciatic nerve are the internal pudendal artery and vien.
- Angle the probe slightly cephalad or caudad to capture the best possible transverse view of the sciatic nerve.

14.2.2.2. *Sonographic Appearance*

- The sciatic nerve in the gluteal region lies lateral to the ischial spine and superficial to the ischial bone (Figure 14.11); if scanned distally, it may be located at about the midpoint between the greater trochanter and ischial tuberosity (i.e., the subgluteal approach block location).
- Vascular landmarks medial to the sciatic nerve and immediately adjacent to the ischial spine are the inferior gluteal artery and internal pudendal artery and vein; it may be difficult to illuminate these vessels with Doppler but it is worth trying.
- Overlying the sciatic nerve lies the large gluteus maximus muscle, which is quite distinct with the usual "starry night" appearance.
- The inner muscle layers (superior and inferior gemellus muscles, obturator internus muscle, quadratus femoris muscle) are often indistinct.
- The sciatic nerve in the gluteal region appears predominantly hyperechoic (bright) and is often wide and flat in short axis on ultrasound.

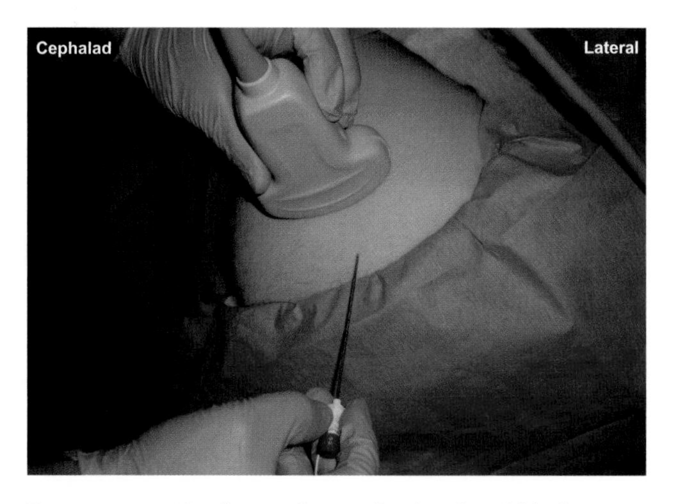

Figure 14.12. Needling technique for the gluteal block using a curved probe and an out-of-plane (OOP) needling alignment.

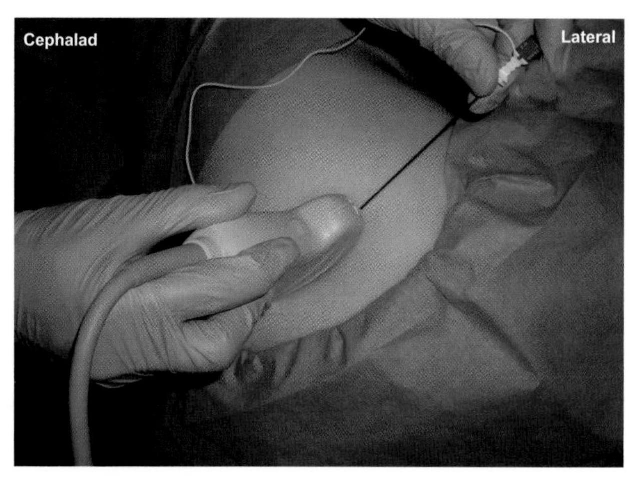

Figure 14.13. Needling technique for the gluteal block using a curved probe and an in-plane (IP) needle alignment with a lateral-to-medial needle insertion.

14.2.2.3. Needle Insertion Technique

- Use an 8-cm, 22-ga insulated needle if nerve stimulation is desired.
- Both the in-plane (IP) and out-of-plane (OOP) approaches (see Chapter 4) are appropriate for ultrasound-guided sciatic nerve block in the gluteal region.
- OOP approach (Figure 14.12)
  - The needle is inserted inferior to the probe in a cephaloanterior direction.
  - A fairly steep angle of insertion will be required, but placing the needle slightly inferior to the probe will reduce the angle somewhat for better visibility of the needle.
  - This approach is often used for catheter insertion and it is important to line up the site of needle insertion at the skin with the target nerve.
  - As with IP technique, electrical stimulation is recommended for confirming needle-to-nerve contact.
- IP approach (Figure 14.13):
  - The needle may be moved in a lateral-to-medial direction to penetrate the gluteus maximus muscle prior to reaching the sciatic nerve above the ischial bone.
  - Needle movement will be observed during advancement and nerve movement may be observed upon contact. Further confirmation by electrical stimulation is recommended.
- For both IP and OOP approaches, scanning prior to needling will determine the angle, distance, and depth of needle penetration.

Clinical Pearl

The angle of needle penetration is often steep (>45°) at the gluteal region, therefore it can be difficult to clearly visualize the needle shaft and tip.

14.2.3. Nerve Stimulation

Table 14.2 shows motor responses associated with nerve stimulation to confirm needle contact to the sciatic nerve.

Table 14.2. Responses and recommended needle adjustments for use with nerve stimulation during the gluteal approach.

Correct Response from Nerve Stimulation
Visible or palpable twitches in any of the hamstring or calf muscles, foot, or toes, at 0.2 to 0.5 mA. Up to 1.0 mA may be required in some patients (elderly, diabetic, peripheral vascular disease, sepsis).

Other Common Responses and Necessary Needle Adjustment

- Muscle twitches from electrical stimulation
  - Gluteus maximus (local twitch from direct stimulation)
    - *Explanation*: Needle tip too superficial
    - *Needle Adjustment*: Advance needle tip
  - Deep muscle layer (local twitch of inferior or superior gemellus, obturator internus, or quadratus femoris muscles)
    - *Explanation*: Needle advanced too deep and beyond the nerve
    - *Needle Adjustment*: Withdraw needle to skin and redirect slightly medially or laterally
- Vascular puncture
  - Inferior gluteal or internal pudendal vessels
    - *Explanation*: Needle tip placed too medially
    - *Needle Adjustment*: Withdraw needle to skin and reinsert more laterally
- Bone contact
  - Iliac bone (close to gluteus insertion)
    - *Explanation*: Needle tip too superior
    - *Needle Adjustment*: Withdraw completely and reinsert according to protocol (check landmarks)
  - Ischial spine
    - *Explanation*: Needle inserted at too medial position or angled in a medial direction
    - *Needle Adjustment*: Withdraw completely and reinsert in a more lateral direction

14.2.4. Local Anesthetic Application

- Performing a test dose with dextrose 5% in water (D5W) is recommended prior to local anesthetic application to visualize the spread and confirm nerve localization (see Chapter 4 sidebar).
- It is generally recommended to deposit the local anesthetic solution completely around the sciatic nerve.

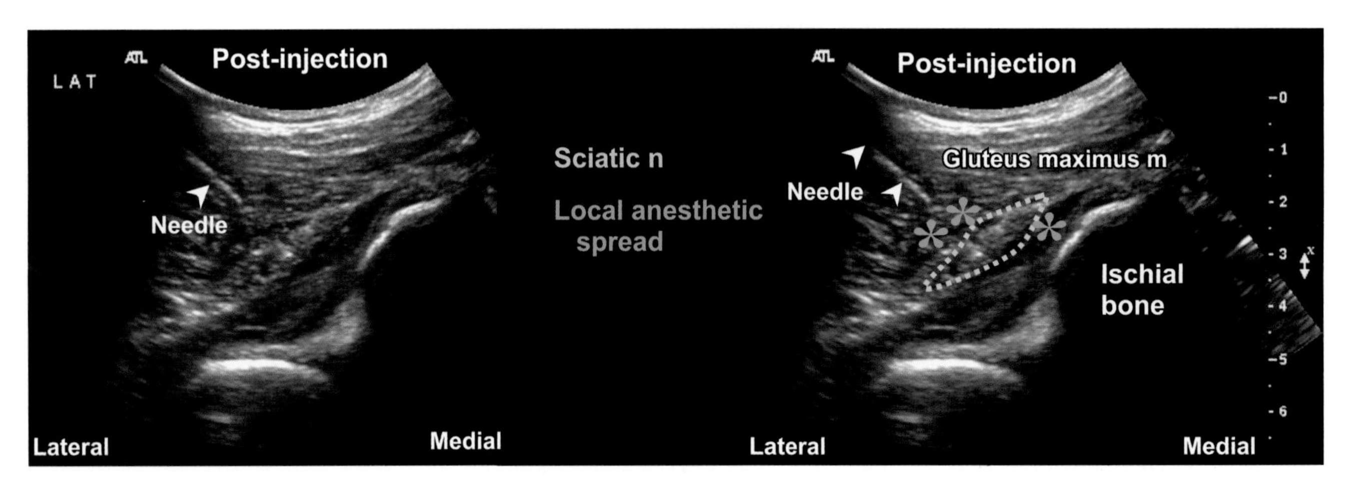

Figure 14.14. Local anesthetic application during the gluteal block using an in-plane (IP) needling approach, as captured by the Phillips ATL HDI 5000 ultrasound system (Philips Medical Systems, Bothell, WA, USA).

- Injection to the deep side of the nerve may require a second needle insertion site.
- A hypoechoic (fluid) expansion can be seen during local anesthetic injection (Figure 14.14).

Clinical Pearls

- Chan (2006) suggests that applying local anesthetic circumferentially around the nerve can be challenging because the sciatic nerve in this region can be flat and thin in cross-section.
- It is therefore common to find local anesthetic on only one side of the nerve (most commonly the superficial/posterior aspect) after injection.

14.3. Subgluteal Sciatic Nerve Block Approach

14.3.1. Patient Positioning and Surface Anatomy

14.3.1.1. Patient Positioning

Place the patient in the lateral or semiprone (Sim's) position, with the hip and knee flexed and the foot resting on the dependent knee. This block is indicated for surgery at and below the knee, including Achilles tendon repair and foot surgery.

14.3.1.2. Surface Anatomy [Figures 14.15(A,B)]

- Horizontal line
  - Joining the medial aspect of the greater trochanter to the ischial tuberosity. The traditional puncture site is located on this line just medial to its midpoint.

14.3.2. Sonographic Imaging and Needle Insertion Technique

Images of the sciatic nerve at the subgluteal location can be seen as captured by MRI (Figure 14.16) and in the corresponding ultrasound image (Figure 14.17).

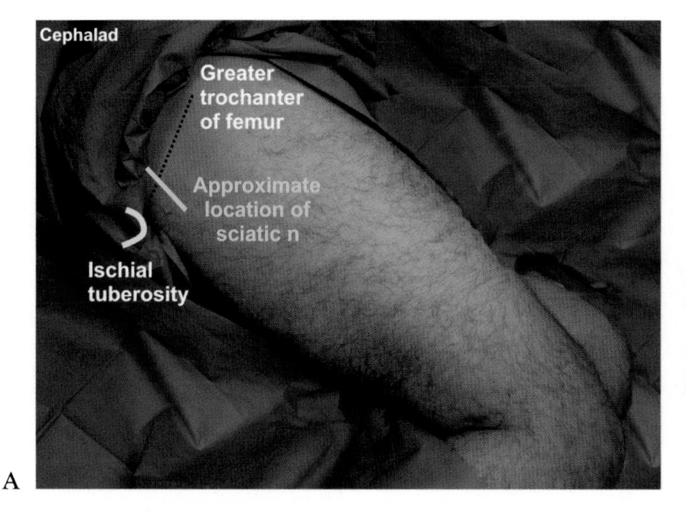

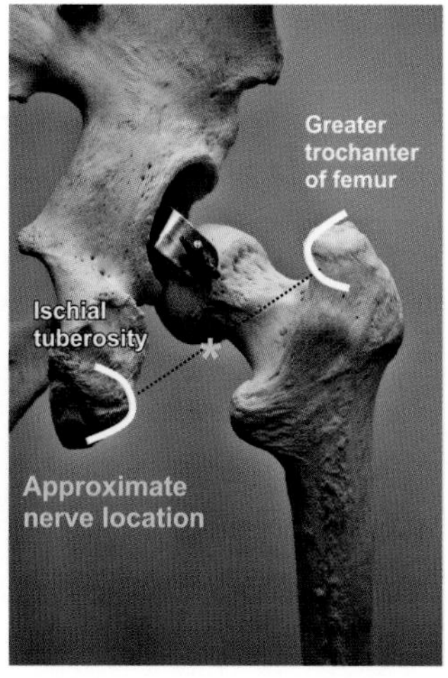

Figure 14.15. Surface anatomy for sciatic nerve blockade at the subgluteal location using (A) a volunteer in the decubitus position and (B) a skeleton model.

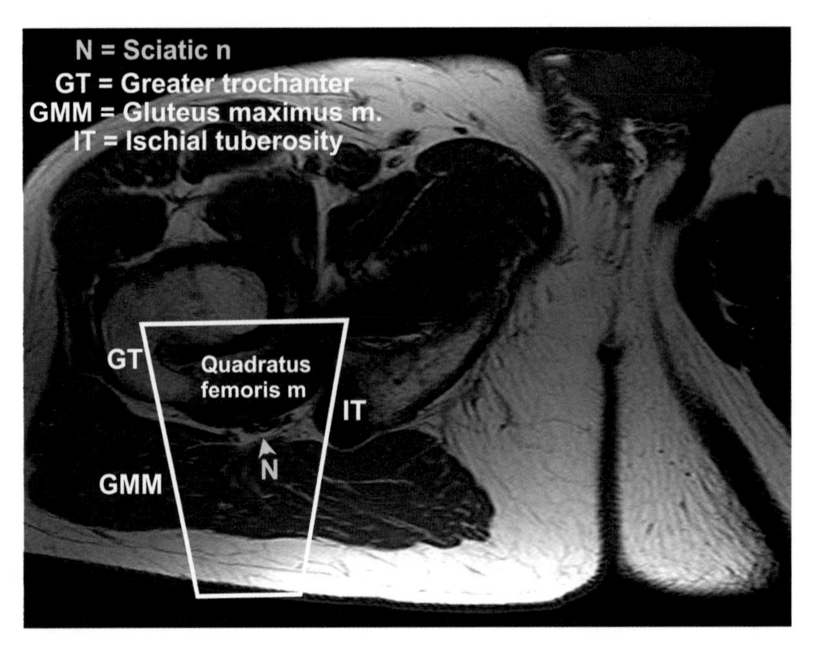

Figure 14.16. MRI image depicting the sciatic nerve at the level of the subgluteal block.

The highly hyperechoic bony structures, ischial tuberosity (medial) and greater trochanter (lateral), with underlying hypoechoic shadows, are excellent landmarks for localization of the sciatic nerve.

Prepare the needle insertion site and skin surface with an antiseptic solution. Prepare the ultrasound probe surface by applying a sterile adhesive dressing to it prior to needling as discussed earlier (see Chapters 3 and 4).

The nerve structures are most visible when the angle of incidence is approximately 90° to the ultrasound beam.

14.3.2.1. *Scanning Technique*

- Use a curved, lower frequency 2- to 5-MHz probe or a linear 4- to 7-MHz probe for scanning the subgluteal region.
- The required depth of penetration is often 3 to 4 cm from the skin surface.
- Align the center of the probe with the midpoint of a line between the ischial tuberosity and the greater trochanter.

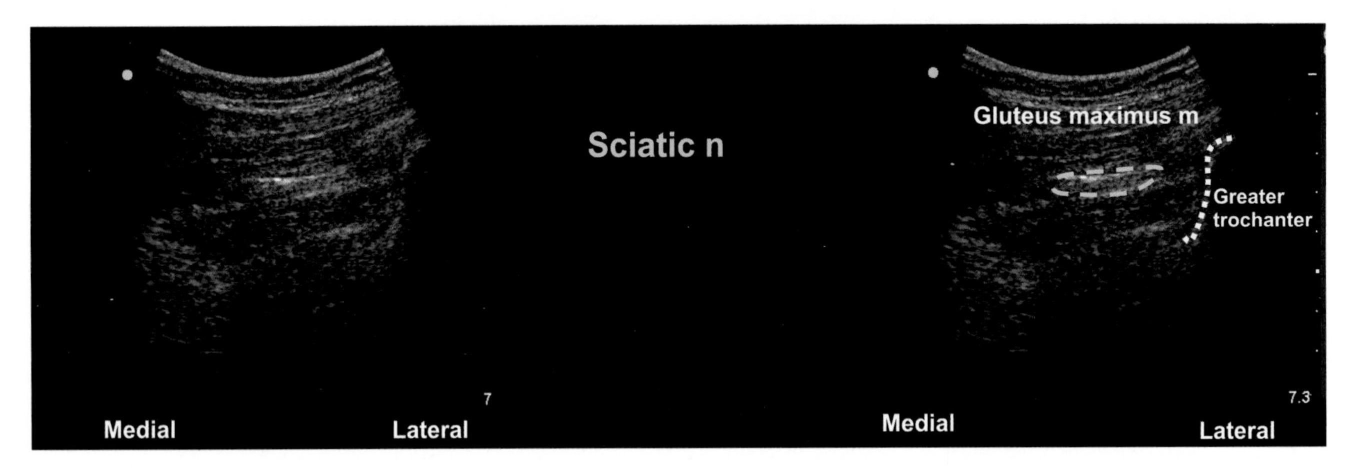

Figure 14.17. Ultrasound image of the sciatic nerve between the greater trochanter and ischial tuberosity.

- In the transverse/short-axis plane the image may show the inner borders of both bony landmarks and the sciatic nerve slightly medial to the midline.
- If the sciatic nerve is hard to localize at the subgluteal region, it can be traced proximally from the bifurcation point at or near the apex of the popliteal fossa (see Section 14.5 for details). Keep in mind the bifurcation of the sciatic nerve may be much higher than expected.

Clinical Pearls

- In obese subjects, it may be necessary to use a curved probe to obtain a wider imaging field of view to show the location of the nerve in relation to the bony landmarks and local anatomy.
- Once satisfied with the anatomical survey, and having marked the expected locations of the bony landmarks and the nerve, one can switch to a higher frequency probe to obtain a clearer image of the nerve.

14.3.2.2. *Sonographic Appearance (2- to 5-MHz Curved Array)*

- On the lateral side of the screen, the medial aspect of the greater trochanter appears almost pear shaped and hypoechoic when using a curved array probe.
- The sciatic nerve in the subgluteal region appears predominantly hyperechoic (bright) and is often elliptical in short axis on ultrasound (Figure 14.17). It may also be wide and flat, almost comet shaped, rendering it difficult to visualize.

14.3.2.3. *Needle Insertion Technique*

- Depending on the depth of penetration [as estimated by the patient's body mass index (BMI)], use a 5- to 8-cm, 22-ga insulated needle if nerve stimulation is desired.
- Both IP and OOP approaches (see Chapter 4) are applicable.
- OOP approach (Figure 14.18):
  - Align the ultrasound probe so the nerve is placed in the center of the screen in order to align the needle insertion site to the location of the nerve.
  - Insert the needle perpendicular to the caudal surface of the probe.
  - Insert the needle 3 to 4 cm inferior to the probe to reduce the angle required to reach the sciatic nerve.
- IP approach (Figure 14.19):
  - Insert the needle at the lateral edge of the probe.
  - Use an angle of insertion of approximately 45° to the skin, although it may be as steep as 60° to 70° in certain obese individuals.
- The authors often use the OOP approach for ultrasound-guided sciatic nerve block in the subgluteal region because indwelling catheters are often inserted in this location for postoperative pain relief.
- With the OOP approach, it is not easy to follow the needle path accurately, particularly with curved array probes.
- Electrical stimulation is recommended as an additional tool to confirm needle-to-nerve contact.

Clinical Pearl

Given the size and depth of the sciatic nerve, it may be advisable to place the needle shaft aganist one side of the nerve, rather than directing the needle tip to contact the nerve, in order to reduce the risk of inadvertent intraneural needle penetration.

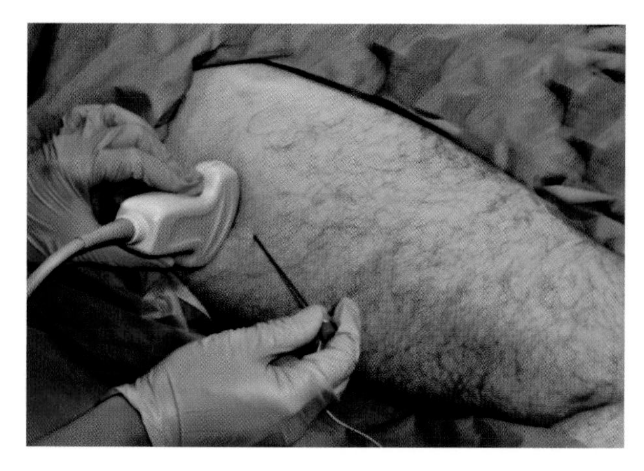

Figure 14.18. Needling technique for the subgluteal block using a curved ultrasound probe and an out-of-plane (OOP) needle alignment.

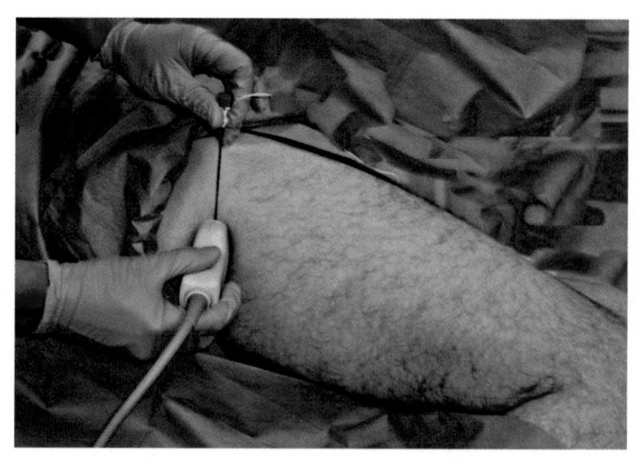

Figure 14.19. Needling technique for the subgluteal block using a curved probe and an in-plane (IP) needle alignment.

14.3.3. Nerve Stimulation

Table 14.3 gives a summary of the correct motor responses to nerve stimulation during subgluteal sciatic nerve block and also recommendations for needle adjustment upon elicitation of other responses. Ultrasound guidance will improve accuracy of needle placement, although nerve stimulation is still recommended at this time for confirming nerve localization.

Table 14.3. Responses and recommended needle adjustments for use with nerve stimulation during the subgluteal approach.

Correct Response from Nerve Stimulation

Twitches (visible or palpable) in any of the hamstring or calf muscles, foot, or toes, at 0.2 to 0.5 mA. Up to 1.0 mA may be required in some patients (elderly, diabetic, peripheral vascular disease, sepsis).

Other Common Responses and Necessary Needle Adjustment

- Muscle twitches from electrical stimulation
  - Gluteus maximus (local twitch from direct stimulation)
    - *Explanation*: Needle tip too superficial
    - *Needle Adjustment*: Advance needle tip
- Bone contact
  - Iliac bone (close to gluteus insertion)
    - *Explanation*: Needle tip too superior
    - *Needle Adjustment*: Withdraw completely and reinsert according to protocol (check landmarks)
  - Ischial or hip joint
    - *Explanation*: Needle missed the plane of sciatic nerve and the tip is placed too far medially (ischial) or laterally (hip)
    - *Needle Adjustment*: Withdraw completely and reinsert with a 5° to 10° angle adjustment
- No response despite deep placement
  - Deep (10 cm) but no response; it is likely that the needle has been placed in greater sciatic notch
    - *Explanation*: Needle tip too inferior and medial
    - *Needle Adjustment*: Withdraw completely and reinsert slightly superiorly

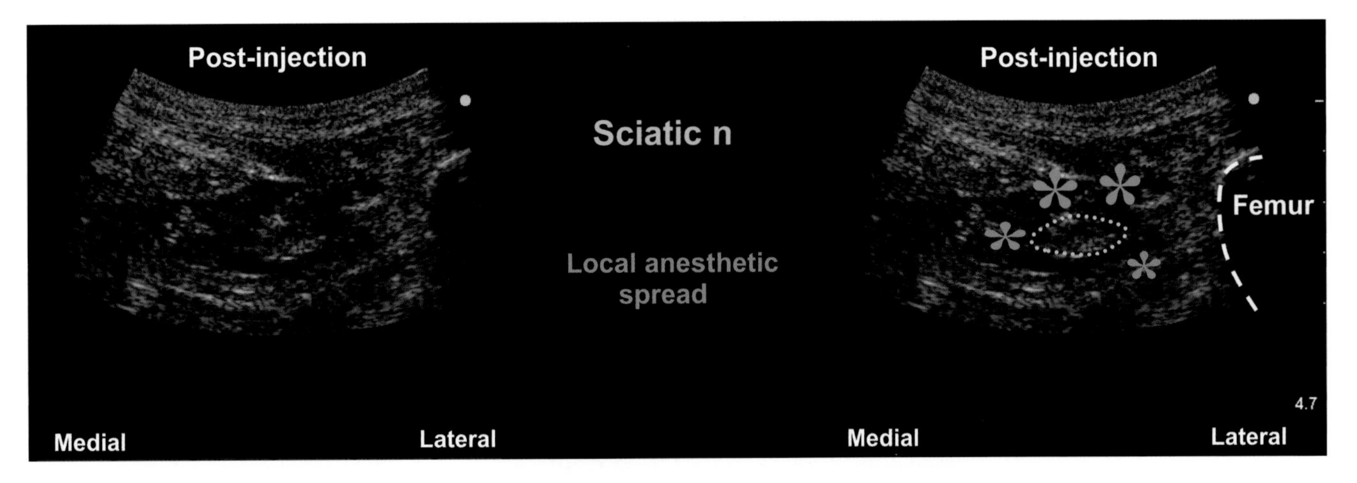

Figure 14.20. Local anesthetic application at the subgluteal location captured by the SonoSite MicroMaxx (Bothell, WA, USA) machine with the curved probe.

14.3.4. Local Anesthetic Application

Confirm sciatic nerve localization with nerve stimulation prior to local anesthetic application. This will also distinguish the tibial and common peroneal (fibular) components of the nerve. Performing a test dose with D5W is recommended prior local anesthetic application to visualize the spread and confirm nerve localization (see Chapter 4 sidebar).

- The goal is to deposit local anesthetic (20–30 mL) next to, but not directly within, the sciatic nerve structure in the subgluteal region.
- A hypoechoic local anesthetic fluid collection is often seen around the hyperechoic nerve within the sheath compartment during injection (Figure 14.20).

14.4. Anterior Sciatic Nerve Block Approach

14.4.1. Patient Positioning and Surface Anatomy

14.4.1.1. Patient Positioning

This block is generally reserved for those patients who cannot be positioned laterally. The block is indicated for surgery below the knee, with the only sensory deficiency being the medial strip of skin supplied by the saphenous nerve.

Position the patient supine with the hip and knee flexed and the hip externally rotated approximately 45°.

14.4.1.2. Surface Anatomy [Figure 14.21(A,B)]

- Femoral crease
  - Natural skin fold on the upper anterior thigh approximately 2 to 3 cm inferior to the inguinal ligament (extending from anterior superior iliac spine to pubic tubercle)
- Femoral artery pulse
  - At intersection of lateral two thirds and medial one third of femoral crease

The anterior block is performed on a short portion of the sciatic nerve close to the lesser trochanter of the femur. To avoid needle contact with bone, the lower extremity can be internally rotated or externally rotated to move the lesser trochanter away from the sciatic nerve.

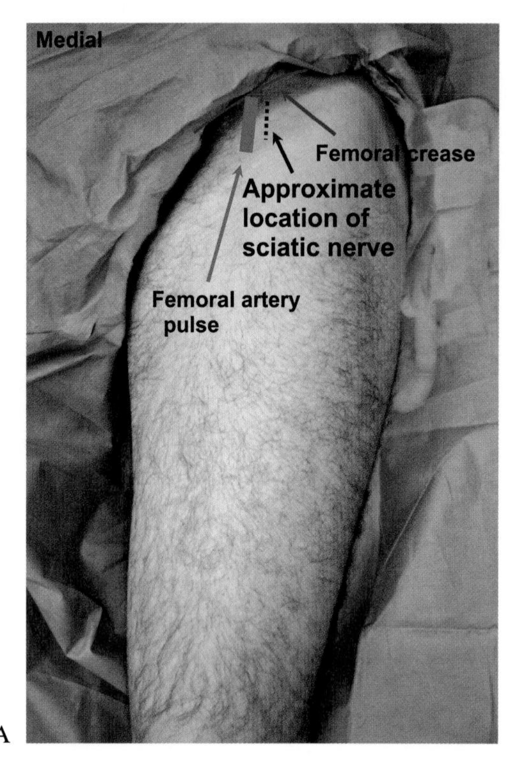

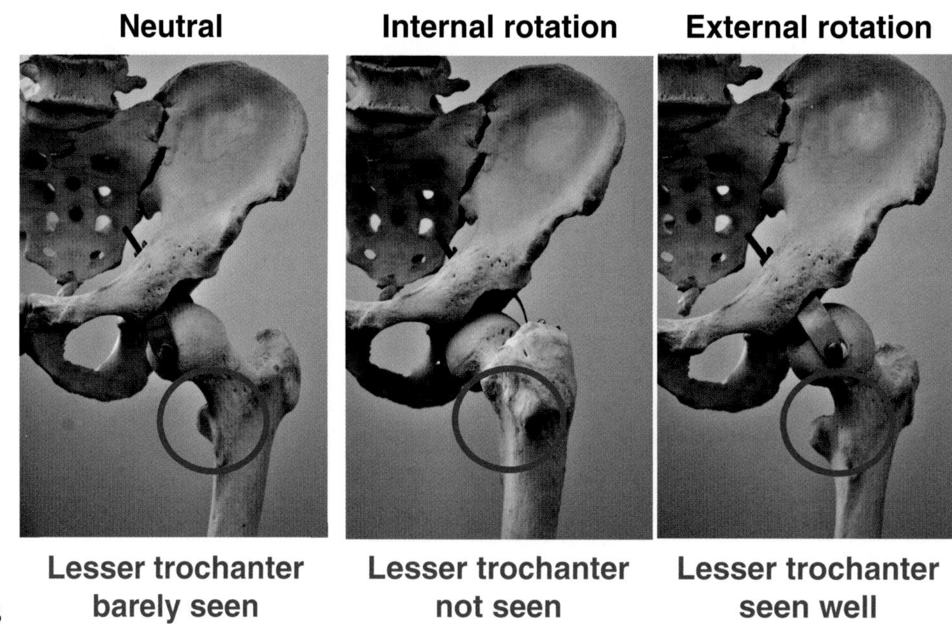

Figure 14.21. (A) Surface anatomy for sciatic nerve blockade from the anterior approach and (B) a skeleton model illustrating the appearance of the lesser trochanter with neutral, internal, and external rotation of the hip.

14.4.2. Sonographic Imaging and Needle Insertion Technique

Images of the sciatic nerve in the proximal thigh captured by MRI are shown (Figure 14.22) and the corresponding ultrasound image is shown in Figure 14.23.

Prepare the needle insertion site and skin surface with an antiseptic solution. Prepare the ultrasound probe surface by applying a sterile adhesive dressing to it prior to needling as discussed earlier (see Chapters 3 and 4).

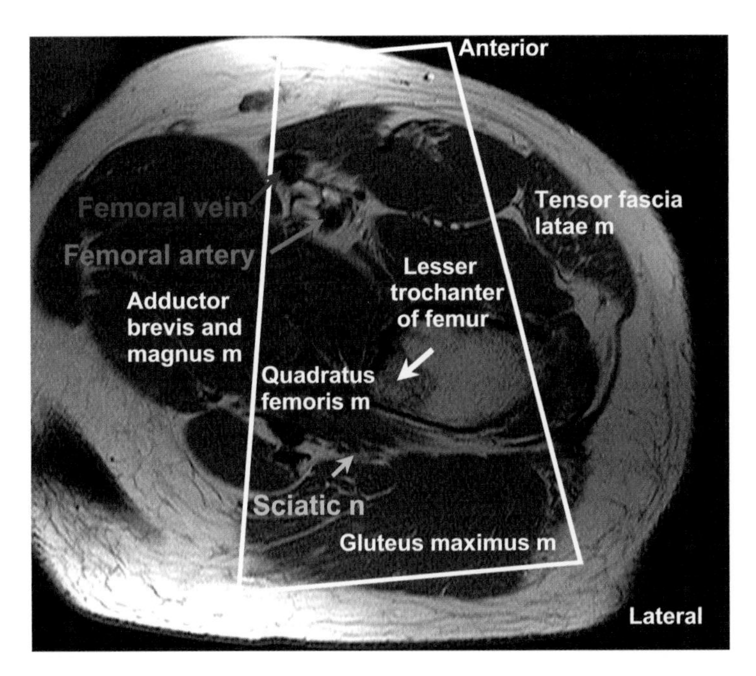

Figure 14.22. MRI image depicting the anterior sciatic nerve block location.

The nerve structures are most visible when the angle of incidence is approximately 90° to the ultrasound beam.

14.4.2.1. *Scanning Technique*

- It is most common to utilize a curved, lower frequency 2- to 5-MHz probe for scanning the sciatic nerve in the proximal anterior thigh.
- Place the probe over the proximal thigh approximately 8 cm distal to the femoral crease.
- The required depth of penetration is often more than 6 cm from the skin surface.
- In the proximal thigh, the sciatic nerve courses posterior to the femur and is often difficult to reach from the front at the level of the lesser trochanter. However, the nerve can be visualized when ultrasound scanned from the medial aspect of the thigh.

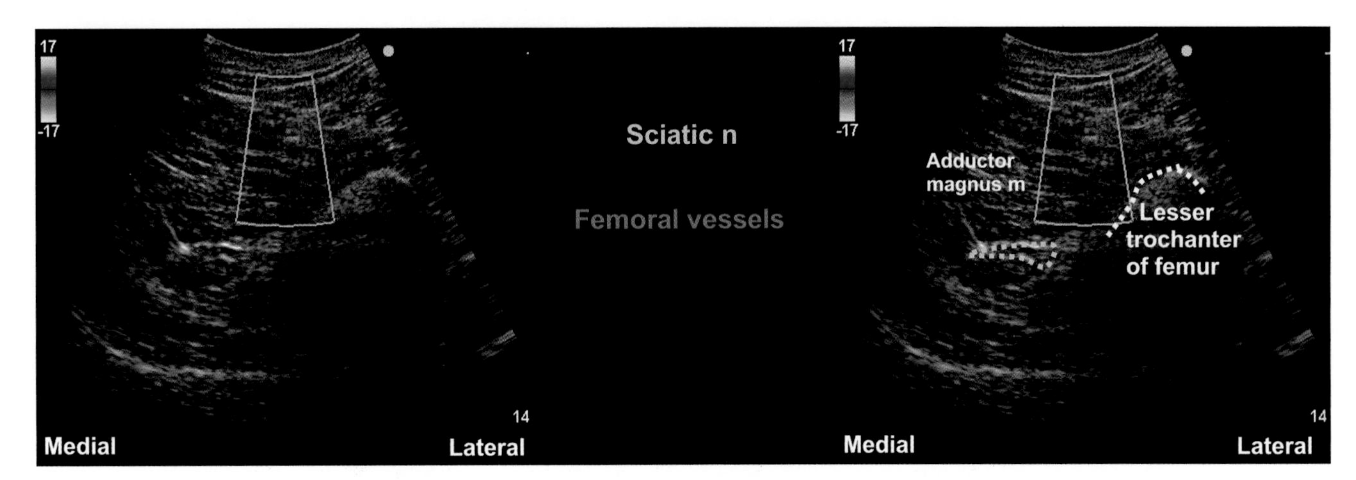

Figure 14.23. Ultrasound image at the anterior sciatic nerve block location.

Clinical Pearls

- The lesser trochanter often obstructs visibility of the sciatic nerve. In this case, one can move the probe to a more medial position where the sciatic nerve is located posterior to the femur.
- The leg can also be internally (commonly) or externally rotated to move the lesser trochanter away from the sciatic nerve [Figure 14.21(B)].

14.4.2.2. *Sonographic Appearance*

- The sciatic nerve is often oval or round, predominantly hyperechoic, medial and posterior to the lesser trochanter, and deep to the adductor magnus and quadratus femoris muscles (Figure 14.23).
- If using Doppler, the femoral neurovascular structures are seen superficial below the hyperechoic fascial tissue and lateral to the sciatic nerve in this projection when the leg is externally rotated.

Clinical Pearls

- Obtaining a clear image of the sciatic nerve during the anterior approach can be challenging due to the deep location of the nerve.
- It is advisable to use an ultrasound machine with higher resolution (e.g., Phillips ATL) to obtain reliable imaging.

14.4.2.3. *Needle Insertion Technique*

- Use an 8- to 12-cm, 22- or 20-ga insulated needle for combined ultrasound and nerve stimulation guidance. The depth of the needle will vary depending on the width of the thigh muscles.
- Both the IP and OOP approaches (see Chapter 4) are appropriate (Figures 14.24 and 14.25).

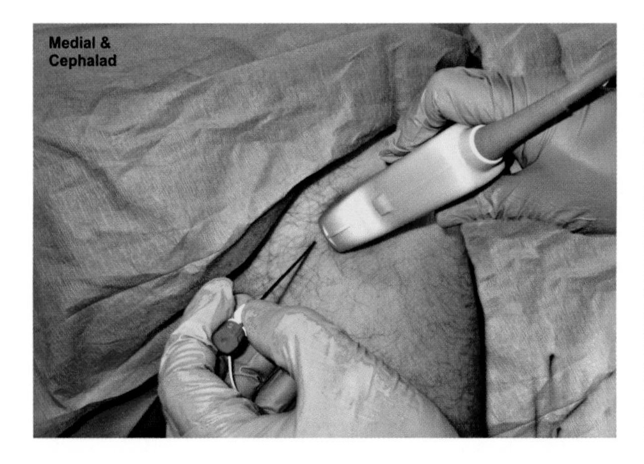

Figure 14.24. Needling technique using a curved probe and an in-plane (IP) needle alignment from anteromedial to posterolateral.

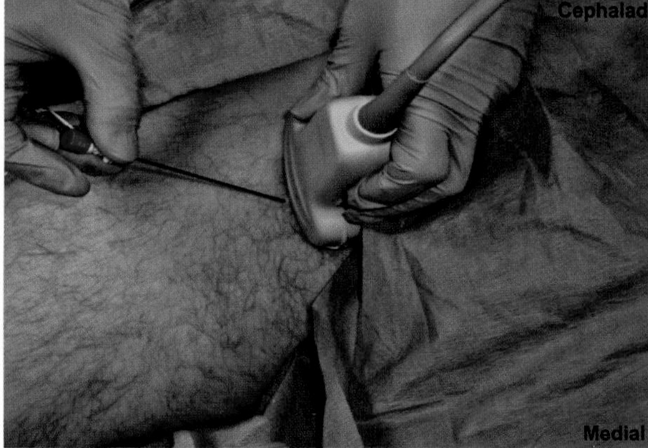

Figure 14.25. Needling technique using a curved probe and an out-of-plane (OOP) needle alignment in a cephalad direction.

- IP approach:
  - Advance the needle in a medial-to-lateral and anterior-to-posterior direction.
  - The femoral neurovascular bundle is lateral to the needle insertion site.
  - Because of the steep angle of needle advancement, needle and tissue (muscle) movement is often observed without a clear view of the needle shaft and tip.
  - Needle-to-nerve contact is often indicated by nerve movement and confirmed by electrical stimulation.
- OOP approach:
  - Place the nerve in the middle of the ultrasound screen in order to align the needle insertion site (in the midline of the probe) to the nerve location site.
  - Insert the needle at the midline of the probe.

14.4.3. Nerve Stimulation

Table 14.4 describes the correct motor responses associated with nerve stimulation for the anterior approach to the sciatic nerve. Recommended adjustments upon obtaining other motor responses are included.

14.4.4. Local Anesthetic Application

- Performing a test dose with D5W is recommended prior to local anesthetic application to visualize the spread and confirm nerve localization (see Chapter 4 sidebar).
- The goal is to deposit local anesthetic circumferentially around the sciatic nerve. However, it is technically challenging to reposition the needle on both sides of the nerve because of its depth within the muscle layers.

Table 14.4. Responses and recommended needle adjustments for use with nerve stimulation during the anterior approach.

Correct Response from Nerve Stimulation
Twitches obtained (visible or palpable) from the calf, foot, or toe muscles at 0.2 to 0.5 mA current. Twitches of the quadriceps muscles will likely occur during advancement.

Other Common Responses and Necessary Needle Adjustment
- Muscle twitches from electrical stimulation
  - Quadriceps (patella twitch)
    - *Explanation:* Needle placement too superficial
    - *Needle Adjustment:* Continue to advance the needle
  - Iliopsoas or pectineus (local twitch at femoral crease area)
    - *Explanation:* Needle tip placement is too superior
    - *Needle Adjustment:* Withdraw needle completely and reinsert more inferiorly
  - Hamstrings (branches of the sciatic nerve or direct stimulation of muscles)
    - *Explanation:* Needle possibly too inferior and caudally directed, although often this is not specific
    - *Needle Adjustment:* Withdraw needle completely and reinsert in a slightly more medial or lateral direction (5°–10° in transverse plane)
- Bone contact
  - Femur (usually lesser trochanter)
    - *Explanation:* Needle tip directed too laterally or excessive lateral rotation of the femur
    - *Needle Adjustment:* Withdraw needle 2 to 3 cm and internally rotate leg, then continue; if this fails withdraw the needle to the subcutaneous tissue and reinsert it in a more medial direction
- No response despite deep placement
  - Deep (12–15 cm) needle advancement but no response
    - *Explanation:* Needle tip is often too medial
    - *Needle Adjustment:* Withdraw completely and reinsert at a slightly more lateral position

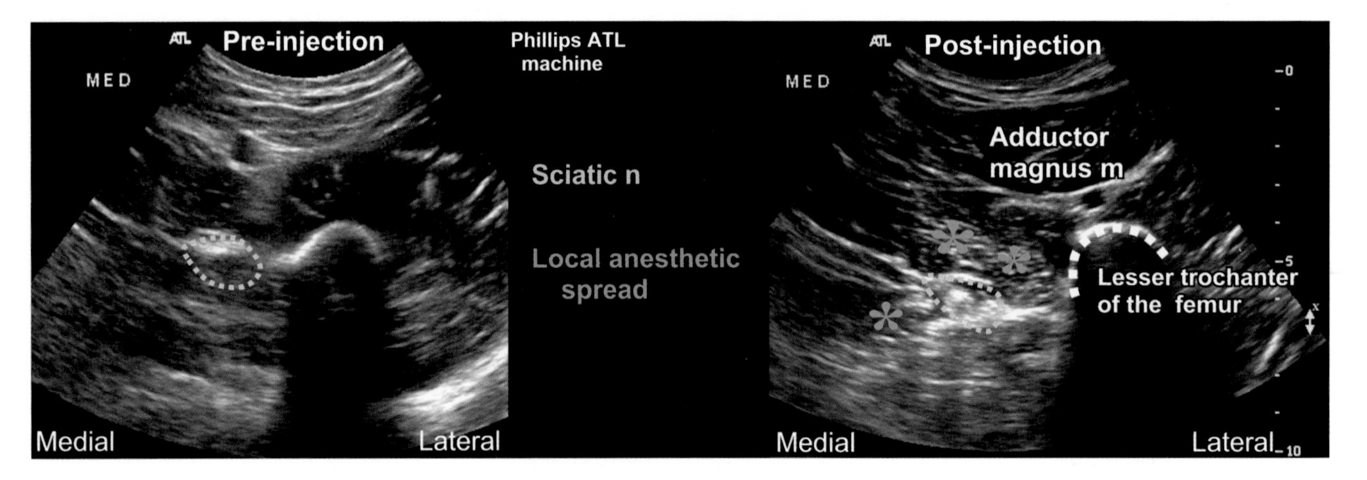

Figure 14.26. Ultrasound image using the Philips ATL machine at the anterior block location. The local anesthetic application can be visualized surrounding the nerve.

- The injection of local anesthetic is often seen as a hypoechoic collection and will often cause the sciatic nerve to be more distinct and luminous (Figure 14.26).

14.5. Popliteal Sciatic Nerve Block (Posterior Approach)

14.5.1. Patient Positioning and Surface Anatomy

14.5.1.1. Patient Positioning (Figure 14.27)

Position the patient laterally or prone with the operative leg slightly flexed. Ideally, the ankles should be positioned beyond the end of the table so that motor responses to nerve stimulation can be readily observed. The landmarks become more visible when the knee is flexed against resistance.

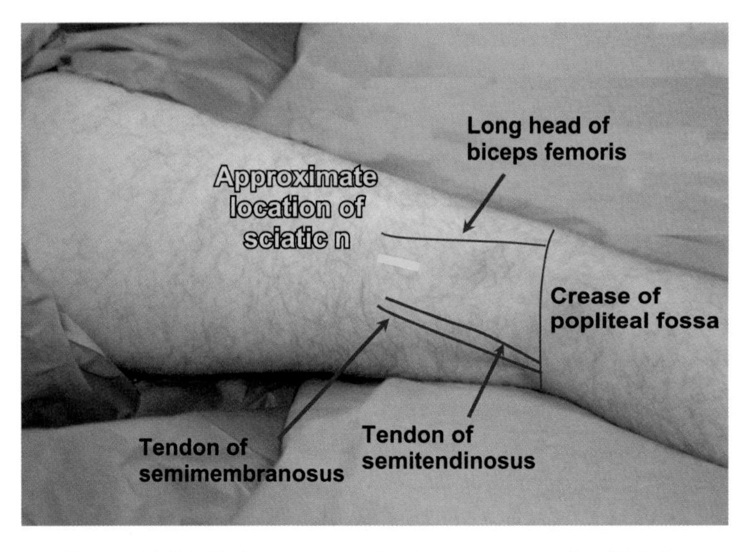

Figure 14.27. Surface anatomy for the posterior popliteal block.

14.5.1.2. *Surface Anatomy*

- Base of popliteal fossa
  - Crease at back of knee
- Lateral side
  - Biceps femoris tendon
- Medial side
  - Semimembranosus tendon (medial to semitendinosus)

The puncture site is often located at the tip of a triangle formed by the popliteal crease at the base and the muscles (above) on the sides. Alternatively, drawing lines 8 cm long in the cephalad direction, from the insertion site of the medial and lateral tendons, the puncture point is at the midpoint of a line attaching the two (almost parallel) lines (Figure 14.27).

14.5.2. Sonographic Imaging and Needle Insertion Technique

The MRI images in Figures 14.28 and 14.29(A–C) show the sciatic nerve and its termination into tibial and common peroneal (fibular) nerves within the popliteal fossa. Figures 14.30 and 14.31 show the ultrasound images of the tibial and common peroneal (fibular) nerves, with emphasis on the distal to proximal course within the popliteal fossa and convergence into the sciatic nerve.

Prepare the needle insertion site and skin surface with an antiseptic solution. Prepare the ultrasound probe surface by applying a sterile adhesive dressing to it prior to needling as discussed earlier (see Chapters 3 and 4). The nerve structures are most visible when the angle of incidence is approximately 90° to the ultrasound beam.

Administering local anesthetic proximal to the bifurcation point of the sciatic nerve is optimal for blocking both components of the nerve with a single injection.

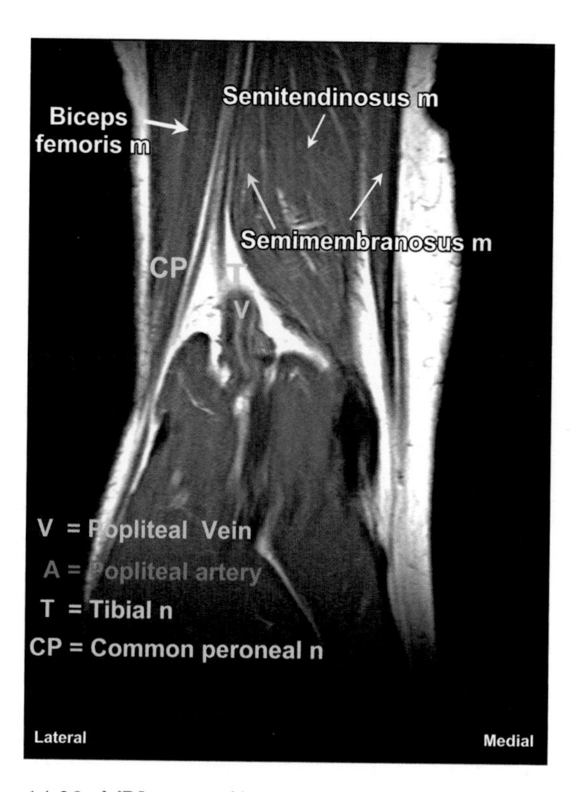

Figure 14.28. MRI image of longitudinal scan showing the popliteal fossa.

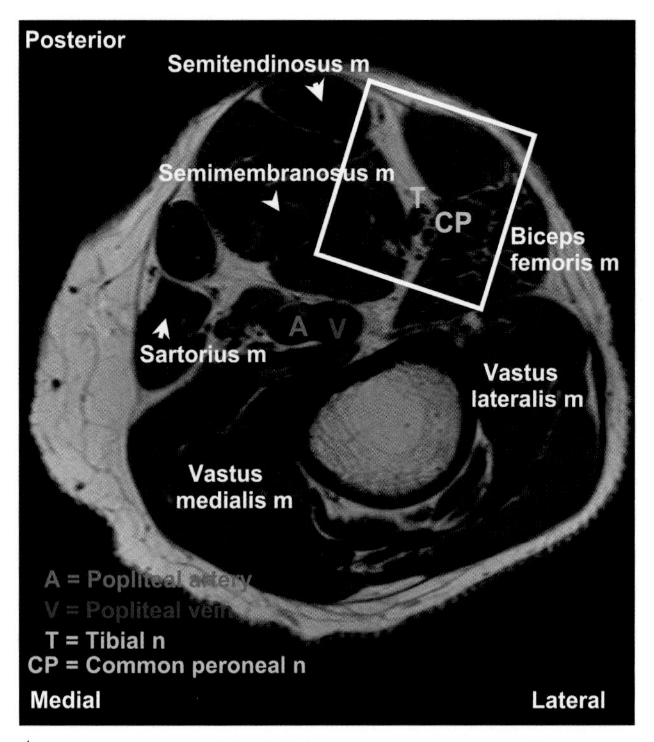

A

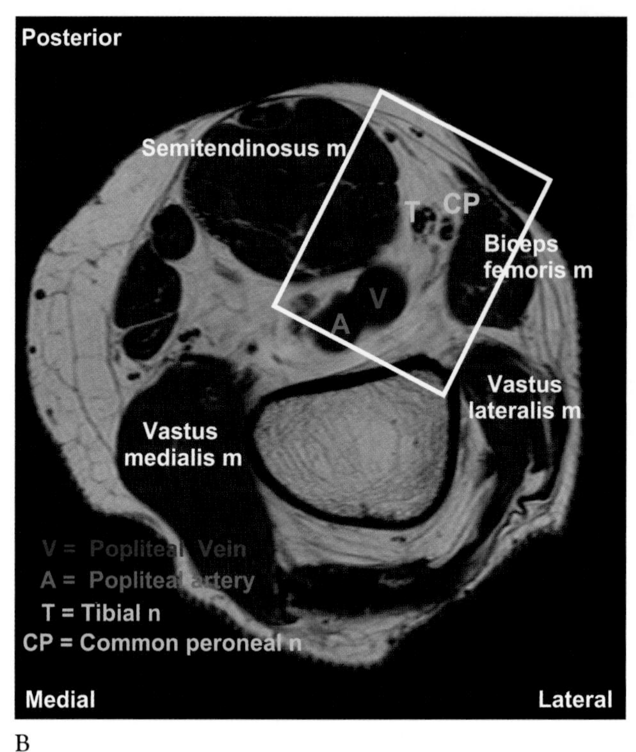

B

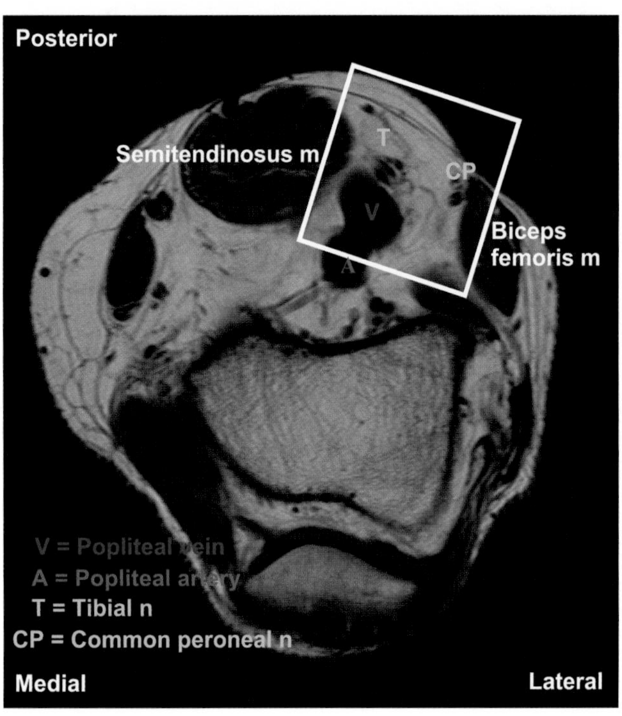

C

Figure 14.29. MRI images of transverse scans at the (A) proximal point of sciatic nerve bifurcation, (B) midlevel in the popliteal fossa, and (C) distal location in the fossa.

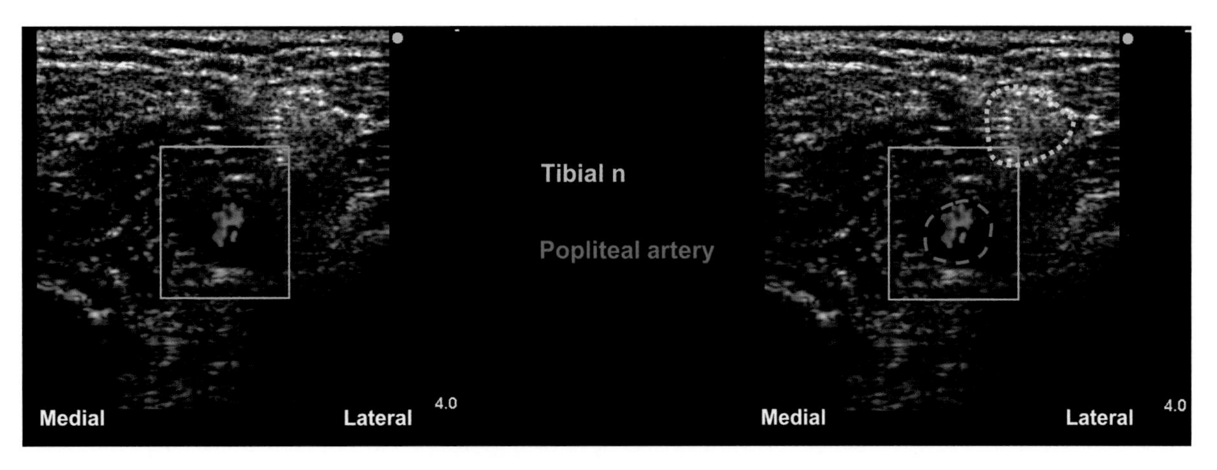

Figure 14.30. Ultrasound image using color Doppler and a linear probe at the popliteal crease.

14.5.2.1. *Scanning Technique*

- A linear higher frequency 10- to 15-MHz probe is commonly used for scanning the sciatic nerve transversely in the popliteal fossa.
- A broadband curved array transducer (4–7 MHz) can be used for patients with a high BMI (depending on the amount of subcutaneous tissue). An OOP needling technique, however, will be more challenging as the needle tip will be harder to view with this curved image.
- The required depth of penetration varies; the general recommendation is to use a higher frequency probe for penetration within 2 to 3 cm and a lower frequency probe for penetration >4 cm.
- If the sciatic nerve is not readily visualized after locating the femur and popliteal vessels, slowly angle the probe in a caudad direction. This often brings the sciatic nerve into view.
- Scan the sciatic nerve along its course to locate the site where it bifurcates into the tibial and peroneal (fibular) components [Figures 14.31(A–C) depict the proximal scan of the tibial and common peroneal nerves].
- The probe may be rotated 90° to show the sciatic nerve in long axis. This is helpful to differentiate the sciatic nerve from other non-neural structures.

14.5.2.2. *Traceback Approach* (see Chapter 4 for Details; Figure 14.31)

- Place the ultrasound probe transversely on the skin surface of the base of the popliteal fossa.
- First identify the popliteal blood vessels in the popliteal fossa. This provides a clearly visible landmark as reference (can easily use color flow Doppler for confirmation; Figure 14.30).
- The small, round hypoechoic tibial nerve can easily be identified lying in the midline, superficial and lateral to the popliteal artery and vein.
- Locate the sciatic nerve by moving the probe in a cephalad direction, tracing proximally along the tibial nerve.
- The ultrasound image changes from that of the distinct lateral common peroneal (fibular) and medial tibial nerves to form one bilobular structure.

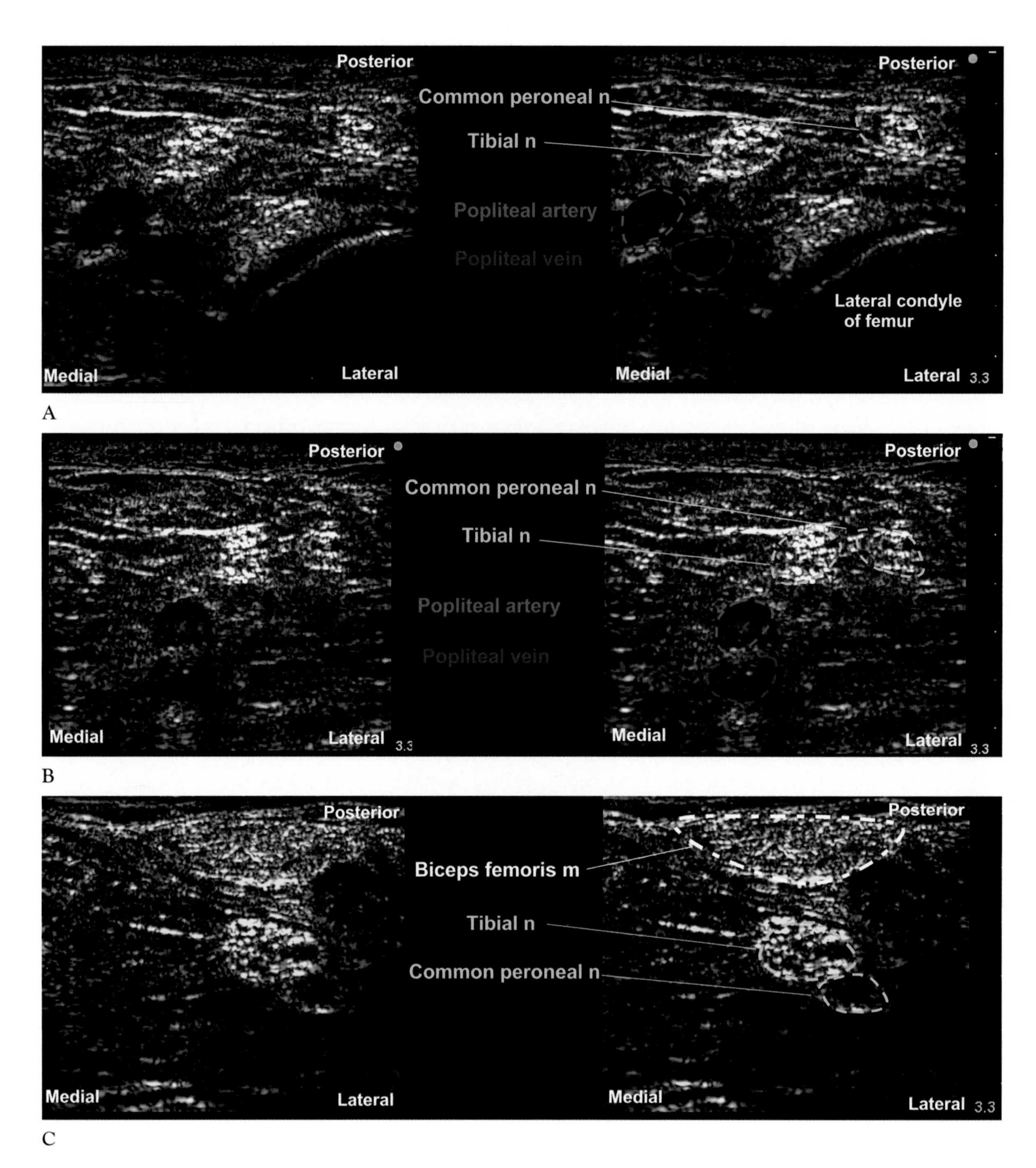

Figure 14.31. Ultrasound images of the tibial and common peroneal nerves during a proximal scan showing (A) the popliteal crease, (B) proximal to the crease as the nerves leave the vessels, and (C) just prior the sciatic nerve bifurcation point.

14.5.2.3. Sonographic Appearance

- At the level of the popliteal crease, the tibial and common peroneal (fibular) nerves lie superficial and lateral to the popliteal vessels (common peroneal nerve is most lateral); both nerves appear round-to-oval and hyperechoic compared to the surrounding musculature [Figure 14.31(A)].
- The nerves often contain small internal hypoechoic areas interspersed between hyperechoic connective tissue (perineurium).

- More cephalad in the posterior thigh, the biceps femoris muscle lies superficial to the nerves and appears as a larger oval-shaped structure with less internal punctuate areas (hypoechoic spots) than the nerves [Figure 14.31(C)].
- Moving the transducer proximally from the popliteal fossa, the sciatic nerve appears as a large round to flat-oval hyperechoic structure (see Figure 14.34).
- The popliteal vessels become deeper and farther away from the tibial nerve, while the common peroneal (fibular) nerve moves toward the tibial nerve forming the sciatic nerve as the scan moves in the proximal direction.

Clinical Pearls

- The sciatic nerve may be difficult to characterize at the apex of the popiteal fossa. Figure 14.31(C) illustrates that the fascicular-appearing biceps femoris muscle and the large sciatic nerve can look similar and may be easily mistaken for each other at this proximal location. It is advisable to use a traceback approach, with a scan from caudad to cephalad along the course of the sciatic nerve terminal components, to confirm and identify the nerve structure at this location (see Chapter 4).
- The traceback approach is very useful for locating the optimal needle insertion site just proximal to the bifurcation of the sciatic nerve. Color Doppler helps to identify the popliteal vessels and to characterize the tibial nerve through the following distinct imaging features while scanning proximally (Figure 14.31).
  - First, the images of surrounding structures (e.g., muscle and other soft tissues) change constantly, whereas the appearance of the tibial nerve remains unchanged.
  - Second, the common peroneal (fibular) nerve can be visualized as it converges with the tibial nerve, forming the sciatic nerve.
  - Third, the popliteal vessels become deeper and farther away from the tibial nerve as the scan moves proximally.
- Some experts suggest that a useful ultrasound sign to confirm localization of the tibial and common peroneal (fibular) nerves is the "seesaw" sign as the nerve components slide up and down when the patient is asked to plantar flex and dorsiflex the foot. However, the value of this sign is often limited as most of the patient's movements have been limited due to their injury.

14.5.2.4. *Needle Insertion Technique*

- Depending on the skin-to-nerve distance, use a 5- to 8-cm, 22-ga insulated (if using nerve stimulation) needle.
- Both the IP and OOP approaches (see Chapter 4) are appropriate for ultrasound-guided sciatic nerve block in this region (Figures 14.32 and 14.33).
- For placement of an indwelling catheter, it is common to perform an OOP needling approach:
  - Position the probe directly above the sciatic nerve at or slightly cephalad to its bifurcation point and place the nerve in the center of the image.
  - Insert the needle at the caudal surface of probe, with the needle tip contacting the skin approximately 2 to 4 cm caudal to the probe surface.
    - The needle puncture site is usually 5 to 7 cm proximal to the popliteal crease and slightly lateral to the midline.
  - Insert the needle in an incremental walk down manner (see Chapter 4) in order to track the needle tip.
  - The block needle is advanced to contact either side of the sciatic nerve; nerve contact is indicated by nerve movement (often two injections are required). Needle placement can be further confirmed by electrical stimulation.

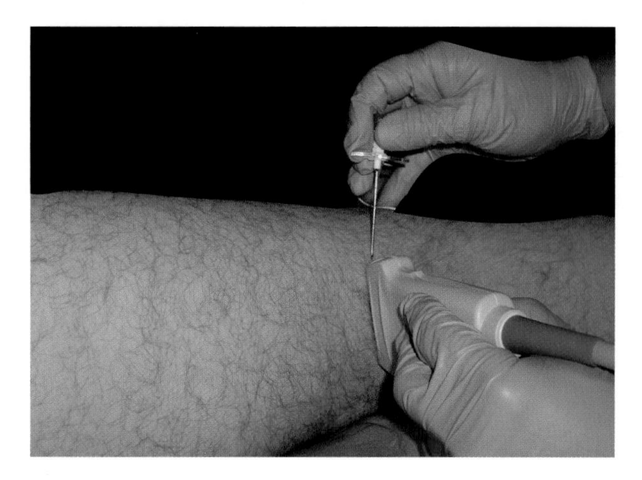

Figure 14.32. Needling technique using a linear probe and an in-plane (IP) needle alignment at the sciatic nerve bifurcation point.

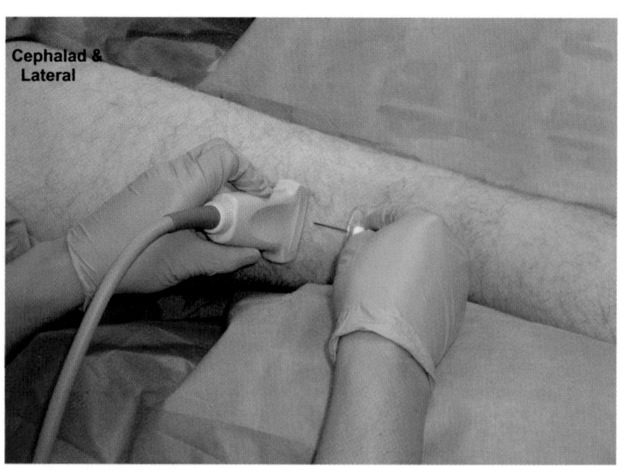

Figure 14.33. Needling technique using a linear probe and out-of-plane (OOP) needling alignment with a needle insertion in a caudad-to-cepalad direction.

14.5.3. Nerve Stimulation

Common motor responses to confirm nerve contact through electrical stimulation are summarized in Table 14.5. Recommended needle adjustments are listed in relation to common responses during the procedure.

Table 14.5. Responses and recommended needle adjustments for use with nerve stimulation during the posterior popliteal approach.

Correct Response from Nerve Stimulation

Twitches (visible or palpable) in the foot or toes with 0.3 to 0.5 mA current. Either a common peroneal (fibular) or tibial nerve response may result and both indicate correct needle positioning even slightly below the sciatic nerve bifurcation as the large volume of local anesthetic will spread within the sheath. The common peroneal (fibular) response is ankle dorsiflexion and eversion; the tibial is ankle plantar flexion and inversion. If eliciting a response is difficult in this current range, 0.7 mA may be used reliably with a tibial nerve response.

Other Common Responses and Necessary Needle Adjustment

- Muscle twitches from electrical stimulation
  - Biceps femoris (local twitch)
    - *Explanation:* Needle placement too lateral
    - *Needle Adjustment:* Withdraw needle completely and reinsert slightly more medial
  - Semimembranosus or semitendinosus (local twitch)
    - *Explanation*: Needle placement too medial
    - *Needle Adjustment*: Withdraw needle completely and reinsert slightly more laterally
  - Calf muscles without foot or toe movement (muscular branches of sciatic nerve)
    - *Explanation:* Needle probably too superficial
    - *Needle Adjustment:* Continue advancement
- Bone contact
  - Femur
    - *Explanation*: Needle tip advanced too deeply
    - *Needle Adjustment*: Withdraw needle to look for response at more superficial location; withdraw if not seen
- Vascular puncture
  - Popliteal artery or vein
    - *Explanation*: Needle tip too medial
    - *Needle Adjustment:* Withdraw completely and reinsert at slightly more lateral position

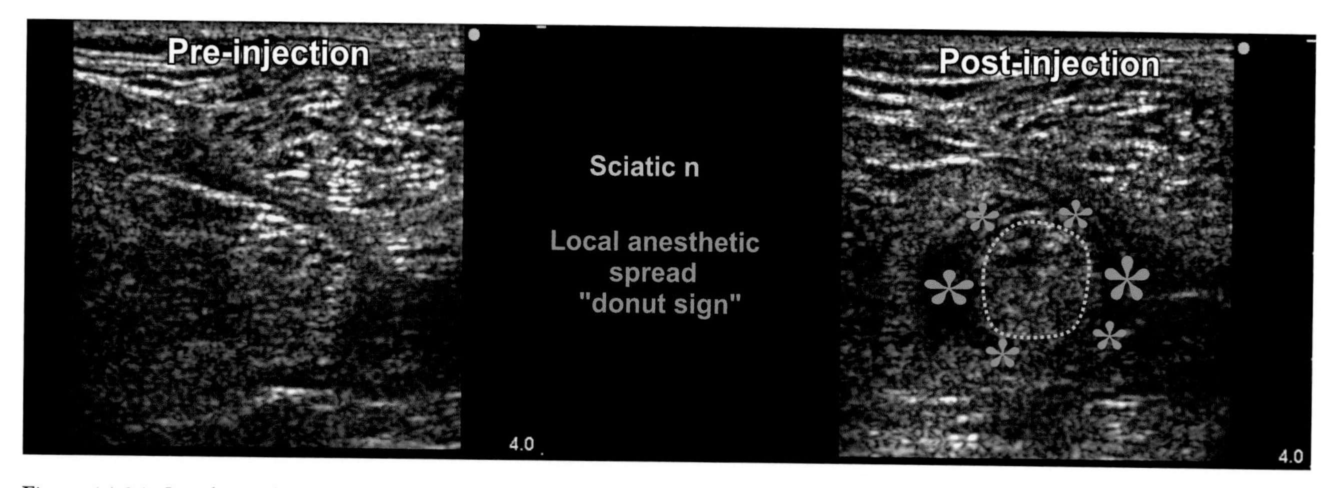

Figure 14.34. Local anesthetic application to the sciatic nerve at the posterior popliteal location; the hypoechogenicity appears in a complete circumferential fashion ("donut" sign), which often requires two separate injections.

14.5.4. Local Anesthetic Application

Nerve stimulation is recommended to confirm needle placement prior to local anesthetic application. Performing a test dose with D5W is recommended prior to local anesthetic application to visualize the spread and confirm nerve localization (see Chapter 4 sidebar).

- The correct response to proper injection is an expansion of hypoechoic fluid completely around the hyperechoic nerve structure and a "donut" sign (Figure 14.34); two separate injections (medial and lateral) may be required for complete circumferential spread.
- Occasionally, the two sciatic nerve components appear more distinct after injection (Figure 14.35).

Clinical Pearls

- Circumferential spread of local anesthetic seen within the sheath may indicate a block of quick onset and good quality.
- This is often achieved by two separate injections (medial and lateral) around the nerve.

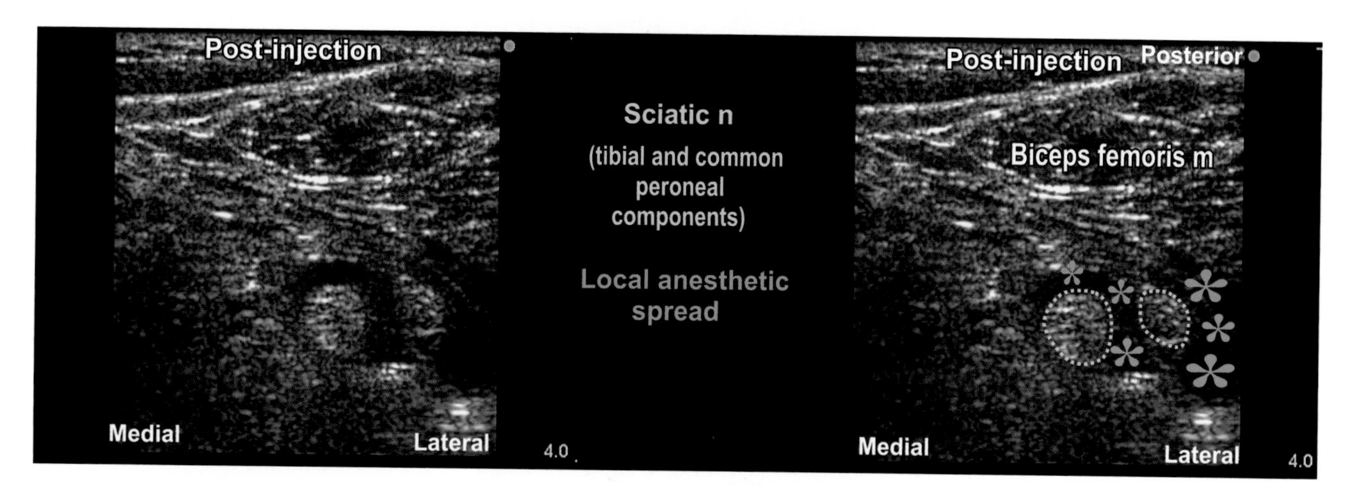

Figure 14.35. Local anesthetic application to the sciatic nerve with postinjection illumination of the two components (tibial and common peroneal) of the nerve.

14.6. Popliteal Sciatic Nerve Block (Lateral Approach)

14.6.1. Patient Positioning and Surface Anatomy

14.6.1.1. Patient Positioning

The patient lies supine with the leg elevated on a large foam pillow to allow sufficient room for ultrasound probe manipulation on the posterior surface of the thigh. Alternatively, the patient lies semiprone. Foot and knee movement should be possible to facilitate nerve stimulation. The landmarks can be accentuated by asking the patient to support the leg off the table, with the knee extended.

14.6.1.2. Surface Anatomy (Figure 14.36)

- Anterolateral
  - Vastus lateralis muscle
- Posterolateral
  - Biceps femoris muscle
- Caudal
  - Lateral epicondyle of femur

14.6.2. Sonographic Imaging and Needle Insertion Technique

The popliteal approach to the sciatic nerve can be challenging because the sciatic nerve divides at a variable level in the posterior thigh. Ultrasound may increase the accuracy of nerve localization and thus improve the success rate of this approach. With ultrasound guidance, there is no need to estimate nerve depth by first contacting the femur. A single needle pass is often adequate.

With the lateral approach (essentially IP approach), the needle and probe are not in contact, which may be advantageous as sterility with the probe will not be as critical.

Prepare the needle insertion site and skin surface with an antiseptic solution. Prepare the ultrasound probe surface by applying a sterile adhesive dressing to it prior to needling as discussed earlier (see Chapters 3 and 4).

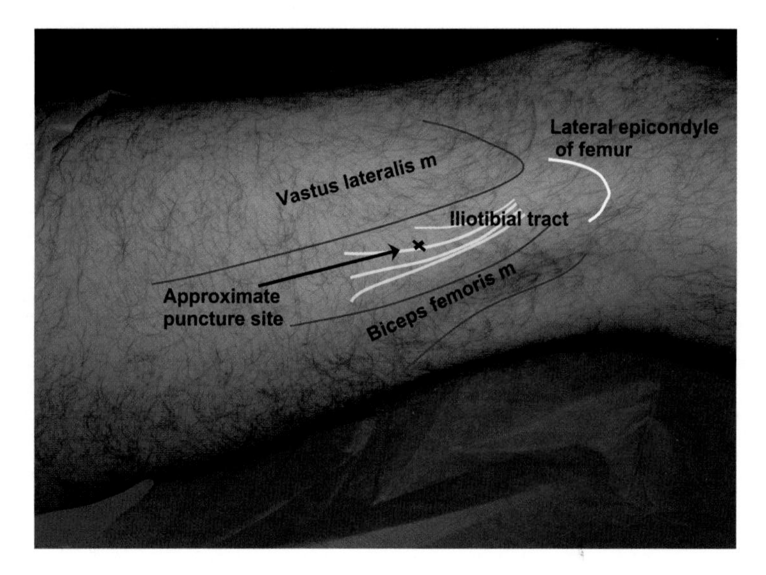

Figure 14.36. Surface anatomy for the lateral popliteal block.

14.6.2.1. *Scanning Technique*

- The scanning technique is essentially the same as the one described for the posterior approach.
- Obtain a short-axis view of the sciatic nerve proximal to its bifurcation point, with a high-frequency linear probe if possible.
- Manipulate the transducer until the tibial and common peroneal (fibular) components are seen (see Section 14.5 for details on how to localize the sciatic, tibial, and common peroneal nerves).

14.6.2.2. *Sonographic Appearance*

- Similar to the posterior approach, round hyperechoic images of the nerves are seen deep to the subcutaneous tissue and muscle (Figures 14.30 and 14.31).
- The traceback method, described in detail in Chapter 4, is very helpful to find the two nerves as they merge together (also see Section 14.5 for details on how to localize the sciatic, tibial, and common peroneal nerves).

14.6.2.3. *Needle Insertion Technique*

- This approach is an IP technique, but the probe and needle are separate from each other (not in contact), with the probe on the posterior and the needle on the lateral thigh (Figure 14.37).
- Insert a 5- to 8-cm insulated needle at the lateral aspect of the leg, at the depth indicated by ultrasound.
  - The approximate puncture location will be in line with the prominence of the lateral epicondyle and at a location approximately 7 to 8 cm above the popliteal crease.
  - The needle puncture site is typically 2 to 4 cm anterior to the probe.
  - The needle is inserted parallel to the probe and in the groove between the vastus lateralis and bicep femoris muscles.
  - The needle is directed with a posterior angle to reach the sciatic nerve, often going through the bicep femoris muscle.
- Move the transducer with fine adjustments to view the needle trajectory.

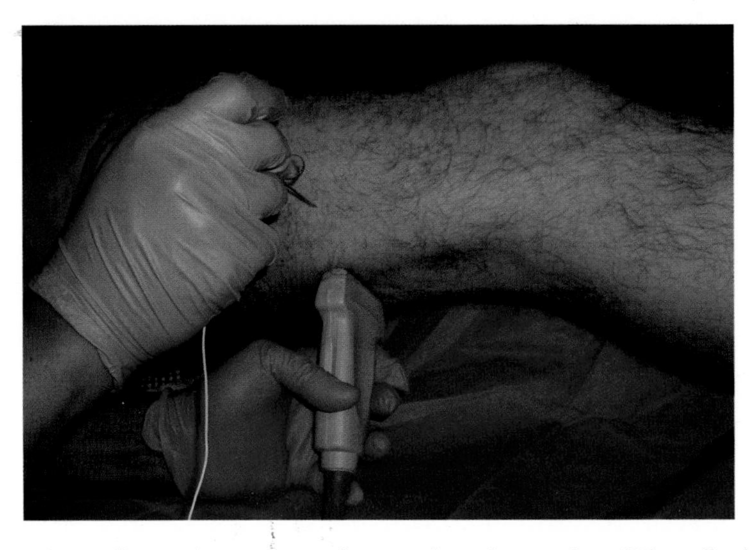

Figure 14.37. Needling technique using a linear probe and an in-plane (IP) needle alignment.

Clinical Pearls

- Good eye–hand coordination is more demanding for this approach.
- Patient sedation is often necessary to decrease procedural-related discomfort because the block needle often penetrates the biceps femoris muscle to reach the sciatic nerve.
- This approach can be difficult for beginners as the needle and probe are placed in completely separate locations (i.e., probe at posterior aspect and the needle at lateral aspect).

14.6.3. Nerve Stimulation

Common motor responses associated with nerve stimulation are described in Table 14.6. Other responses are characterized, with recommendations for needle adjustment included.

14.6.4. Local Anesthetic Application

- Performing a test dose with D5W is recommended prior to local anesthetic application to visualize the spread and confirm nerve localization (see Chapter 4 sidebar).
- Gray, Huczko, and Schafhalter-Zoppoth (2004) describe using a V-shaped redirection of the block needle to place local anesthetic on both the anterior and posterior sides of the nerves.
- Applying local anesthetic circumferentially around the sciatic nerve is important.

Table 14.6. Responses and recommended needle adjustments for use with nerve stimulation during the lateral popliteal approach.

Correct Response from Nerve Stimulation

- Twitches (visible or palpable) in the foot or toes at 0.3 to 0.5 mA current.
- It is common to encounter a biceps femoris twitch at a location superficial to the sciatic nerve. Once this ceases, proceed slowly and the sciatic response should be detected at about 2 cm beyond this location.
- With this approach, it is common to stimulate the common peroneal portion (i.e., dorsiflexion) of the sciatic nerve first.

Other Common Responses and Necessary Needle Adjustment

- Muscle twitches from electrical stimulation
  - Biceps femoris (local twitch)
    - *Explanation:* Needle placement too superficial
    - *Needle Adjustment:* Advance needle slowly, approximately 2 cm
  - Vastus lateralis (local twitch)
    - *Explanation*: Needle placement too anterior
    - *Needle Adjustment*: Withdraw needle completely and reinsert slightly more posterior
  - Calf muscles without foot or toe movement (muscular branches of sciatic nerve)
    - *Explanation:* Needle probably too superficial
    - *Needle Adjustment:* Continue advancement
- Vascular puncture
  - Popliteal artery or vein
    - *Explanation*: Needle tip too deep and anterior
    - *Needle Adjustment:* Withdraw completely and reinsert posteriorly with less depth
- Bone contact
  - Femur
    - *Explanation*: Needle tip too anterior and deep
    - *Needle Adjustment:* Withdraw completely and reinsert at slightly more posterior location

Suggested Reading and References

Chan VWS. The use of ultrasound for peripheral nerve blocks. In: Boezaart AP, ed. Anesthesia and orthopaedic surgery. New York: McGraw-Hill; 2006; pp. 283–290.

Chan VWS, Nova H, Abbas S, McCartney CJL, Perlas A, Xu D. Ultrasound examination and localization of the sciatic nerve: a volunteer study. Anesthesiology 2006;104:309–314.

Elstraete V, Poey C, Lebrun T, Pastureau F. New landmarks for the anterior approach to the sciatic nerve block: imaging and clinical study. Anesth Analg 2002;95:214–218.

Gray AT, Huczko EL, Schafhalter-Zoppoth I. Lateral popliteal nerve block with ultrasound guidance [letter]. Reg Anesth Pain Med 2004;29:507–509.

Jan van Geffen G, Gielen M. Ultrasound-guided subgluteal sciatic nerve blocks with stimulating catheters in children: a descriptive study. Anesth Analg 2006;103:328–333.

Ricci S. Ultrasound observation of the sciatic nerve and its branches at the popliteal fossa: always visible, never seen. Eur J Vasc Endovasc Surg 2005;30:659–663.

Sites BD, Gallagher JD, Tomek I, et al. The use of magnetic resonance imaging to evaluate the accuracy of a handheld ultrasound machine in localizing the sciatic nerve in the popliteal fossa. Reg Anesth Pain Med 2004;29:413–416.

15

Ankle Blocks

Ban C.H. Tsui

Ultrasound guidance may be most useful for blocking the posterior tibial and deep peroneal (fibular) nerves as their location can be easily identified next to reliable landmarks (i.e., bones and vessels) that are clearly visible. The sural, superficial peroneal, and saphenous nerves can be blocked reliably in the usual manner without ultrasound guidance.

15.1. Clinical Anatomy

- Deep nerves at the ankle (Figures 15.1 and 15.2)
  - Deep peroneal (fibular): originates from L5, S1; lies anterior to the tibia and interosseous membrane and lateral to the anterior tibial artery and vein at the ankle; is deep to and between the tendons of the extensor hallucis longus and extensor digitorum longus muscles; beyond the extensor retinaculum it branches into medial and lateral terminal branches.
    - The medial branch passes over the dorsum of the foot and supplies the first web space through two terminal digital branches.
    - The lateral branch traverses laterally and terminates as the second, third, and fourth dorsal digital nerves.
  - Tibial nerve (often called posterior tibial nerve): originates from S1 to S3; on the posterior aspect of the knee joint, it joins the posterior tibial artery and then runs deep until the lower third of the leg, where it emerges at the medial border of the calcaneal tendon (Achilles tendon).

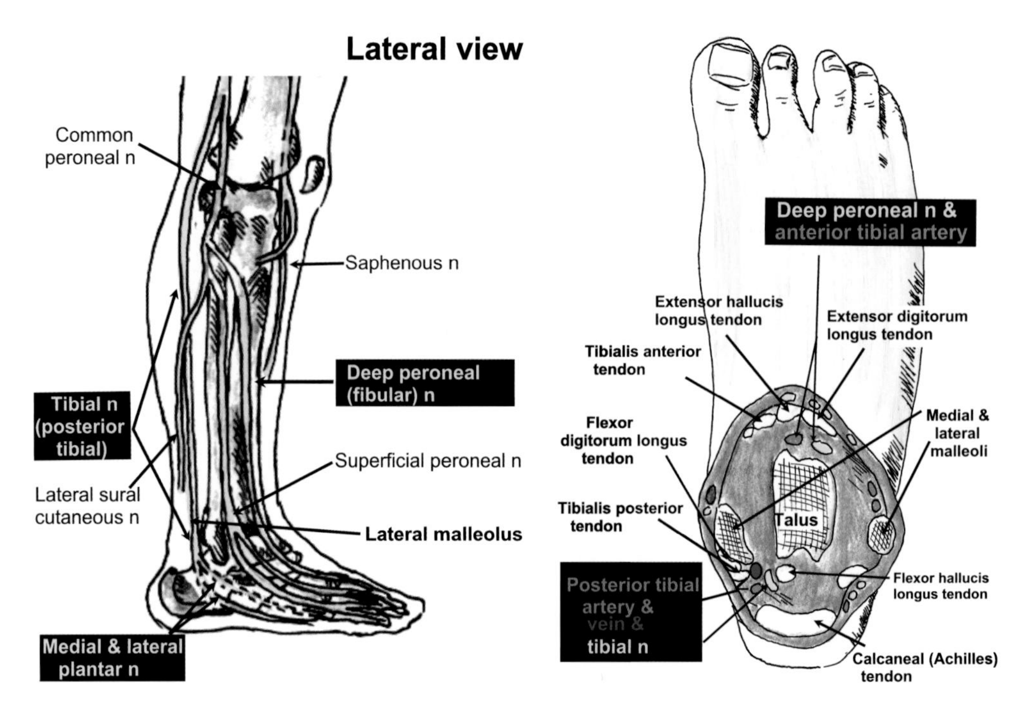

Figure 15.1. Peripheral nerves of the leg and foot.

Figure 15.2. Cross-section at the ankle.

- Behind the medial malleolus it lies beneath several layers of fascia and is separated from the Achilles tendon only by the tendon of the flexor hallucis longus muscle; the nerve is posteromedial to the posterior tibial artery and vein, which in turn are posteromedial to the tendons of the flexor digitorum longus and tibialis posterior muscles (Figure 15.3).
- Just below the medial malleolus, the nerve divides into the lateral and medial plantar nerves.
- The nerve innervates the ankle joint through its articular branches and the skin over the medial malleolus, the inner aspect of the heel (including Achilles tendon),

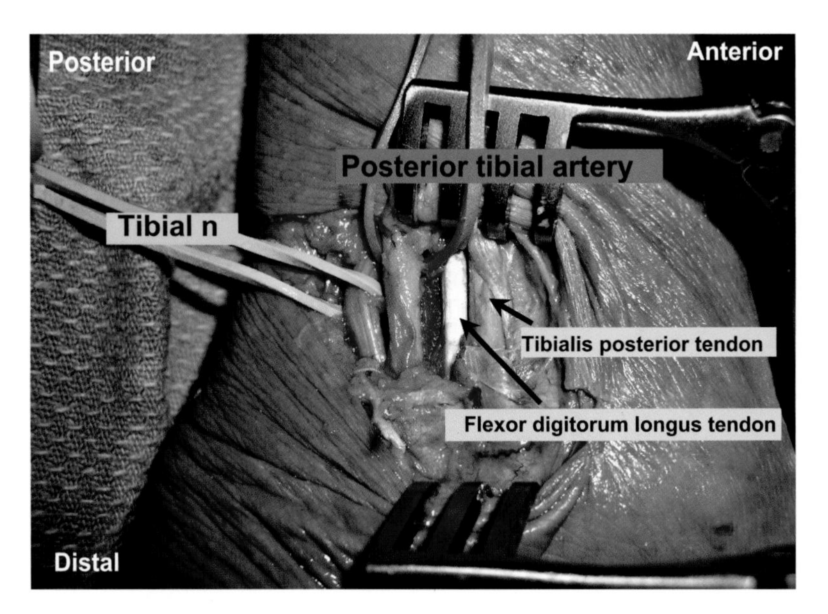

Figure 15.3. Dissection at the medial surface of the ankle.

Table 15.1. Terminal nerves of the sacral plexus blocked at the ankle: origin and motor responses associated with nerve stimulation.

Movement	Nerve	Root
Ankle and toe extension	Deep peroneal	L5 & S1
Foot eversion (peroneus longus and brevis)	Superficial peroneal	L5 & S1
First toe abduction	Medial plantar (tibial)	S1, 2
Fifth toe abduction	Lateral plantar (tibial)	S1, 2, 3

and the dorsum of the foot (through the medial and lateral plantar nerves) with its cutaneous branches.

Chapter 14 provides some detail regarding the superficial nerves at the ankle. Table 15.1 summarizes the origin of the terminal nerves of the sacral plexus that are targets of the ankle blocks and the related movements.

15.2. Patient Positioning and Surface Anatomy

15.2.1. Patient Positioning

The patient lies supine with the foot extended beyond the footrest. Dorsiflexion of the foot will bring the deep peroneal (fibular) nerve into a more superficial position between the prominent extensor hallucis longus and extensor digitorum longus tendons. Identification of the (posterior) tibial nerve does not require any particular positioning as it can be located by palpating its accompanying artery.

15.2.2. Surface Anatomy

- Tibial (posterior tibial) (Figure 15.4)
  - Medial malleolus
  - Flexor digitorum longus and tibialis posterior tendons lie anterior to the nerve
- Deep peroneal (fibular) (Figure 15.5)
  - Extensor hallucis longus tendon, coursing straight towards the big toe
  - Extensor digitorum longus tendon, just lateral to the extensor hallucis longus tendon and coursing towards the second and third toes

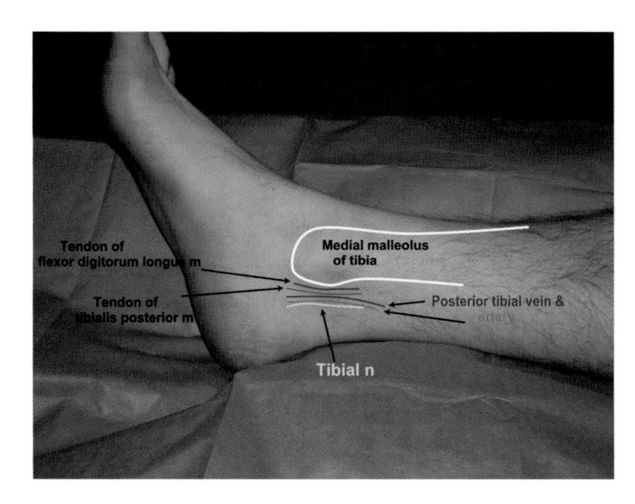

Figure 15.4. Surface anatomy for the tibial nerve block.

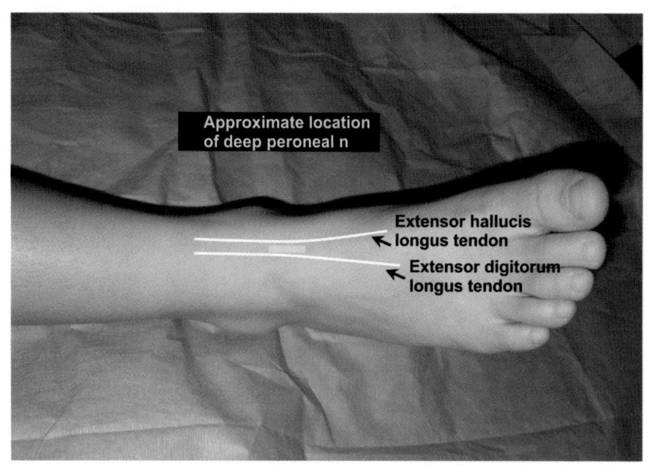

Figure 15.5. Surface anatomy for the deep peroneal nerve block.

15.3. Sonographic Imaging and Needle Insertion Technique

Figure 15.6 shows a magnetic resonance imaging (MRI) scan of the medial and lateral plantar branches of the (posterior) tibial nerve taken at the medial aspect of the ankle distally. The ultrasound images in Figure 15.7(A,B) represent probe placement at (a) the medial malleolus (prior to the branching point of the tibial nerve) and (b) proximally about 3 to 5 cm. The block should be performed at a point before the nerve divides to ensure block completeness. The ultrasound images in Figure 15.8(A,B), taken at distal and proximal sites, will assist with ultrasound scanning for the deep peroneal (fibular) block.

Prepare the needle insertion site and skin surface with an antiseptic solution. Prepare the ultrasound probe surface by applying a sterile adhesive dressing to it prior to needling as discussed earlier (see Chapters 3 and 4).

15.3.1. Scanning Technique

- Tibial (posterior tibial)
  - Position a linear ("hockey stick") 10-MHz probe with a small footprint in transverse (short) axis to the nerve just posterior and inferior to the medial malleolus.
  - Alternatively, the nerve can be identified 3 to 5 cm above the malleolus.
  - Color Doppler is helpful to localize the nerve at the above locations, with the nerve posterior and deep to the posterior tibial artery at both (Figure 15.7).
  - Localize the nerve before it branches into the medial and lateral plantar nerves (Figure 15.6).
- Deep peroneal (fibular)
  - Position a small footprint linear ("hockey stick") 10-MHz probe in transverse (short) axis to the nerve at the anterior surface of the ankle joint. Alternatively, the nerve can also be found 3 to 5 cm above the ankle joint. However, the nerve itself can be difficult to see and only the artery can be consistently located.

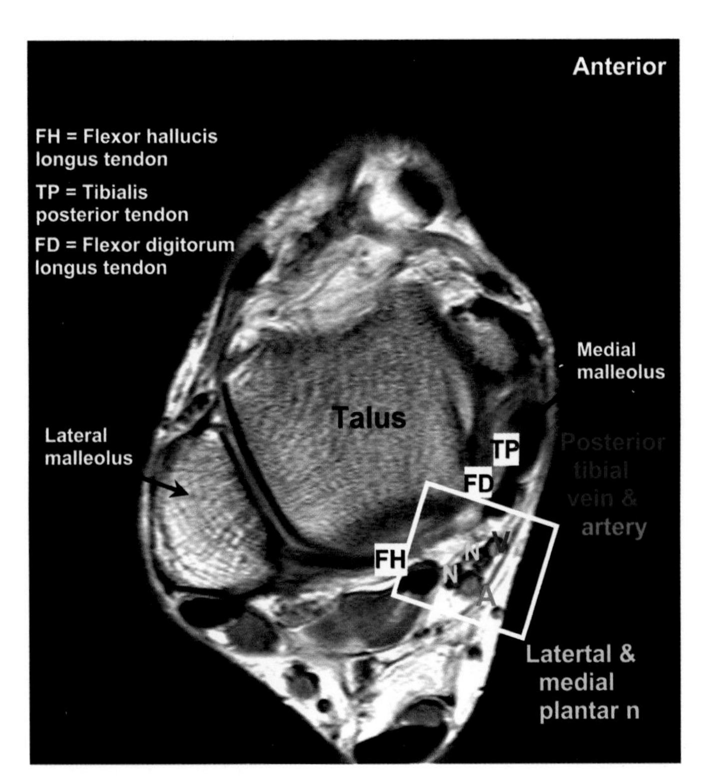

Figure 15.6. MRI image from transverse scan at the ankle showing the terminal nerves (medial and lateral plantar) of the tibial nerve.

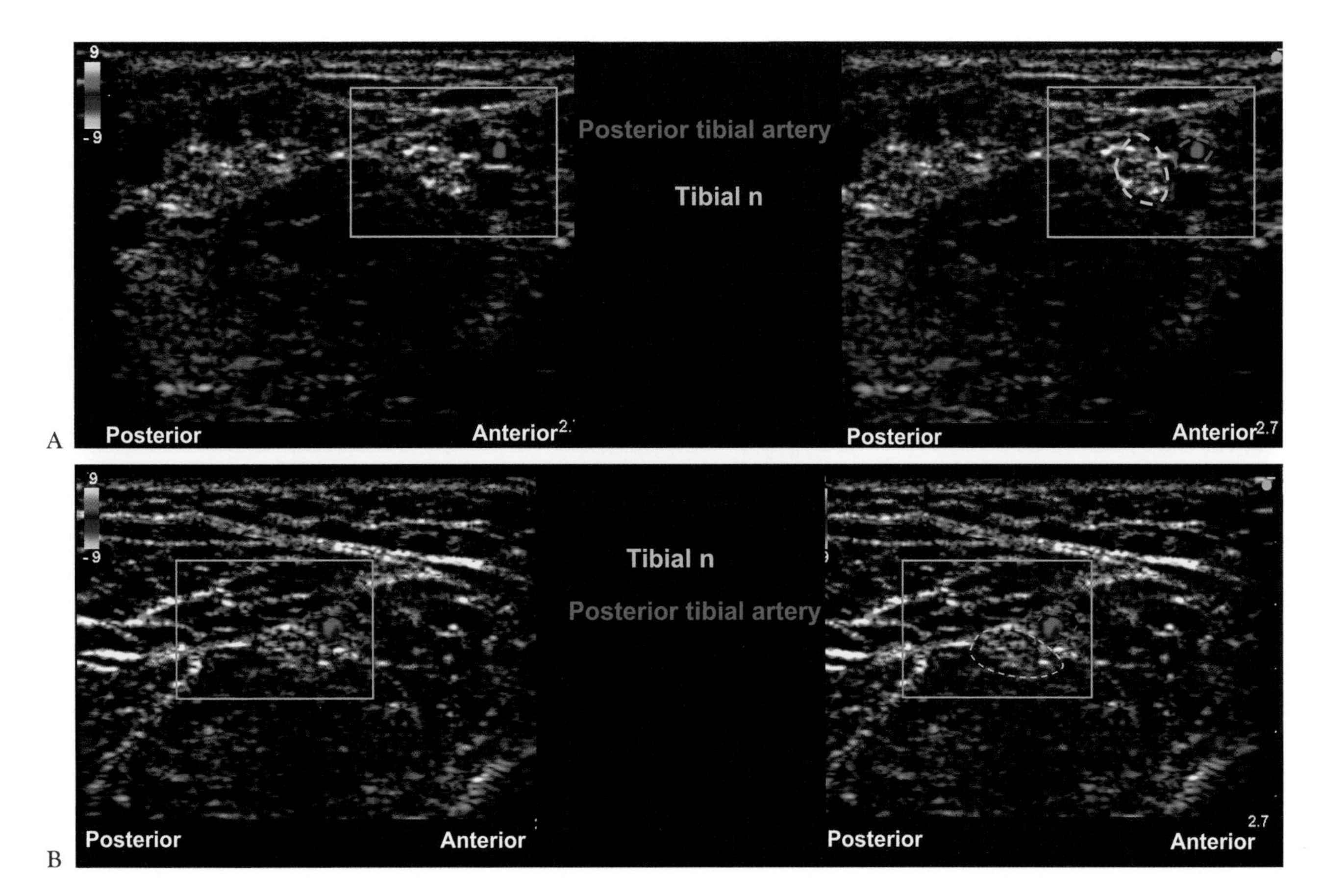

Figure 15.7. Ultrasound image from scanning the medial ankle in a transverse plane at the levels of (A) the medial malleolus and (B) 3 to 5 cm proximally. Occasionally, it may be difficult to identify the tibial nerve at the ankle level. However, it can be confirmed as it remains posterior to the artery when traced back proximally.

- Color Doppler can be used at both locations to illuminate the anterior tibial artery lying medial to the nerve (Figure 15.8).

15.3.2. Sonographic Appearance

- Tibial (posterior tibial) (Figure 15.7)
  - The mass of fascial tissue and tendons at the medial malleolus area may make the identification of the nerve difficult; color Doppler illumination of the posterior tibial vessels [Figure 15.7(A)] will be of assistance.
  - Immediately anterior to the artery lies the hypoechoic circular posterior tibial vein; this may be compressed and not apparent on the screen.
  - Posterior to the artery, the nerve appears slightly more hyperechoic than the surrounding tissues and looks like a condensed honeycomb-appearing structure.
  - Superficial to the neurovascular bundle lies striated appearing and hyperechoic connective tissue including the flexor retinaculum.
  - At the proximal (3–5 cm proximal to the ankle joint) location, the nerve will be in the same position relative to the artery and vein and color Doppler will be helpful [Figure 15.7(B)].
- Deep peroneal (fibular)
  - Similarly to the tibial nerve, color Doppler helps to identify the anterior tibial artery lying medial and deep to the deep peroneal nerve at the ankle joint [Figure 15.8(A)] and proximally [Figure 15.8(B)].

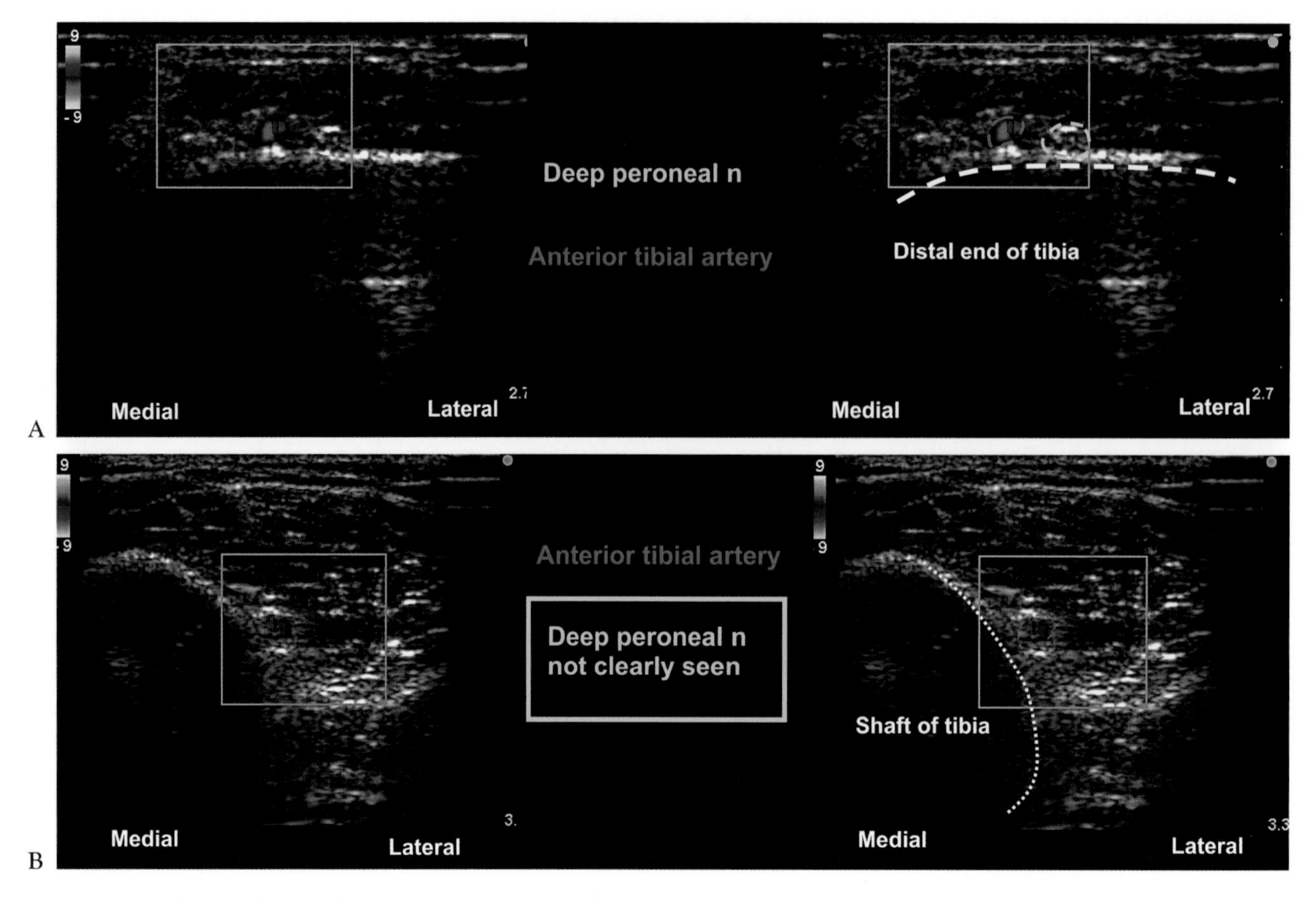

Figure 15.8. Ultrasound image from scanning anterior ankle in transverse axis at the level of (A) the anterior ankle deep to the superior extensor retinaculum and (B) 3 to 5cm proximally. The deep peroneal nerve may be difficult to visualize at both locations.

- Both artery and vein (if seen) appear hypoechoic.
- The nerve appears as a small cluster of hyperechoic fascicular-appearing fibers immediately lateral to the artery, with both adjacent to the well-demarcated distal end of the tibia. However, the nerve itself can be difficult to see and only the artery can be consistently located easily.

15.3.3. Needle Insertion Technique

- Tibial (posterior tibial)
  - Insert a 3.5- to 5-cm insulated needle either out-of-plane (OOP) and distal (Figure 15.9) or in-plane (IP) and posterior (Figure 15.10) to the transversely positioned probe.
- Deep peroneal (fibular)
  - Insert a 3.5- to 5-cm insulated needle either OOP and distal (Figure 15.9) or IP and lateral [Figure 15.11(A,B)] to the transversely positioned small footprint probe at either the anterior ankle or distal leg.

Clinical Pearls

- Due to the limited and compact space at the ankle, OOP needling approaches are easier to perform than IP approaches.
- Alternatively, the probe can scanned proximally 3 to 4cm cephalad to the ankle and either IP or OOP needling may be possible.

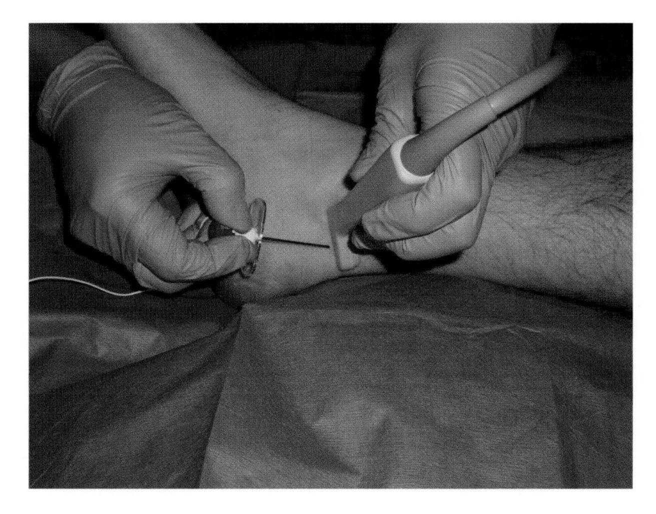

Figure 15.9. Needling technique for the tibial nerve using a small footprint ("hockey stick") probe with an out-of-plane (OOP) needle alignment in a cephalad direction.

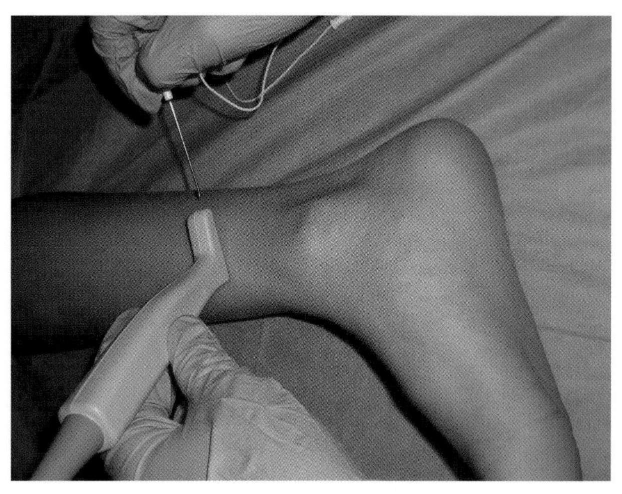

Figure 15.10. Needling technique for the tibial nerve using a small footprint ("hockey stick") probe with an in-plane (IP) needle alignment at a proximal location.

15.4. Nerve Stimulation

- Nerve stimulation is rarely used clinically for ankle blocks; however, the two deep nerves (tibial and deep peroneal) can theoretically be identified with nerve stimulation as follows:
  - Correct motor responses during the (posterior) tibial and deep peroneal (fibular) blocks will be (1) twitches of the first (medial plantar branch) and fifth (lateral plantar branch) toes with the (posterior) tibial and (2) toe extension with the deep peroneal.
  - Twitches of the ankle and foot (dorsiflexion, extension, or inversion) may be unreliable as they may indicate local muscle twitches from the respective tendons in the medial and anterior regions in the foot.
  - Contact with bone indicates that needle placement is too deep; withdraw the needle and localize by ultrasound prior to repeating nerve stimulation.

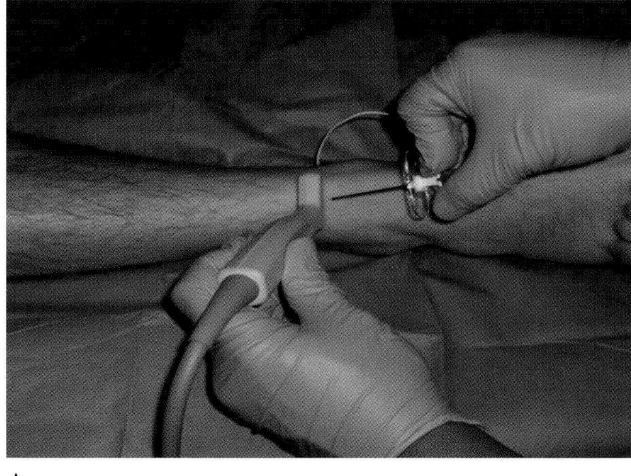

A

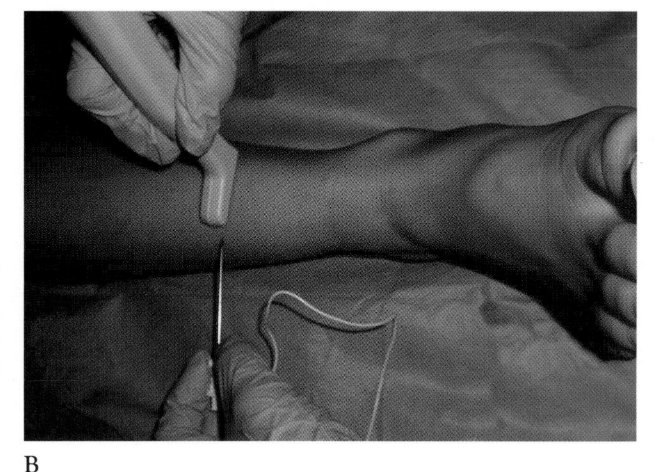

B

Figure 15.11. Needling technique for the deep peroneal nerve using a small footprint probe and (A) an OOP needle alignment in a cephalad direction and (B) an IP needle alignment at a proximal location.

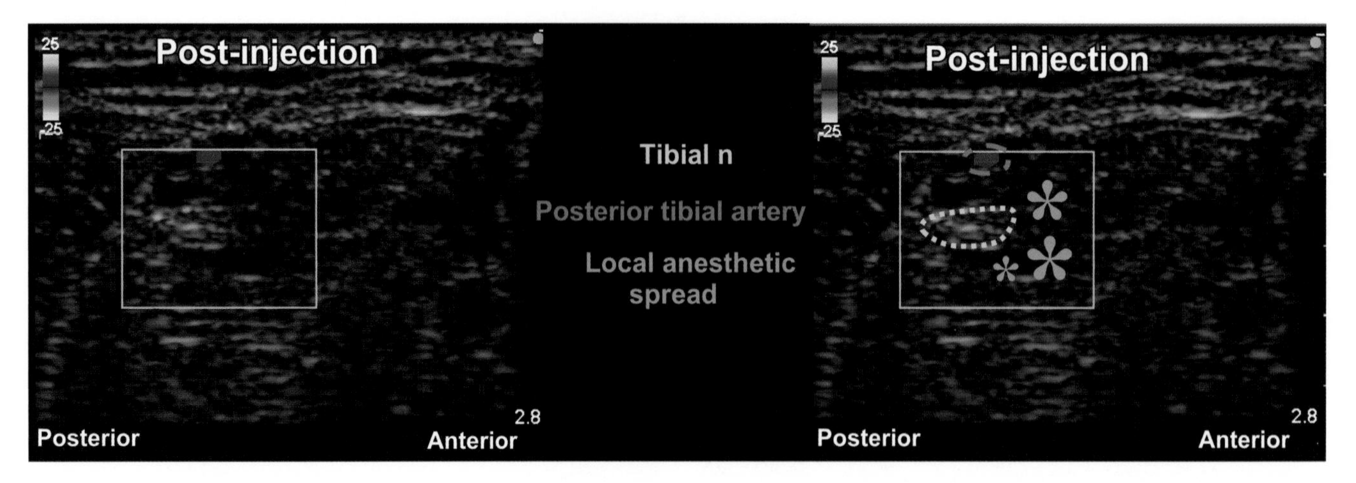

Figure 15.12. Local anesthetic application during a tibial nerve block 3 cm above the ankle. After local anesthestic injection posterior to the artery, the nerve is seen to move to a slightly deeper location with respect to the artery.

15.5. Local Anesthetic Application

- Ultrasound guidance may alleviate the need for both needle contact to the bone and a multiple fan injection technique as with blind approaches to the blocks.
- Performing a test dose with dextrose 5% in water (D5W) is recommended prior to local anesthetic application to visualize the spread (see Chapter 4 sidebar).
- Inject 4 to 5 mL of local anesthetic next to the nerve.
  - With an OOP technique, the local anesthetic can be applied posterior and deep to the (posterior) tibial nerve and lateral to the deep peroneal (fibular) nerve in order to avoid the arteries.
  - During an IP technique at the (posterior) tibial location, it is important to avoid the posterior tibial artery by placing the needle tip deep and posterior to the artery.
- Local anesthetic appears as a hypoechoic collection around the nerves and may separate the nerves from their adjacent artery (Figures 15.12 and 15.13).

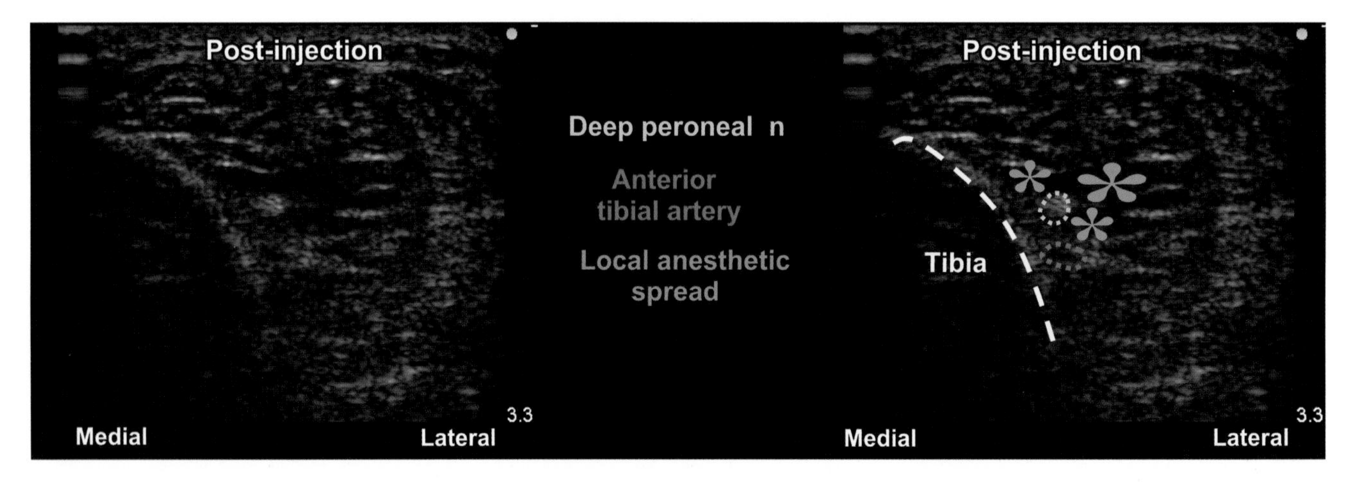

Figure 15.13. Local anesthetic application during a deep peroneal nerve block 3 cm above the ankle. The nerve can also be difficult to visualize prior to injection, but is expected to be lateral to the artery. After injection of local anesthetic lateral to the artery, the nerve is seen to be pushed up from a lateral location to a slightly anterior position with respect to the artery.

Suggested Reading and Reference

Silvestri E, Martinoli C, Derchi LE, Bertolotto M, Chiaramondia M, Rosenberg I. Echotexture of peripheral nerves: correlation between US and histologic findings and criteria to differentiate tendons. Radiology 1995;197:291–296.

16

Regional Block Catheter Insertion Using Ultrasonography and Stimulating Catheters

Sugantha Ganapathy

16.1. Introduction

Continuous catheter regional anesthesia has been well documented to provide excellent quality of pain relief, with reduced incidence of side effects, and an improved quality of life. Traditionally, catheters are introduced blindly after the neural structures are identified using the peripheral nerve stimulator and the initial local anesthetic dose is injected via the needle. This method has been associated with at least 20% to 40% secondary block failure, due to the catheters being in a suboptimal location. This high failure rate resulted in the development of stimulating catheters to aid in positioning the catheters close to the nerve, thus resulting in improved success. Stimulating catheter insertion requires technical expertise and increased time to achieve ideal positioning. Needle insertion with stimulating catheters is still a blind procedure with the aid of neurostimulation and anatomical landmarks.

Recently, ultrasonography is being used extensively to initiate regional blocks. In a recent abstract we documented shorter insertion times, with improved primary block success and reduced secondary catheter failure rates, using ultrasound-guided insertion of stimulating catheters for infraclavicular blocks. There is very little in the literature concerning techniques of insertion of catheters using ultrasound. This chapter will detail the technique of inserting a regional block catheter using ultrasonography and nerve stimulation to verify the catheter tip location.

16.2. Equipment and Injectates

16.2.1. Stimulating Catheters

Although nonstimulating catheters can be used to initiate regional blocks using ultrasonography, we recommend starting with stimulating catheters as this has resulted in the highest success rates in our hands. There are three commercial varieties of catheters available with different lengths of needles required for various blocks.

Arrow StimuCath (Arrow International, Inc., Reading, PA, USA; Figure 16.1)

- The needle has a Tuohy tip and is available in two lengths: 4 cm and 8 cm.
- The catheter is made more rigid by a steel stylet, which has a female adaptor to accept the stimulating cable from the nerve stimulator.
- A significant amount of the metal extends beyond the catheter tip.
- The catheter hub has a stimulating cable that can be used to stimulate the catheter at the end of insertion.
- Liquids cannot be injected via the catheter until the stylet is removed.
- The catheter can kink if it encounters resistance on insertion.

Pajunk stimulong (Pajunk, Germany; Figure 16.2)

- Includes insulated Tuohy needles in 50-mm, 100-mm, and 110-mm lengths.
- The catheter can be stimulated and has a gold tip, which was reported to require a higher current to achieve stimulation.
- The catheter is relatively soft without stylet.
- There is also a specially designed hub through which solutions can be injected via the catheter as it is advanced. This allows one to generate a potential space with an injectate (i.e., space dilation) as the catheter is advanced.

Clinical Pearl

It is beneficial to perform preprocedural ultrasound imaging of the region to assess the depth of the neural structure in order to select the appropriate length of the needle system.

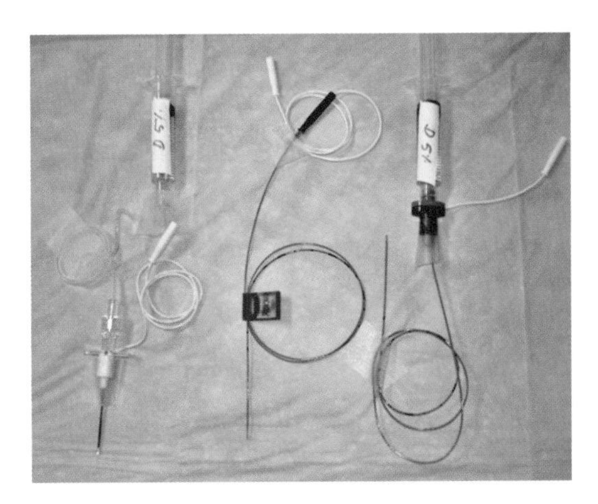

Figure 16.1. Arrow StimuCath (Arrow International, Inc., Reading, PA, USA). Note that the catheter has a stylet and therefore it is impossible to inject during its advancement (middle). It is only possible to inject through the catheter after removal of the stylet (right).

Pajunk StimuLong-Tsui (Pajunk GmbH Medical Technology, Geisngen, Germany; Figure 16.3)

- This product has just recently been introduced but there has been no clinical experience with this product to date.
- Insulated Tuohy needles are available in 50-mm and 100-mm lengths (Figure 16.2).
- This StimuLong-Tsui catheter is suggested to have two distinct features to facilitate advancing the catheter into the nerve sheath:
  - The stiffness of the catheter can be adjusted by manipulating the length that the steel stylet is advanced within the catheter. Depending on the anatomical characteristics (i.e., composition of soft/connective tissue) of the region through which the distal tip of the catheter is advancing, the final length of the stiffening stylet will be affected during its axial introduction.
    - Once the desirable stiffness is achieved, the stylet position can be locked or unlocked by tightening and loosening the hemostatic valve.
  - During the forward advancement of the catheter, a solution can be injected into the catheter via the sideport tubing of the catheter, which will emerge from the tip of the catheter.

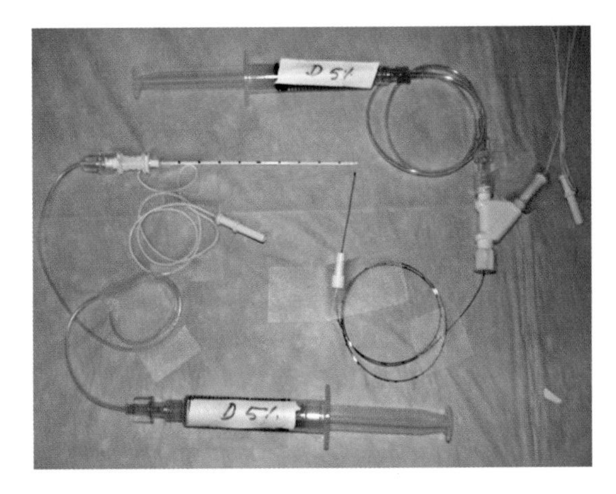

Figure 16.2. Pajunk StimuLong set (Pajunk GmbH Medical Technology, Geisingen, Germany). The assembled catheter hub has an injection port for dextrose injection during advancement. Note the gold tip of the catheter.

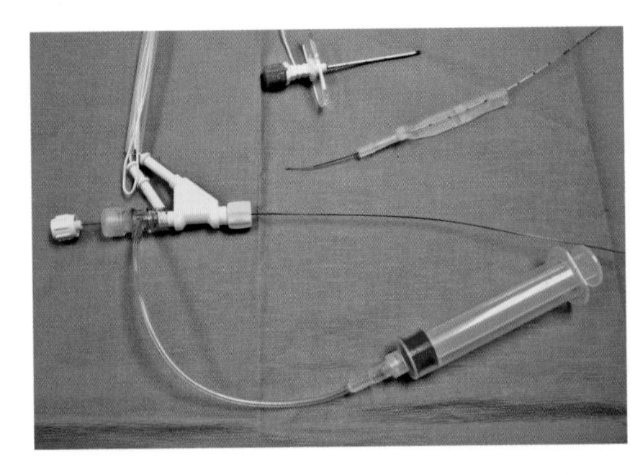

Figure 16.3. Pajunk StimuLong-Tsui (Pajunk GmbH Medical Technology, Geisingen, Germany). This stimulating catheter has an adjustable stylet which is locked into place by the hemostatic valve. Note the presence of sideport tubing for injecting solution, for example, D5W, to maintain the electrical characteristics of the catheter.

- This liquid can serve to dilate the space through which the catheter advances, essentially forming a liquid cushion, and will make the advancement of the catheter tip easier.
- Once the catheter is properly placed, the presence of fluid will also facilitate stylet removal by reducing friction between the surfaces of the stylet and catheter.
- Using the aqueous 5% dextrose solution (D5W) for space dilation is optimal, as it allows for both mechanical lubrication surrounding the catheter and maintenance of electrical stimulation conditions (see Chapter 2 and the following section in this chapter).

16.2.2. What Injectate Should One Use?

- Use of either local anesthetic or electrically conducting solutions such as normal saline will abolish the capacity to electrically stimulate the nerves.
- The use of D5W will allow the creation of the potential perineural space prior to advancing the catheter without losing the capacity to apply stimulation until ideal positioning of the catheter tip is achieved.
- Despite the benefits of D5W, injection of large volumes of dextrose can also create a mechanical barrier to stimulation.

16.3. Technique

All sterile precautions should be used for catheter insertion to avoid infections. Key points are summarized as follows:

- The procedure cannot be done singlehandedly. A nurse or assistant will be required to handle the nerve stimulator, sedation, and monitoring.
- Routine monitoring includes pulse oximetry, noninvasive blood pressure monitoring, and electrocardiogram.
- Patients receive supplemental oxygen and intravenous sedation using titrated doses of fentanyl and midazolam.
- Prior to skin preparation with poviodine or chlorhexidine, a scout (preprocedural) ultrasound scan of the nerves of interest should be performed to optimize the machine settings for the best view of the structures. This includes depth, dynamic range, gain, and scanning mode.
- After skin preparation with a sterile solution the drapes are applied.

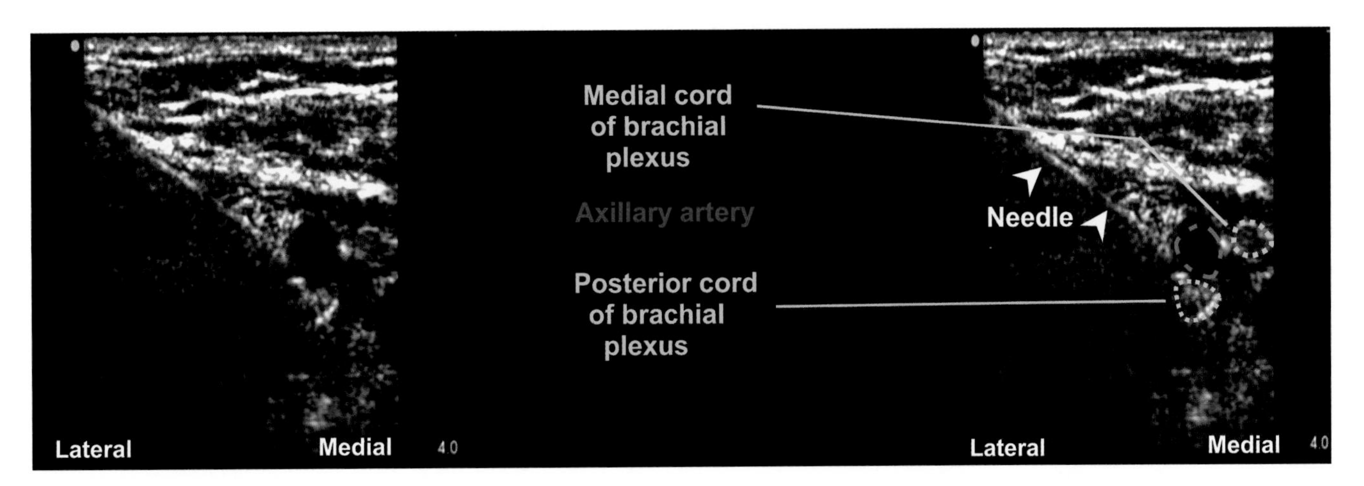

Figure 16.4. Infraclavicular block using an in-plane (IP) needling approach. The needle can be tracked during this alignment, in this case in a position near the posterior cord of the brachial plexus. In other block locations, the out-of-plane (OOP) technique is more suitable for smooth catheter insertion.

- The probe must be covered entirely with a sterile probe cover and with sterile gel. It is important to ensure that there are no air bubbles entrapped between the probe and the plastic cover.
- The catheter is assembled and kept inside a towel close to the block site over the drapes. The needle is connected to the extension tubing and flushed with a 5% dextrose solution. A small amount of sterile ultrasonographic gel is applied on the skin.
- The assistant can perform skin infiltration once the probe is positioned and the image is optimized.
- The needle may be inserted out of plane (OOP) or in plane (IP) with respect to the probe axis (also see Chapter 4).
  - An IP approach allows the needle to be visualized as it advances towards the nerve, but the needle will contact the nerve at an angle that may inhibit smooth catheter advancement (except with infraclavicular blocks; Figure 16.4).
  - When the needle is advanced OOP, the tissue movement that is associated with the needle advancement will be seen, but most often the needle tip will not be directly identified. To assist visibility of the needle tip:
    - Inject small quantities of D5W, which will appear as a hypoechoic shadow near the tip of the needle.

16.3.1. Confirming the Catheter Tip Location with Nerve Stimulation Technique

- The nerve stimulator should be set to deliver current at 0.5 to 0.6 mA.
- Higher currents result in vigorous muscle twitches that can displace the probe and the needle.
- Once the needle tip is confirmed to be in good position, an additional injection of 1 mL of D5W will often increase the amplitude of the motor response. The nerve will also appear more hyperechoic.
- At this point, the ultrasound probe is kept aside in the sterile field and the extension tubing is removed from the needle hub. Insert the catheter while still applying stimulation.
- Insert 5 to 10 cm of the catheter past the needle tip as long as motor responses are observed. Changes in the twitch pattern may be seen depending on the course the catheter takes. For example, even if the initial stimulation elicits a twitch of the deltoid with the interscalene block, upon catheter advancement a biceps brachii muscle twitch

followed by a triceps brachii muscle twitch will signify that the catheter tip is advancing towards the lower roots of the brachial plexus.

- Ideally, one should aim to stimulate the specific motor root pertaining to the area to be anesthetized, thereby allowing one to use the least amount of local anesthetic that will provide the most effective analgesia.
- Occasionally, the twitch may show distal advancement but may change back to higher root stimulation, signifying that the catheter is coiling up in the perineural area.

16.3.2. Confirmation of Catheter Tip Location with Ultrasonography

- There are two techniques using ultrasound that are used to identify the catheter tip before local anesthetic injection.
- One method is to inject additional dextrose, and see the lake of hypoechogenicity develop around the neural structures making the nerves appear more hyperechoic.
- The second method is useful if the block site is close to a vessel: color Doppler can capture the tissue movement where the injectate is delivered. The color Doppler window is positioned over the estimated location of the catheter and the gain is adjusted until the vessel pulsations are just seen.
  - An injection of agitated dextrose is performed in aliquots and a medley of colors is seen, which confirms where the injectate is being delivered (Figure 16.5).
  - It is important to keep the probe steady, as movement of the probe can also result in a medley of colors. If the entire area is embellished with color, the gain is too high or large amounts of injectate are being injected. The gain may be altered by adjusting the gain button or by reducing the pulse repetition frequency (PRF). Occasionally, with certain blocks such as the femoral, the catheter may track proximally and the tip may be outside of the color Doppler window at the level of the groin.
- We recommend performing at this time an electrical stimulation using stimulating catheters for objective confirmation of catheter placement prior to injection of local anesthetic.
- Injection of the local anesthetic can be visualized with the ultrasound probe as a hypoechoic lake developing around the nerve. Once the catheter is positioned well, it is tunneled for an inch and fixed to the skin with occlusive dressing. The ultrasonographic gel often makes the skin wet and slippery. This needs to be removed and we use a skin glue, such as mastisol or cyanacrylate glue, to make the occlusive dressing adhere to the skin.

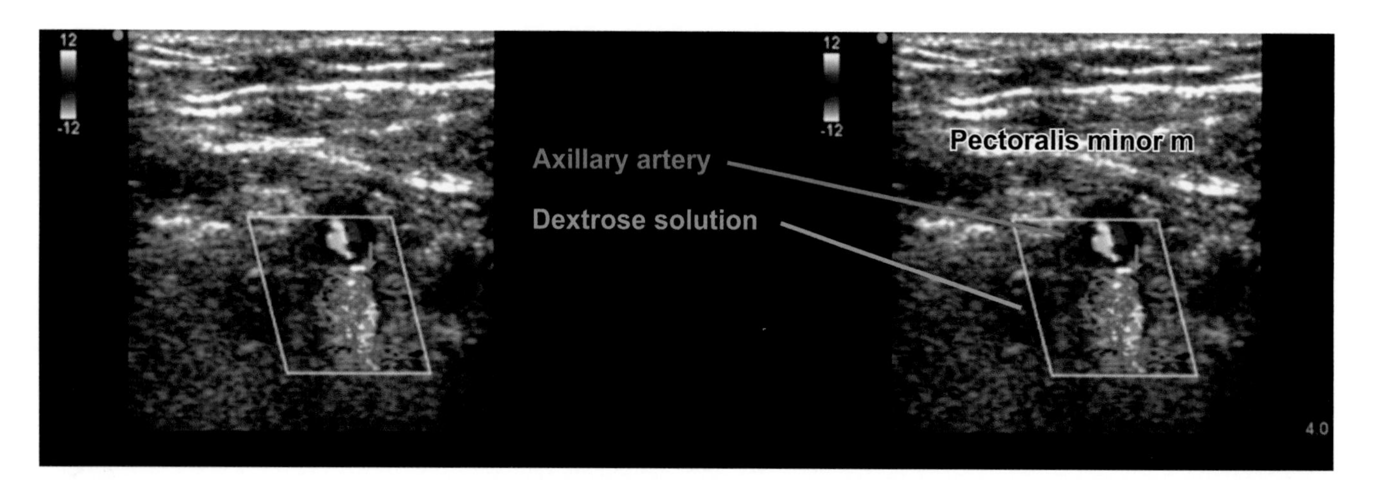

Figure 16.5. Infraclavicular block using color Doppler. The delivery of dextrose is between the artery and the chest wall and appears as a medley of colors.

- Ultrasound guidance has allowed us to accomplish almost 100% success with catheter placement. Using ultrasonic identification of the needle tip and an estimation using the color Doppler, we can confidently apply local anesthetic solutions close to the nerve. Furthermore, it may be possible to perform catheter insertion with high success without stimulation. However, no studies making this comparison have been documented to date.

16.4. Examples of Specific Blocks

16.4.1. Interscalene Catheterization

- A linear 38-mm 7- to 12-MHz probe is used.
- The probe is applied perpendicular to the interscalene groove at the level of the cricoid cartilage.
- The C4/C5 root appears to be the most superficial root observed in the interscalene groove.
- The needle is inserted perpendicular to the probe (OOP) to contact this root (see Chapter 4 for a discussion of OOP needling technique).
- When one advances the needle IP, the contour of the needle is optimally visualized; however, in doing so the catheter makes an acute turn in the grove, frequently resulting in occlusion.
- After distending the perineural space with dextrose, the stimulating catheter is advanced 5 cm beyond the tip of the needle, tunneled, and secured.
- Ensure that the shoulder and biceps twitches are maintained as the catheter is advanced (vide supra).

16.4.2. Infraclavicular Catheterization

- A linear 38-mm probe is used and positioned parasagitally just medial to the coracoid process.
- The needle tip and catheter are positioned at the 6 o'clock position in relation to the artery, between the artery and the chest wall, close to the posterior cord.
- This increases the success rate with the block as the drug spreads around the artery surrounding all the three cords (Figures 16.4 and 16.5).

16.4.3. Femoral Nerve

- The linear 38-mm probe is positioned parallel to the inguinal ligament.
- One can often see the profunda femoris artery if the imaging is performed lower in the thigh.
- The probe should be moved proximally until only one artery is seen.
- The probe may have to be toggled to get the best view of the nerve and the fascia iliaca.
- For stimulation, we currently accept medial or midline thigh (quadriceps) twitches.
- Often as the dextrose is injected or as the catheter is advanced, the medial twitches change to midline quadriceps contractions.
- Occasionally as the dextrose is injected, one can see the two branches of the femoral nerve and the needle can be rotated to direct the catheter towards the deeper branch of the femoral nerve.
- If the catheter advances proximally, color Doppler may not be successful, but one can still see the hypoechoic lake of local anesthetic around the nerve.

16.4.4. Sciatic Nerve

- It is common to use the subgluteal or the popliteal sciatic approach to initiate continuous sciatic block.

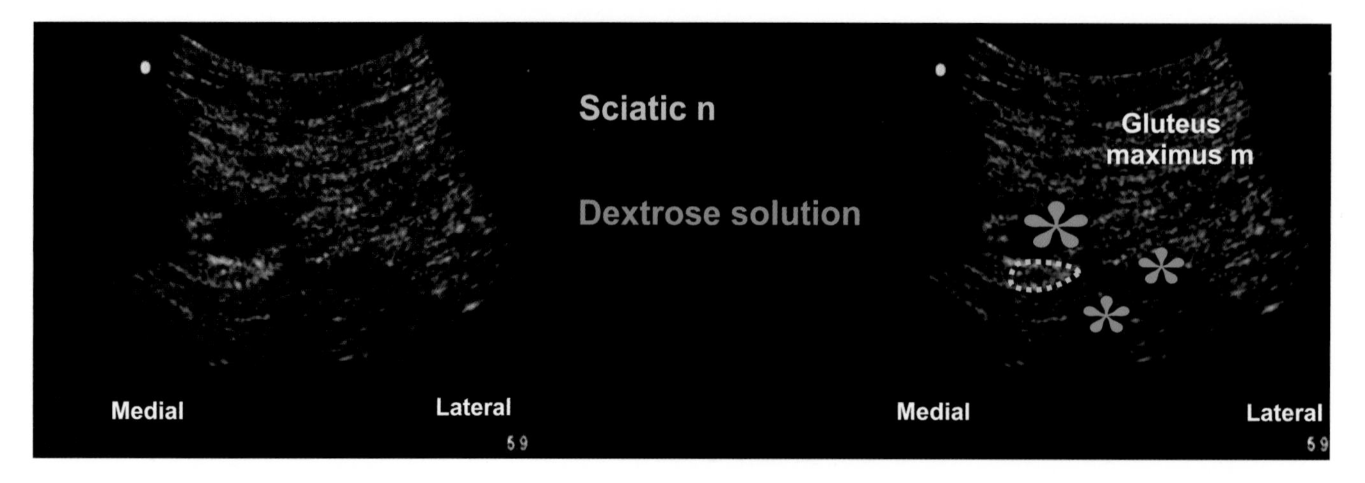

Figure 16.6. Subgluteal sciatic block. The injection of dextrose forms a hypoechoic lake around the nerve.

- For the subgluteal block, a curved array 60-mm 2- to 5-MHz probe can be used.
- The patient is placed in the lateral position for the popliteal block, as it is difficult to stabilize the probe in the supine position and maintain sterility.
- It is beneficial to first scan between the greater trochanter of the femur and the ischial tuberosity to identify the sciatic nerve.
- Subsequently, the nerve can be traced about 4 cm inferior down the posterior aspect of the thigh.
- The needle is inserted perpendicular to the probe as this allows the catheter to glide along the sciatic nerve.
- As with the femoral nerve, it is difficult to see the needle tip and the injection of dextrose makes a hypoechoic lake around the nerve making it more visible (Figure 16.6). Color Doppler can also be used in this location (Figure 16.7).
- When using the popliteal approach to the sciatic block, the nerve is identified at the apex of the popliteal fossa. At the level of the popliteal crease, the tibial nerve lies posterior to the artery and vein. This nerve is traced up proximally to the apex of the popliteal fossa, where the common peroneal nerve joins the tibial nerve. The needle is inserted with the bevel facing cephalad to facilitate proximal catheterization of the sciatic nerve. One can often visualize the sciatic nerve longitudinally after the injection is made, which will show a fusiform hypoechoic lake around the nerve. The medley of colors with the color Doppler will appear within this lake.

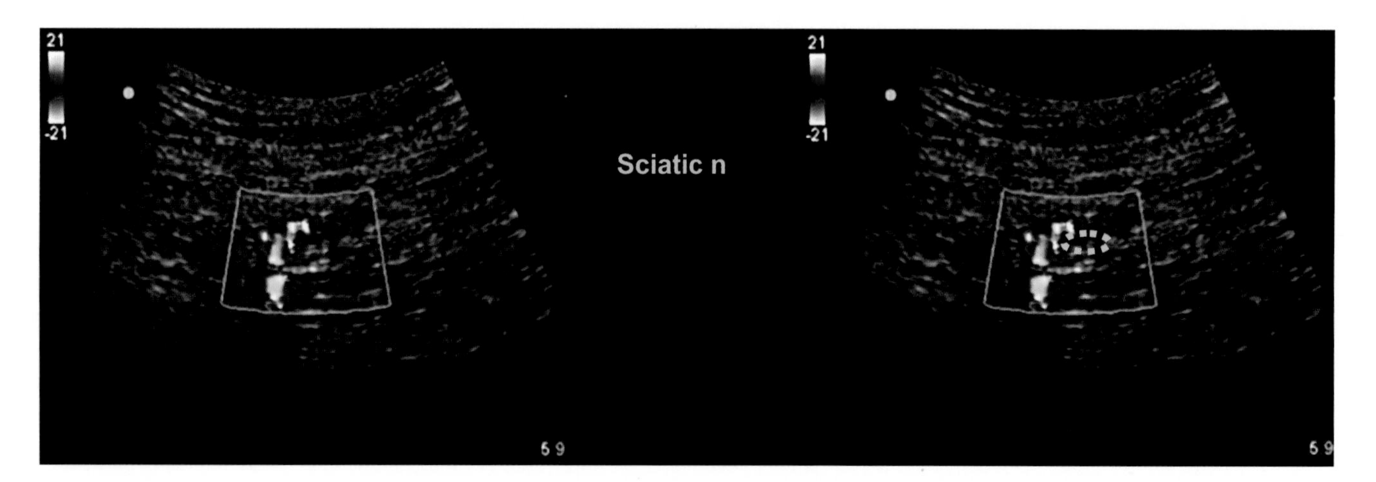

Figure 16.7. Subgluteal sciatic catheterization using color Doppler. Note the medley of colors to the right of the sciatic nerve.

16.5. Summary and Advantages

Ultrasonography can allow precise visibility of the position of needle tips and catheters that are close to nerves. Color Doppler can be useful for identification of the catheter in the vicinity of the vessels. In our experience, use of this technique can increase the success rate of these blocks in a range close to 100%. Injection and spread of local anesthetic around the nerves can be visualized with ultrasonography. With practice, traditional nonstimulating catheters may be used successfully using ultrasonography. This will be particularly useful in patients with fractures, where motor twitches can be painful.

Suggested Reading and References

Dalens B. Some current controversies in paediatric anaesthesia. Curr Opin Anaesthesiol 2006;19:301–308.

Plunkett AR, Brown DS, Rogers JM, Buckenmaier CC. Supraclavicular continuous peripheral nerve block in a wounded soldier: when ultrasound is the only option. Br J Anaesth 2006;97:71–717.

Swenson JD, Bay N, Loose E, Bankhead B, Davis J, Beals TC, Bryan NA, Burks RT, Greis PE. Outpatient management of continuous peripheral nerve catheters placed using ultrasound guidance: an experience in 620 patients. Anesth Analg 2006;103:1436–1443.

Tsui BC, Wagner A, Finucane B. Electrophysiologic effect of injectates on peripheral nerve stimulation. Reg Anesth Pain Med 2004;29:189–193.

Tsui BCH, Kropelin B, Ganapathy S, Finucane B. Dextrose 5% in water: fluid medium for maintaining electrical stimulation of peripheral nerves during stimulating catheter placement. Acta Anaesthesiol Scand 2005;49:1562–1565.

Van Geffen GJ, Mathieu G. Ultrasound-guided subgluteal sciatic nerve blocks with stimulating catheters in children: a descriptive study. Anesth Analg 2006;103:328–333.

17

Anatomy of the Trunk for Paravertebral, Intercostal, and Epidural Blocks

Ban C.H. Tsui

17.1. Vertebral Column

The anatomy related to the normal adult vertebral column is not covered here in any depth as this is assumed well understood by anesthesiologists. Instead, this section focuses on an overview of the developmental anatomy of the vertebral column in order to provide a basis for appreciating the improved visibility of vertebral, paravertebral, and related structures in the pediatric patient.

17.1.1. Developmental Anatomy of the Thoracic and Lumbar Spine

- At birth, the vertebrae of the thoracic and lumbar spine consist of three bony masses: a centrum anteriorly and two neural arches posteriorly.
- Development of the thoracic spine:
  - The laminae typically unite in a caudocranial (upwards, T12 through T1) fashion, usually by the end of the first or beginning of the second year.
  - The centrum (body) fuses with the neural arches, also in a caudal to cranial manner, generally by the end of the fifth year (neurocentral fusion).
  - The vertebral canal in young infants is quite small, with the epidural space as narrow as 1–2 mm.
- Development of the lumbar spine:
  - The lamina fuse at levels L1 to L4 by the first year, but not until the fifth year at L5.
  - Neurocentral fusion is generally complete by the fourth year.
  - The transverse processes begin to develop at the end of the first year.
  - The secondary compensatory curve (through intervertebral disc modification) at the lumbar spine does not start to form until the infant begins to sit upright (6–8 months).
- In children, most vertebrae contain secondary ossification centers (at the transverse and spinous processes as well as at the inferior and superior surfaces of the bodies), which allow continual growth and remodeling of the vertebral column.
- In adults (early 20s), the vertebral column is essentially complete with the exception of fusion between the bodies of S1 and S2.
- In adults:
  - Thoracic vertebral bodies are of medium size and heart shaped (Figure 17.1); vertebral (spinal) canals are small and nearly circular in shape; laminae are relatively small; spinous processes are long and oriented inferiorly (Figures 17.2 and 17.3); transverse processes are relatively broad and robust for articulation with the ribs and generally face posterolaterally.

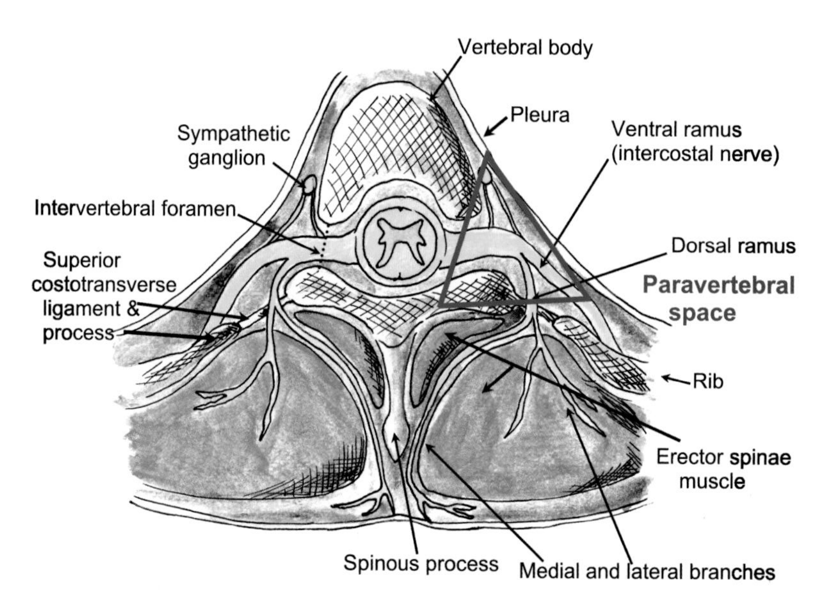

Figure 17.1. Cross-section of a vertebral segment with a simplified spinal nerve and the paravertebral space (only right side shown).

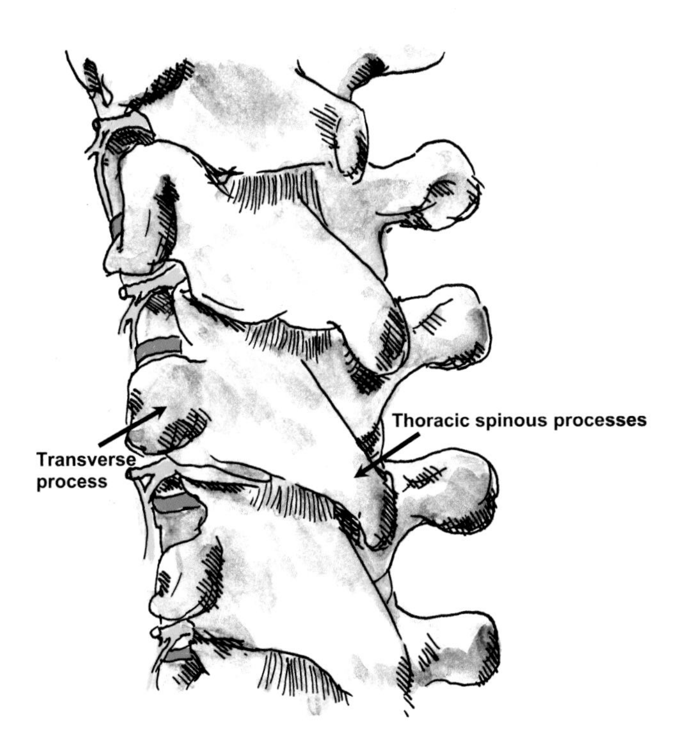

Figure 17.2. Vertebrae of the thoracic spine with their inferiorly orientated spinous processes.

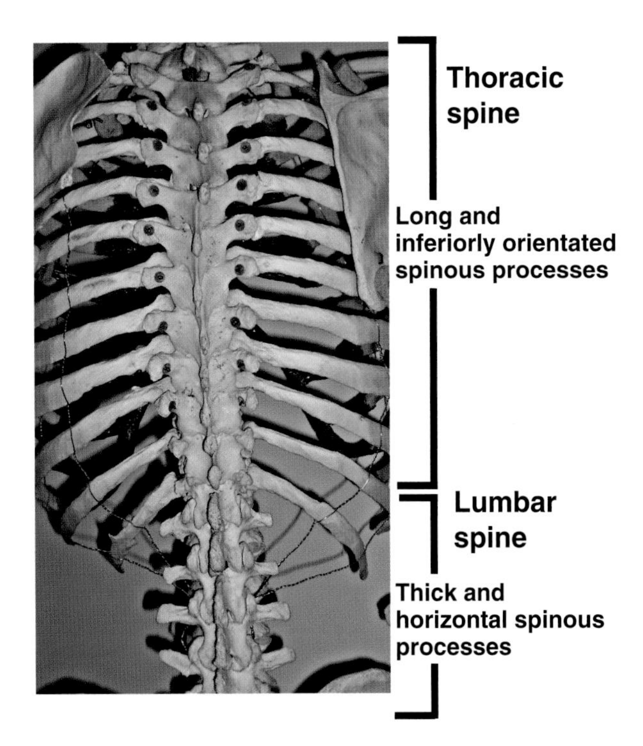

Figure 17.3. The spinal column in the thoracic and lumbar regions.

- Lumbar vertebral bodies are large and kidney shaped; vertebral (spinal) canals are triangular in shape; laminae are thick; spinous processes are short and stout with a posterior (horizontal) orientation (Figure 17.3); intervertebral discs are thickest with respect to the rest of the spine; and transverse processes are long, slender and directed laterally.

17.1.2. Developmental Anatomy of the Sacrum

- In infancy and childhood, the sacrum is highly variable with respect to its shape and ossification, and therefore also its visibility (Figure 17.4).
  - The sacral vertebrae and sacroiliac joints are oriented almost vertically until weight bearing commences around age 1.
  - All (approximately 21) of the primary centers of ossification of the sacrum are present at birth, but fusion does not generally take place until puberty (S1–S2 ventral fusion may not be completed until 25 years of age).
  - At birth, the sacral (and most other) vertebrae are composed of two half neural arches and a centrum (called bodies once neurocentral fusion is complete); S1 and S2 also contain lateral elements which will form the articular surfaces of the sacro-iliac joints.
  - The centrums fuse with the neural arches on both sides between the second and sixth years of life.
  - Fusion of the neural arches to form spinous processes, is usually not complete until 7 to 15 years of age.
  - The posterior aspect of the sacrum is not completed until puberty, although continual fusion and ossification occurs throughout development.
- Beyond puberty, the sacral hiatus is an inferiorly placed opening into the caudal epidural space, below the fifth sacral vertebra and between it and its inferior horns or cornua (this

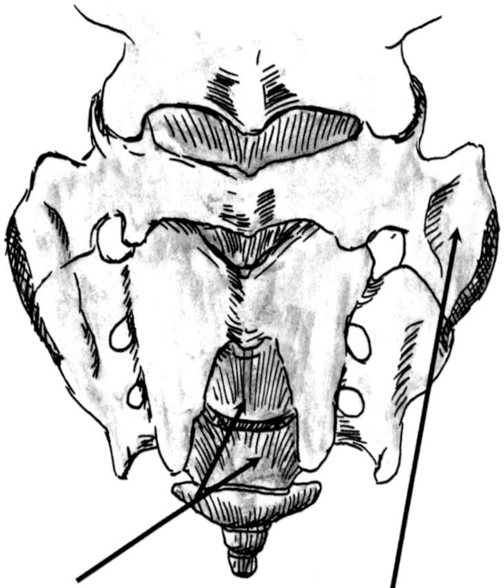

Incomplete fusion of vertebral bodies and neural arches

Caudal epidural space

Lateral elements to form articular surfaces of sacrum

Figure 17.4. Posterior view of a pediatric sacrum illustrating incomplete fusion of the sacral neural arches and anterior vertebral bodies, as well as the incorporation of lateral elements that form the articular surfaces to form the sacro-iliac joints.

is because the S5 laminae fail to fuse; see Figure 20.3). In young infants, the sacral hiatus is generally lower, below the fifth sacral vertebra, and because there is much less ossification of the sacrum, ultrasound imaging in infants is generally rendered easier and generates superior image quality.

- The posterior sacrococcygeal membrane covers the sacral hiatus externally and requires penetration for epidural needle entry (see Figure 18.1).

17.2. Costovertebral Articulations

The costovertebral articulations (Figure 17.5) are primarily relevant for paravertebral and intercostal blockade, although practitioners will encounter these joints during ultrasound-guided epidurals as the imaging technique will incorporate these structures. The ribs articulate through two synovial joints with the vertebral column:

- Costovertebral joint: The head of the rib articulates through a synovial joint with demi-facets on adjacent thoracic vertebral bodies and the corresponding intervertebral disc of the upper vertebral joint, for example, seventh rib with bodies of T6, T7, and T6 to T7 disc (except for 1st, 10th–12th ribs, which articulate with a single vertebral facet). The joints are enclosed in fibrous capsules that are reinforced by ligaments.
- Costotransverse joint: Articular facets on the tubercles of the ribs articulate through synovial joints with the transverse processes of the thoracic vertebrae (the 11th and 12th ribs lack this articulation because they do not possess tubercles). The joints are enclosed in fibrous capsules that are reinforced by ligaments.

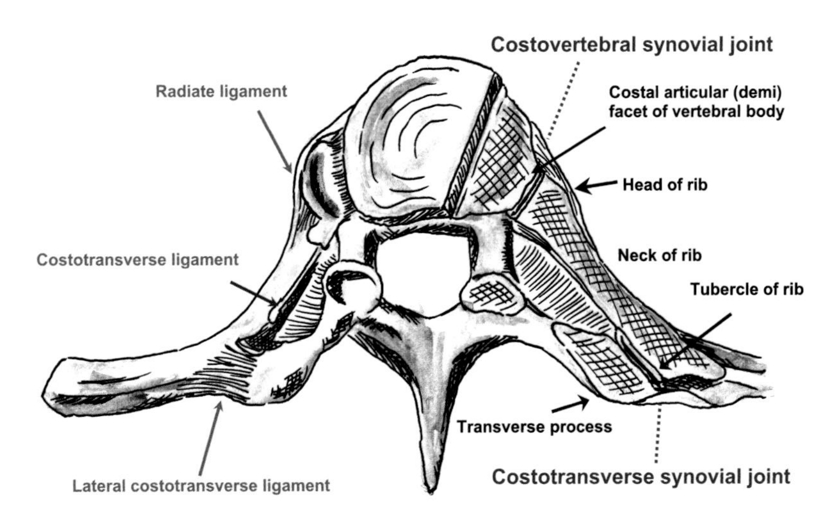

Figure 17.5. Costovertebral articulations: costovertebral and costotransverse synovial joints with left side illustrating the exterior surfaces with ligamentous coverings and the right side illustrating a section through the synovial joints.

17.3. Paravertebral Space

This is a bilateral wedge-shaped space on either side of the vertebral column between the individual vertebrae, extending its entire length, through which the spinal nerves exit from the intervertebral foramina. In the thoracic region, its boundaries are as follows (Figure 17.1):

- Medially: Vertebral body, intervertebral disc and foramen.
- Anterolaterally: Parietal pleura.
- Posteriorly: Costotransverse process; approximately 2.5 cm from the tip of the transverse process, often in a slightly caudal orientation.

17.4. Spinal Membranes (Meninges) and Nerves Above the Sacrum

- Three membranes (meninges) cover the spinal cord within the vertebral (spinal) canal. Immediately on the surface of the spinal cord and inseparable from it is the single cell-layered pia mater. Just superficial to the pia is the spider web–like arachnoid mater, which sends fine trabeculae down to the pia. Between the pia and the arachnoid is the subarachnoid space, containing cerebrospinal fluid, blood vessels of the cord, and filaments of the spinal nerve roots. The third layer of the meninges, the outermost tough dura mater, is superficial to the arachnoid mater, and continues as a sheath over the ventral and dorsal roots of the spinal nerves and for a short distance over the spinal nerves, where it blends with the epinurium.
- The spinal epidural space (Figure 17.6) is a real space between the dura mater and the periosteum lining the vertebral (spinal) canal. This space is richly vascularized (internal vertebral venous plexus) and filled with epidural fat which surrounds the dura mater. It is bordered posteriorly by the ligamentum flavum and anteriorly by the posterior longitudinal ligament, which lies on posterior aspect of the vertebral body within the vertebral canal.
- The ventral and dorsal roots (dorsal roots containing the dorsal root ganglion at this location) of the spinal nerves join as they leave the spinal cord, forming the spinal nerve, which exits the vertebral canal through the intervertebral (spinal, neural) foramen.
- Grey and white rami communicantes (Figure 17.1; not labeled) connect the spinal nerves to the sympathetic chain ganglia to allow preganglionic sympathetic fibers leaving the

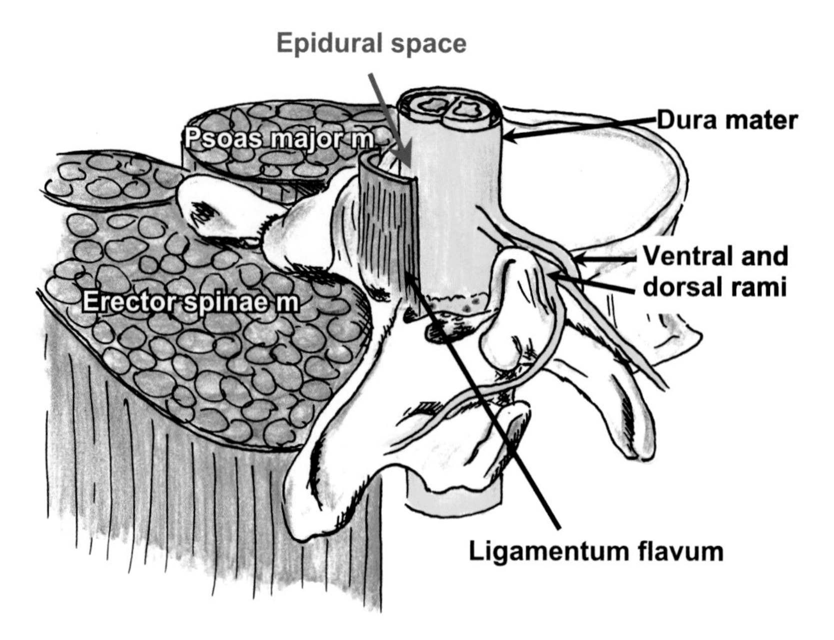

Figure 17.6. Spinal epidural space.

spinal cord (T1 to L2/L3) to enter the chain and leave it again to be distributed with spinal nerves at all levels.

- The spinal nerves divide into ventral and dorsal rami (Figures 17.1 and 17.6); the dorsal rami supply the paravertebral muscles and skin near the midline of the back; the ventral rami form the intercostal nerves (T1–T12) in the thorax and the cervical, brachial, lumbar, and sacral plexuses, which supply the muscles and skin of the trunk and extremities.

17.5. Intercostal Nerves (Figure 17.7)

- Thoracic spinal nerves emerge from the intervertebral (spinal) foramina, between superior and inferior articulations of the vertebral bodies and ribs.
- The spinal nerves divide to supply paraspinal muscles and skin of the back (dorsal ramus or branch) and the intercostal spaces (ventral ramus or branch; Figure 17.1).
- The ventral rami of the thoracic spinal nerves form 11 pairs of intercostal nerves (T1–T11) for the 11 intercostal spaces and the subcostal nerve (T12; not shown in Figure 17.7), which courses below the 12th rib.
- The intercostal nerves give off cutaneous branches at the anterior and lateral aspects of the thoracic wall.
- Thoracic spinal nerves T2 through T12 and lumbar spinal nerve L1 can be blocked for surgical intervention.

17.6. Caudal Epidural Space

- The spinal cord ends at the conus medullaris, usually at the L1–L2 disc in the adult. The spinal cord decreases in length significantly throughout prenatal and antenatal development, with the cord reaching as far as S1 or S2 in the first few intrauterine months and as low as L2 or L3 at birth (Figure 17.8). This results from the greater growth rate of the spinal column as compared to the cord.
- The dural sac extends beyond this level, to approximately the second sacral vertebral level (lower prenatally); within the sac, the cauda equina runs vertically from the conus

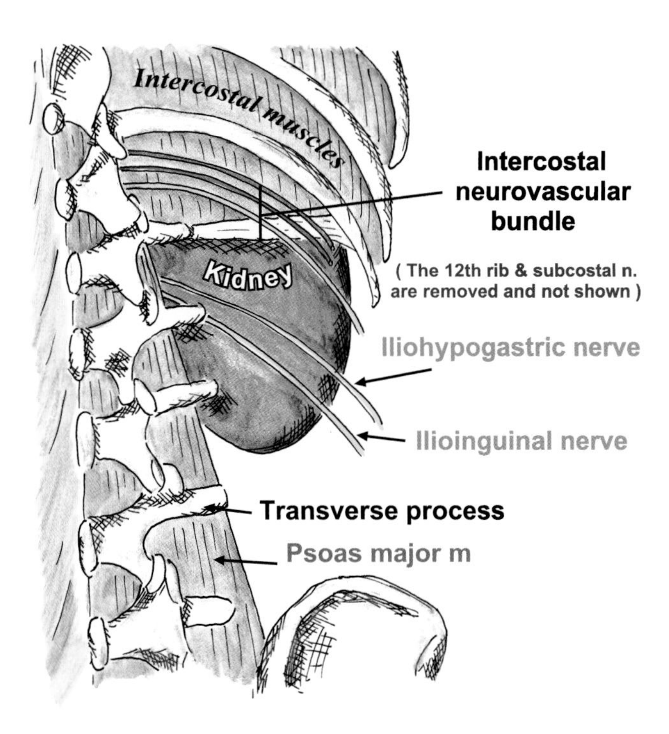

Figure 17.7. Ventral rami of the thoracic spine form the intercostal nerves to supply the intercostal spaces after leaving the intervertebral foramina between the transverse processes.

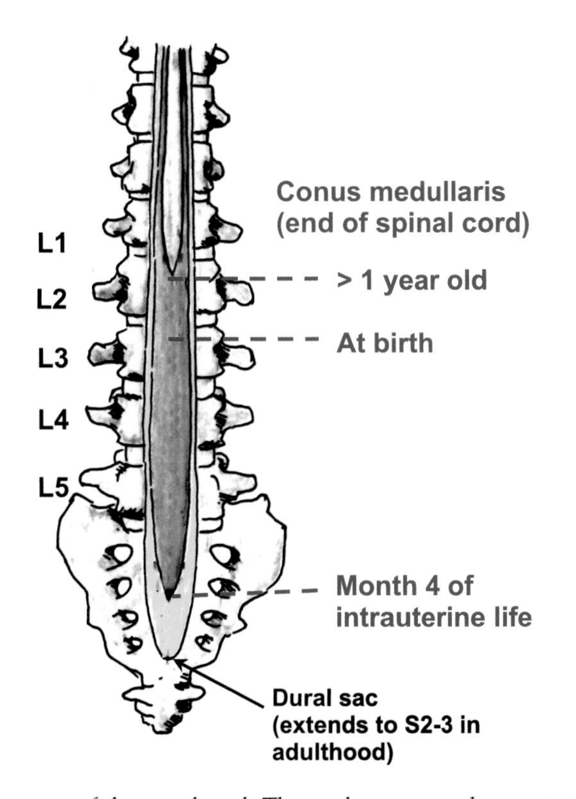

Figure 17.8. Development of the spinal cord. The cord appears to decrease in length significantly throughout early development because the vertebral column grows at a faster rate.

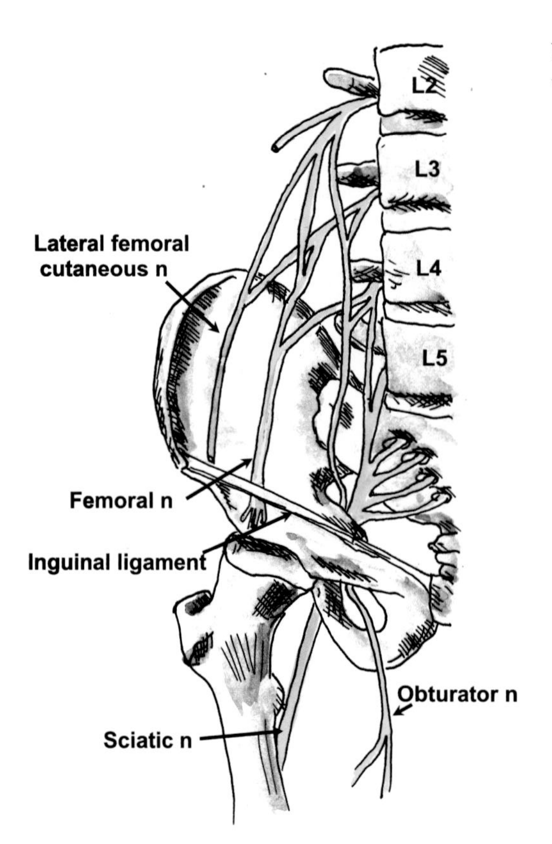

Figure 17.9. Lumbar and sacral plexuses within the skeletal system.

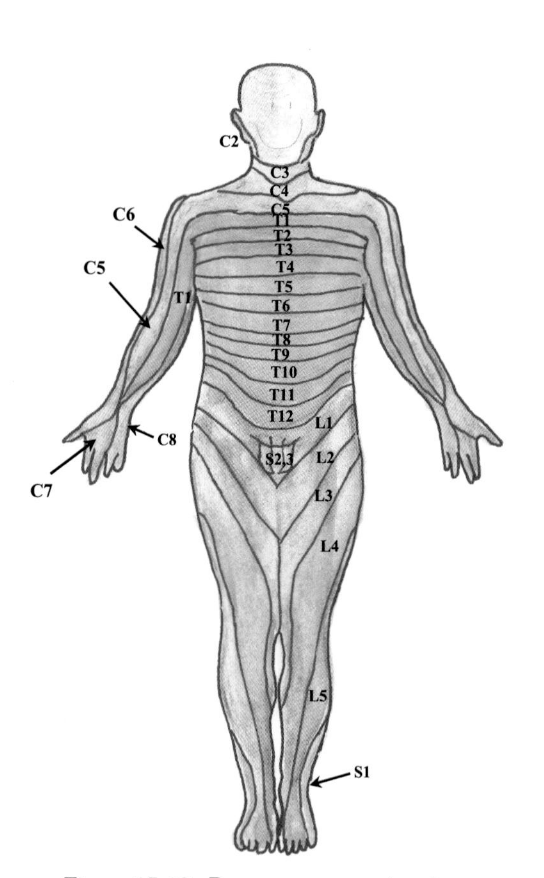

Figure 17.10. Dermatomes: anterior view.

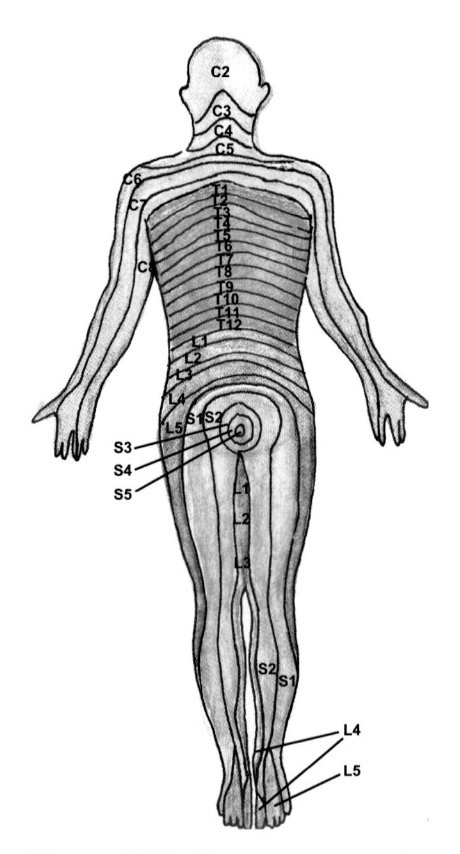

Figure 17.11. Dermatomes: posterior view.

medullaris in the canal between the posterior surface of the sacrum and the fused pedicles (intervertebral foramina in infants).
- The dura mater ultimately ends as the external filum terminale and the pia mater as the internal filum terminale.
- The lumbar plexus forms from the anterior primary rami of L1 to L3, with some of the L4 spinal nerve. The sacral plexus incorporates lower lumbar nerves (L4 and L5) with sacral nerves 1 through 5 (Figure 17.9).

17.7. Dermatomes

With the exception of C1 (which does not have a sensory component), dorsal fibers of the spinal nerves supply a specific segment or band of skin. This skin segment is termed a *dermatome*. C5 to T1 spinal nerves provide cutaneous innervation to the upper extremity; T1 through L1 to the trunk and L1 through S2 to the lower extremity. There is considerable overlap between contiguous dermatomes and adjacent dermatomes are generally arranged as consecutive horizontal bands on the surface of the axial skeleton, and more or less vertical projections on the extremities (Figures 17.10 and 17.11). The paravertebral and intercostal blocks (Chapter 19) will target the dermatomes of the trunk, while epidural anesthesia can target various segmental levels.

Each intercostal or trunk spinal nerve dermatomal region forms an essentially horizontal band (of approximately 2–4 cm width) on the anterior of the body and a broad inverted V shape on the back, with caudal levels less angulated and T12 being almost horizontal.

- T1: Anteriorly it covers the upper aspect of the pectoralis major muscles, anteroinferior shoulder, and anteromedial arm down to the wrist. Posteriorly it covers the mid- to upper aspects of the scapula with the peak at the level of the T1 through T2 spinous processes.
- T2: Anteriorly it supplies the skin on the upper pectoral region (at the level of the axilla); posteriorly, the dermatome is approximately 4 to 6 cm below the spine of the scapula.
- T3: Anteriorly it supplies a 3- to 4-cm band of skin across the upper pectoral level through to the anterior surface of the axilla and immediately superior to the nipples; posteriorly the dermatome is a 3- to 4-cm band at the lower one third of the scapula.
- T4: This dermatome covers the nipples anteriorly; posteriorly, the band is located at the inferior tip of the scapula.
- T5: Anteriorly, the T5 dermatome supplies the skin between and just under the pectoralis muscles at the level of the zyphoid process; posteriorly, it extends across the back at approximately midhumeral level.
- T6 to T12: These dermatomal bands extend around the thorax and abdomen with broad but subtle U shapes anteriorly and a broad but slightly inverted V shape posteriorly; T10 lies approximately at the umbilical level anteriorly.
- L1: The L1 dermatome supplies the anterior aspect of the pelvic (hypogastric, suprapubic) region and the groin (inguinal region) except for the scrotal/labial area (supplied by S2, S3), including the skin over the anterior portion of the iliac crest.

The myotomes and osteotomes within the body are described in Chapters 5 (upper extremity) and 11 (lower extremity) and will be important for epidural anesthesia.

Suggested Reading and References

Netter FH. Atlas of human anatomy. Summit, NJ: CIBA-GEIGY Corporation; 1989.

Saint-Maurice C, Steinberh OS. Regional anaesthesia in children. Switzerland: Mediglobe; 1990. [See Chapter 1.]

Scheuer L, Black S. The juvenile skeleton. London: Elsevier; 2004:181–227.

Snell RS, Katz J. Clinical antomy for anesthesiologists. Stamford, CT: Appleton & Lange; 1988. [See Chapters 4–6.]

18

Epidural Anesthesia Using Electrical Epidural Stimulation and Ultrasound Guidance

Ban C.H. Tsui

18.1. Introduction

Recently, many approaches have been described for use with regional anesthesia of the neuraxis. There is still some room for improvement in the success rates of epidural anesthesia and any approach we can use to improve the safety of this technique is desirable. Continuous epidural analgesia has become popular, as single-injection epidural blocks are associated with limited duration and segmental effects. Several new methods are being examined to benefit epidural catheter introduction and advancement. Precise placement of needles and catheters in the epidural space is essential and can potentially reduce adverse effects of local anesthetic and opioid administration, in addition to reducing the risks of serious systemic complications. This is particularly relevant in pediatric patients, where maximizing effect with minimal doses of local anesthetic is of paramount importance. Furthermore, the risk of spinal cord damage with these techniques is real and, therefore, it is far more desirable to insert epidural needles/catheters at sites far removed from the spinal cord level (e.g., sacral or lumbar versus thoracic). There have been few advances in this area of regional anesthesia until very recently which makes this an exciting new era for central neuraxial blockade.

Epidural anesthesia and analgesia has many beneficial effects, including

- Improved postoperative pain relief.
- Earlier ambulation.
- Rapid weaning from mechanical ventilators.
- Reduction in the catabolic state.
- Reduction in circulating stress hormone levels.
- Reduction in cardiovascular events.
- Reduction in thromboembolic complications.
- Improved gastrointestinal function.
- Reduced requirement for blood transfusion.

Despite these potential advantages, there are several challenges related to epidural needle and catheter insertion.

18.1.1. Technical Issues in Epidural Analgesia

- Precise placement of epidural needles/catheters ensures that the dermatomes involved in the surgical procedure are selectively blocked, allowing minimal doses of local anesthetic to be used for maximal analgesia.
- There is always an associated risk of needle trauma to the spinal cord from direct thoracic and high lumbar epidural needle placement.
- Failure to recognize placement of the epidural needle or catheter in the intrathecal space, followed by the injection of the usual epidural dose, could result in a total spinal block or serious neurological complications.
- The thoracic epidural space is particularly challenging as the spinal cord is comprehensively protected by a shield of bone and the epidural space is very narrow in that region. This makes thoracic epidural needle/catheter placement technically difficult while placing the spinal cord at risk from needle trauma.

In response to the above concerns, clinicians have attempted to move the site of needle puncture and catheter entrance caudally, below the level of the spinal cord and often through a caudal route (Figure 18.1), to circumvent the risks from potential direct needle trauma. However, this approach also has limitations that have challenged clinicians to find an innovative way to circumvent these problems.

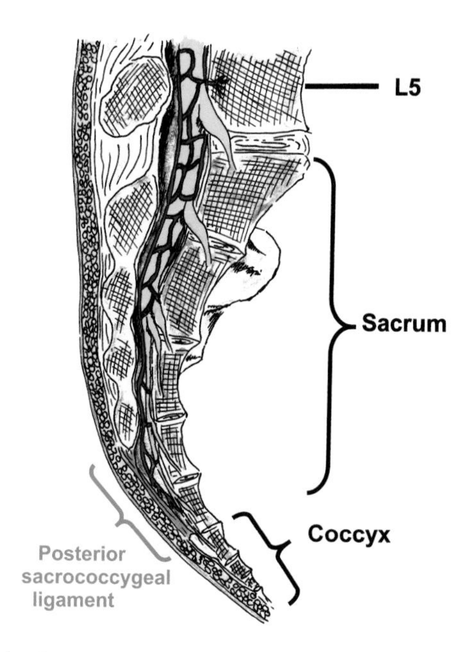

Figure 18.1. Caudal epidural space. At this location of epidural entry, through puncturing the posterior sacrococcygeal ligament, there is minimum risk of potential needle trauma to the spinal cord.

18.1.2. Issues Related to Caudal Needle Puncture and Catheter Advancement

- While the loss-of resistance (LOR) method to identify entry into the epidural space, using saline, is a fairly accurate method for determining needle entry, a reliable method of accurate epidural catheter placement or advancement is needed.
- The risk of the catheter kinking and inaccurate placement discouraged the widespread use of these caudal approaches.
- It is important to be able to control catheter position, especially when advancing catheters long distances into the epidural space, because of the risk of catheter migration.
- It is now generally recommended that catheter tip placement should be verified using either radiography, ultrasound, or nerve stimulation.
  - Real-time X-ray imaging using a contrast or a radiopaque catheter precisely confirms catheter tip position in specific anatomical locations, but it requires additional setup, is increasingly expensive, and, more importantly, increases patients' exposure to ionizing radiation.
  - As a result, fluoroscopy is not for routine use and is usually limited to difficult and/or special circumstances, such as chronic epidural catheter placement.
  - Electrical stimulation of the epidural space is a reliable method of confirming catheter tip location and may be used dynamically to guide epidural catheter placement and advancement.
  - Ultrasound imaging may assist when directing catheters cranially; however, its success depends on the ability to see the catheter tip by observing tissue displacement and disruption from local anesthetic injection during real-time (online) imaging.

Novel techniques for confirming placement of, and oftentimes guiding, catheters include: electrical epidural stimulation, electrocardiographic guidance, epidural pressure waveform analysis, and bedside ultrasound. All of these techniques have their merit; however, this chapter focuses on the basic concepts and the application of electrical epidural stimulation and ultrasound.

18.2. Electrical Epidural Stimulation

Electrical stimulation has been used in epidural anesthesia and for peripheral nerve blocks for many years. The epidural stimulation test (Tsui test) was developed to confirm epidural catheter placement, applying similar principles to those of peripheral nerve blockade, that is, using electrical pulses and the current versus nerve–distance relationship. This test has shown 80% to 100% positive prediction for epidural catheter placement. It has been shown to be effective to guide catheters to within two segmental levels (with radiological confirmation), which can assist smooth placement to appropriate levels and allow adjustments in the event of catheter migration, kinking, or coiling. In addition to confirming and guiding epidural catheter placement, this test has been shown to be useful for detecting intrathecal, subdural, or intravascular catheter placement. Lastly, the test also confirms needle placement during single-injection and continuous and caudal anesthesia (with catheter advancement in the cephalad direction) and direct epidural anesthesia of the lumbar and thoracic spine.

18.2.1. Test Equipment and Procedure

The procedure is performed in addition to standard mechanical tests (i.e., LOR to saline or air) for determining epidural needle placement

- The original setup (Figure 18.2) for testing catheter placement is relatively simple.
- After sterile preparation, connect a nerve stimulator to a metal-containing epidural catheter using an electrode adapter (e.g., Arrow-Johans ECG (electrocardiogram) adapter, Arrow International, Inc., Reading, PA, USA).
- Prime the catheter and adapter with sterile normal saline (0.2–1 mL).
- Attach the cathode lead of the nerve stimulator to the metal hub of the adapter and the grounding anode lead to an electrode on the patient's body surface.
- Set the nerve stimulator to low frequency and pulse width (1 Hz; 0.2 ms).
- Carefully and slowly increase the current intensity until motor activity begins.
- The characteristics of the various responses are compared in Table 18.1. Catheter location is identified and the required adjustments are made.

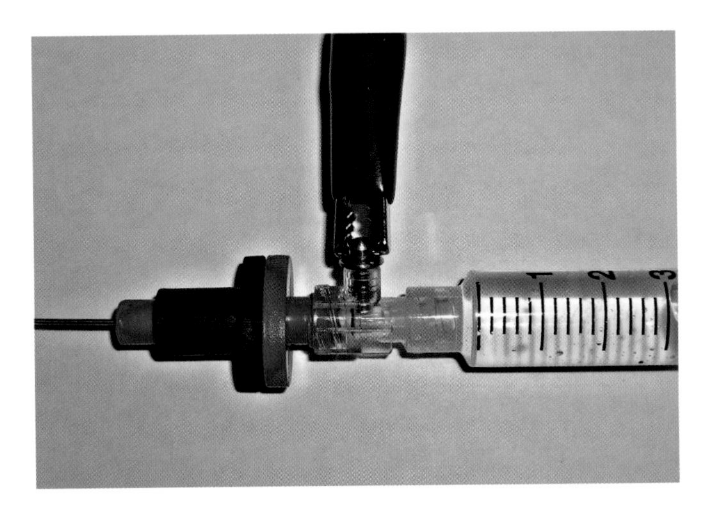

Figure 18.2. Electrical epidural stimulation test original setup. An adapter (Arrow-Johans ECG adapter, Arrow International, Inc., Reading, PA, USA) is attached to the connector of the epidural catheter (19-g FlexTip Plus, Arrow International, Inc., Reading, PA, USA); the adaptor and catheter are filled with normal saline and the cathode lead of the nerve stimulator is attached to the metal hub of the adapter.

Table 18.1. Catheter location determined by motor response and current threshold.

Catheter location	Motor response	Current
Subcutaneous	None	NA
Subdural	Bilateral (many segments)	<1 mA
Subarachnoid	Unilateral or bilateral	<1 mA
Epidural space		
Against nerve root	Unilateral	<1 mA
Non-intravascular	Unilateral or bilateral	1–15 mA (threshold current increases after local anesthetic injection)
Intravascular	Unilateral or bilateral	1–15 mA (no change in threshold current after local anesthetic injected)

Abbreviation: n/a, not applicable.
Needle placement at the caudal and lumbar spine adheres well to these criteria, although placement at thoracic spinal levels may necessitate higher upper limits (up to 17 mA has been shown).
The lower threshold applies to both catheter and needle placement.

For needle confirmation:

- The same procedure applies, with the exception that the nerve stimulator is attached to an insulated needle (e.g., 18- to 24ga insulated needles).
- The current is applied after skin puncture and during advancement; the epidural stimulation test is applied in addition to using a "pop" (at the posterior sacrococcygeal membrane; Figure 18.1) or LOR to saline.
- The test may provide further confirmation during direct epidurals, with the added benefit of warning that a needle is placed intravascularly, intrathecally, or near a nerve root.
- The threshold current range for determining correct needle placement is similar for the lumbar or caudal routes, but the higher limit of 10 mA may be extended for thoracic placement (up to 17 mA).

The stimulator should be versatile enough to allow the current to be increased in small increments and to be applied for short intervals.

18.2.2. Mechanism of the Test

- Catheter placement is confirmed by stimulating the spinal nerve roots (not spinal cord) with an electrically conducting catheter that conducts a low-amplitude electrical current through normal saline.
- A correct motor response (1–10 mA; Table 18.1) confirms accurate placement of the epidural catheter tip, defined as 1 to 2 cm from the nerve roots (Figure 18.3).
- Responses observed with a significantly lower threshold current (<1 mA), especially if substantially diffuse or bilateral, may warn of catheter placement in the subarachnoid or subdural space (i.e., contacting highly conductive cerebrospinal fluid), or in close proximity to a nerve root.
- The segmental level of the catheter tip may be predicted based on the progressive nature of the motor twitches (i.e., from lower limbs and back to intercostals and upper limb) as the catheter is advanced.
- A local anesthetic test dose helps confirm epidural versus intravascular location, as the motor threshold current should increase after local anesthetic application if the catheter

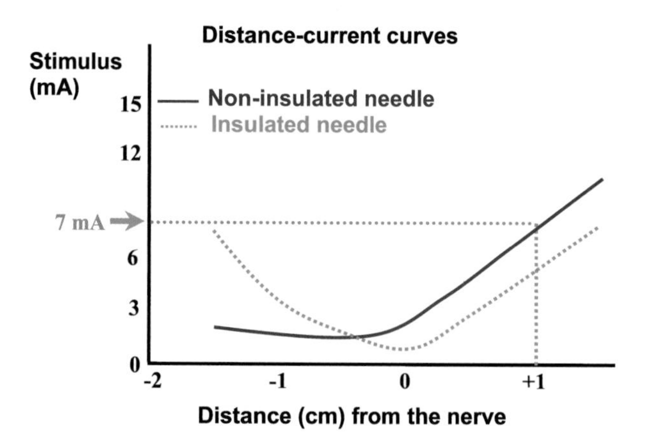

Figure 18.3. Current–distance curve. Using an insulated needle, the required current needed to generate a motor response is about 1 to 10 mA when the needle is placed 1 to 2 cm from the target nerve. By the same reasoning, using a stimulation catheter during epidural stimulation will result in current thresholds generally between 1 to 10 mA when the catheter is placed within 1 to 2 cm of the spinal nerve root. However, insulated epidural needles may require higher threshold currents (up to 17 mA has been observed) at the thoracic region than epidural catheters. This is perhaps due to the minimal insertion of the needle tip into the space whereas the catheter is fully embedded. (Adapted with permission from Pither CE, Ford DJ, Raj PP, Peripheral nerve stimulation with insulated and nuinsulated needles: efficacy and characteristics. Res Anesth 1984;9:42).

is localized to the epidural space, while unintentional injection into the systemic circulation (i.e., removing it from the vicinity of the nerve) will allow subsequent motor stimulation at similar currents.

- When used for needle placement:
  - Insulated needles provide low electrical resistance to current and are required for this test.
  - The upper limit of the threshold current indicating a positive test using needles is similar to catheter placement at the caudal space (mean, 3.7 mA), but higher at the thoracic level (up to 17 mA); the lower limit of >1 mA applies to all segmental levels.
  - The higher threshold currents that may be seen with direct thoracic level needle insertion may be related to the minimal depth of needle penetration that is inherently used for caution at this level.

18.2.3. Considerations for Test Performance and Interpretation

- Because local muscle contraction in the trunk region can be confused with epidural stimulation, it is recommended to place the anode in the upper extremity for lumbar epidurals and the lower extremity for thoracic epidurals.
- The 1- to 10-mA test criteria should be used as a guideline only. Epidural stimulation may occur outside this range. The reason we recommend this range is that it is easy to remember. In addition:
  - It is important to begin using the lowest current to allow detection of intrathecal placement or nerve root proximity; the lower limit of 1 mA applies to all situations (see Section 18.2.6).
  - Some cases will require stimulation upwards of 17 mA, particularly when using insulated needles in the thoracic region.
  - The best predictor of epidural placement is a combination of the threshold current level and the distribution of elicited motor responses (i.e., correlation with approximate segmental location), as subcutaneous placement would not elicit such predictive and segmental responses.

18.2.4. Stimulating Epidural Catheter Requirements

For advancing catheters significant distances, a specialized catheter will be needed. In Canada, positive results have been demonstrated using a special styletted catheter setup, including an injection port system which was previously commercially available (Epidural Positioning System using Tsui Test, Arrow International Inc., Reading PA). Similar results have been obtained abroad by in-house modification of regular metal-containing catheters (see Chapter 16). New products are under development to fulfill the essential requirements, including (1) effective conduction of electrical current, and (2) the correct balance of stiffness and malleability for advancement. Examples of stimulating catheters are shown in Figure 18.4(A–C).

18.2.4.1. Effective Conduction of Electrical Current

- The catheter's electrical resistance must remain low in order to induce electrical pulses.
- Any highly conductive ionic solution (e.g., normal saline) can be used to prime the catheter, but the metal coil in the lumen is still required because of the catheter length and the risk of air trapping, each of which can increase the resistance to current flow.
- A soft metal-containing epidural catheter (e.g., FlexTip Plus from Arrow International; Perifix from B. Braun, Bethlehem, PA; Spirol from Sims, Portex, Markham, Ontario, Canada) is effective for epidural stimulation testing [Figure 18.4(B)].
- Peripheral stimulating catheters (e.g., StimuLong Plus from Pajunk GmbH Medical Technology, Geisingen, Germany) contain a fixed wire internally that extends beyond the distal lumen tip [Figure18.4(C)]; these have been used for the epidural stimulation test without the saline column requirement. However, clinical experience with these catheters in the epidural space is still limited.

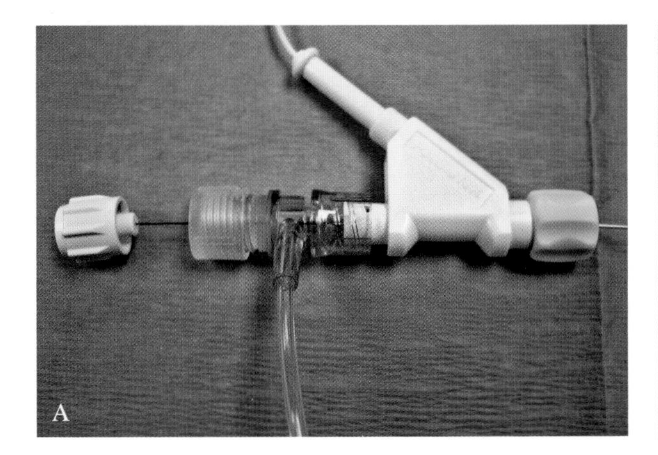

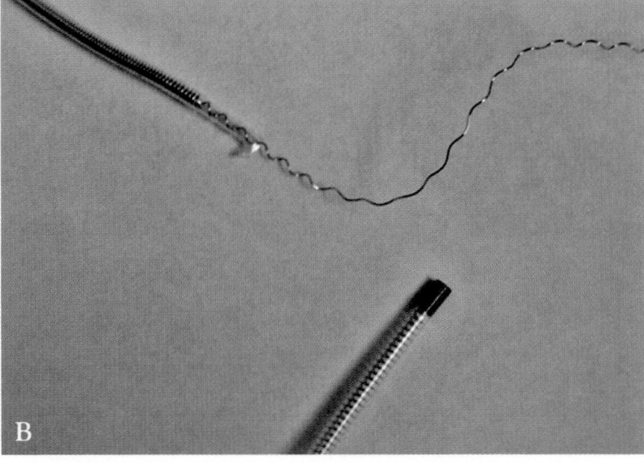

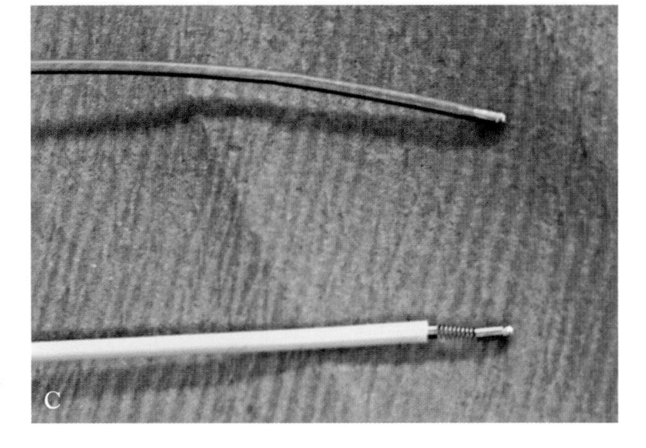

Figure 18.4. (A) Previously available Epidural Positioning System using Tsui test (Arrow International Inc., Reading PA). The setup includes a styletted soft metal-containing epidural catheter and an injection port to inject fluid for lubrication and perineural space expansion; (B) soft metal-containing epidural catheters can be used for the epidural stimulation test; (C) peripheral stimulating catheters, with a wire extension beyond the distal tip, have been used for epidural catheter insertion using electrical stimulation.

18.2.4.2. *Soft and Smooth but Stiff Enough for Advancement*

- Because the regular metal-containing catheters are fairly soft and pliable, when they are threaded long distances they need to be reinforced with metal stylets and modified to allow ejection of fluid for space dilation and lubrication during threading [Figure 18.4(A)].
- The ejected fluid may reduce friction between the catheter and surrounding tissues and thus limit impediments to advancement.
- Minor resistance to the passage of the catheter can be overcome by injecting normal saline through the advancing epidural catheter and/or simple flexion or extension of the patient's vertebral column.
- Recently, the use of multiport catheters has been introduced and shows promise to maximize the lubrication effect.

> Clinicians must remain vigilant because all techniques of epidural catheter placement have the potential for neurological injury. Therefore, under no circumstances should any force be used to advance the catheter.

18.2.5. Safety of Epidural Electrical Stimulation

- Electrical stimulation has been applied to central neural structures for neurophysiological evaluation or pain control for several years.
- Epidural stimulation uses similar current strengths to those used for patients with chronic pain disorders (4–30 mA) and for intra-operative monitoring during spinal surgery (2–40 mA).
- Although no known complications or patient discomfort have resulted, it is recommended that the current remains fairly low (<15–20 mA) and brief (few minutes).
- It is important that the current output is carefully increased from zero to ensure that all motor responses, even those elicited with low current (<1 mA), are detected; the current should also be blunted once motor activity is seen.
- The nerve stimulator must allow current levels to reach at least 10 mA in a gradual manner.

18.2.6. Clinical Applications

18.2.6.1. *Detecting Intrathecal and Intravascular Catheter and Needle Placement* (Table 18.1)

Aspiration should always be performed prior to local anesthetic injection. However, the inability to aspirate blood or cerebrospinal fluid (CSF) is not an absolute indication that an epidural needle/catheter is not in the intravascular or intrathecal space. The threshold current for a motor response during catheter and needle placement with the electrical stimulation test may help predict intrathecal placement. Intravascular placement may be detected with the electrical stimulation test in conjunction with a local anesthetic test dose.

18.2.6.1.1. *Intrathecal*

- When a needle/catheter is situated properly within the epidural space, a current much greater than 1 mA should be required to elicit muscle twitches.
  - From two studies using insulated needles, currents to elicit a motor response in the epidural space (3.84 ± 0.99 mA and 5.2 ± 2.4 mA) are much higher than that for the intrathecal space (0.77 ± 0.32 mA and 0.6 ± 0.3 mA).

- If any motor response is detected with a current less than 1 mA, intrathecal catheter or needle placement should be suspected.

18.2.6.1.2. *Intravascular*

- Repeated injections of local anesthetic into a properly placed epidural catheter results in impairment of nerve conduction and requires a gradual increase in the amplitude of electrical current to produce a positive motor response to the stimulation test. Lack of electrical resistance changes after injection of any solution may also provide a clue of intravascular placement (see Chapter 2).
- If the local anesthetic is inadvertently injected into the intravascular space (i.e., systemic circulation thereby reducing the concentration in the vicinity of the nerves), the threshold will not incrementally increase with repeated application, but remain the same or return to baseline levels.
- Caution is required when extrapolating the intravascular information because this application has only been tested in a few adult obstetric patients and never in the pediatric population.
  - An epinephrine test dose (0.5 μg/kg) should still be administered to identify inadvertent intravascular placement by observing specific ECG changes (i.e., >25% increase in T wave or ST segment changes irrespective of chosen lead).
  - However, when using the test dose in combination with the epidural stimulation test, one can confidently rule out the risk of an accidental intravascular or a subarachnoid injection.

18.2.6.2. *Confirming Needle Placement*

- Insulated needles are used as they allow electrical conductance.
- In a recent study, the epidural stimulation test showed better positive prediction than a "pop" in confirming needle placement in the caudal epidural space; the sensitivity and specificity were shown to be 100%. Electrical stimulation may thus be used as a teaching tool for placing needles during caudal epidural anesthesia.
- For caudal needle placement, an external anal sphincter contraction (S2–S4) is used to indicate appropriate placement; posterior trunk muscle contraction indicates local fiber stimulation only.
- For needle placement in the lumbar and thoracic spines, electrical stimulation has been applied through insulated Tuohy needles (see Chapter 1) after LOR to saline.
  - Although epidural stimulation seems to be a reliable way to detect insulated needle entrance into the lumbar or thoracic epidural space, the merit of using electrical stimulation in addition to LOR for needle entrance has not been studied and established.

18.2.6.3. *Guiding Epidural Catheter Placement*

18.2.6.3.1. *Caudal Approach*

- Caudal catheter anesthesia has been most successful for patients under 1 year of age. Beyond 1 year of age, the lumbar curve becomes more pronounced, preventing easy advancement of epidural catheters from the caudal space. It is this curvature that partly contributes to the kinking of catheters during their cephalad advancement; another contributor may be the change in the type of intrathecal tissue from fluid (cerebrospinal fluid) to solid (spinal cord).
- The introduction of new equipment and techniques (e.g., electrical epidural stimulation) has demonstrated that caudal catheter advancement is possible in older children using epidural stimulation.

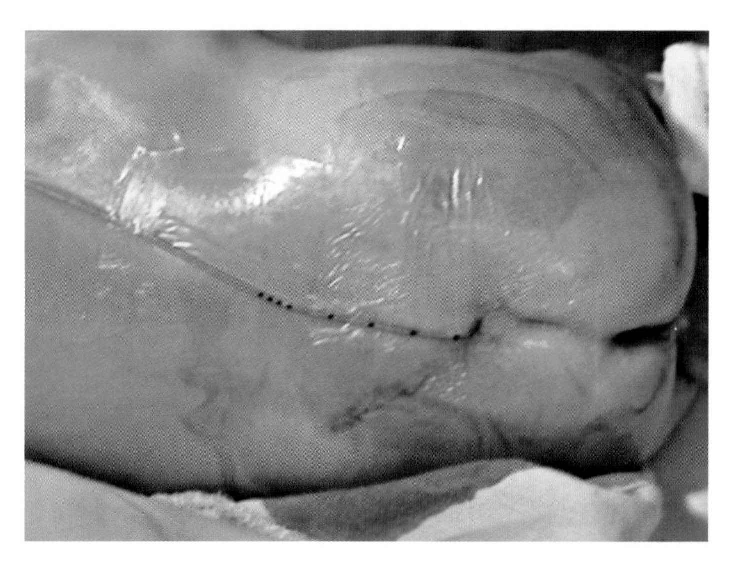

Figure 18.5. The catheter is secured on infants back with sterile occlusive dressing to maintain sterility.

- The improved success rate in older children has been attributed to the inclusion of a stylet in the test setup, which allows the simultaneous injection of saline during advancement and the ability to monitor the advancing catheter tip using stimulation.
- Tunneling caudal catheters or simply fixing the catheter with a sterile occlusive dressing immediately cephalad to the site has been recommended to reduce the risk of contamination by stool and urine (Figure 18.5).

18.2.6.3.2. Lumbar Approach

- Lumbar epidural anesthesia is often used in lower extremity and urological surgery.
- The previously reported lack of success for advancing catheters from lumbar to thoracic epidural spaces may be due to obstruction of the flexible catheter tip caused by the lumbar curve.
- Electrical stimulation testing using a modified styletted catheter has shown potential, but the number of reports on this testing is limited so far.
- Further research and study is warranted.

18.2.6.3.3. Thoracic Approach

- It is not required to advance epidural catheters very far into the epidural space when direct thoracic approaches are used as the introduction of the catheter is in close proximity to the site of required surgical anesthesia.
- Epidural catheter stimulation does not seem to have significant benefit over LOR for improving accuracy in placing epidural catheters at specific nerve root levels.
- However, it has been demonstrated that catheters can be successfully placed, and provide good analgesia, at the cervical spine after advancement from the mid-to-high thoracic spine.
- The primary benefit of the electrical stimulation test with thoracic approaches may be the additional safety feature alerting the clinician of needle proximity to the intrathecal space, spinal cord, or nerve root.

18.2.6.4. Limitations of Epidural Stimulation

- Significant clinical neuromuscular blockade or local anesthetics in the epidural space limit the use of this test.

- One alternative monitoring technique (see Chapter 20), described by Tsui et al., uses ECG monitoring:
  - The amplitude of the QRS complex matches the surface electrode amplitude as it passes the target level.
- Unlike the epidural stimulation test, the ECG technique cannot warn of a catheter placed in the subarachnoid or intravascular space, nor can it predict the catheter placement level when short threading distances are required.
- Ultrasound imaging is an alternative method for catheter placement and guidance in young children (see next section).
- Minor limitations of electrical stimulation include the need for and cost of a "specialized" stimulating catheter, but clearly the cost of ineffective analgesia or intrathecal/intravascular placement would be much higher.

18.3. Ultrasound Imaging in Neuraxial Anesthesia

Ultrasound imaging for regional anesthesia is discussed to a large extent in Chapters 3 and 4, and this chapter will only deal with those aspects relevant to caudal and epidural anesthesia. Generally, two approaches can be used for applying ultrasound imaging for epidural procedures. First, ultrasound-supported epidurals utilize ultrasound imaging preprocedurally to scan the relevant area and determine the puncture site, depth of epidural space, and ideal needle trajectory. These procedures require multiple still images in different planes to capture accurate measurement with the ultrasound device. Second, real-time or online imaging can be used during epidural procedures to observe the needle puncture, catheter placement, and local anesthetic application. There are some challenges with using ultrasound in neuraxial procedures, but it has demonstrable benefits for infants and neonates and may have some efficacy (e.g., reduced needle attempts and visibility of the sacral hiatus for caudal blocks) with older pediatric and adult patients. This book mainly focuses on infant epidurals as these are most amenable to ultrasound guidance.

18.3.1. Visibility Through Ultrasound

Generally, the lower lumbar region has the highest visibility (i.e., ultrasound window) as it is less compact than the more cephalad high-lumbar and thoracic levels. Rapp and colleagues (2005) studied neuraxial imaging in pediatric patients and found a ratio of visible to nonvisible segments to be 2 : 1 at the sacral, 1 : 1 at the lumbar, and 1 : 2 at the thoracic levels. Visibility of neuraxial structures in the lumbar and thoracic regions is best in patients 3 months of age and under, with age-dependant decreases in quality thereafter. There will be variation in the available structures within different planes of ultrasound scanning (i.e., paramedian longitudinal scanning will visualize the dura mater better than median longitudinal; Figures 18.6, 18.7, and 18.8) and different techniques may require separate planes, while many will require two or more for comprehensive assessment.

18.3.1.1. Direct Visiblity

Figures 18.8(A–C), 18.9(A–C), and 18.10(A–D) are high-quality ultrasound images obtained with ultrasound machines having superior resolution than that of the portable machine used for capturing the practical images in Chapter 20 (MicroMaxx, SonoSite, Inc., Bothell, WA, USA; see Chapter 3). The images are shown so the reader can appreciate the structural relations and ideal appearance within the neuraxis, rather than for practical use with portable systems often purchased for regional anesthesia purposes.

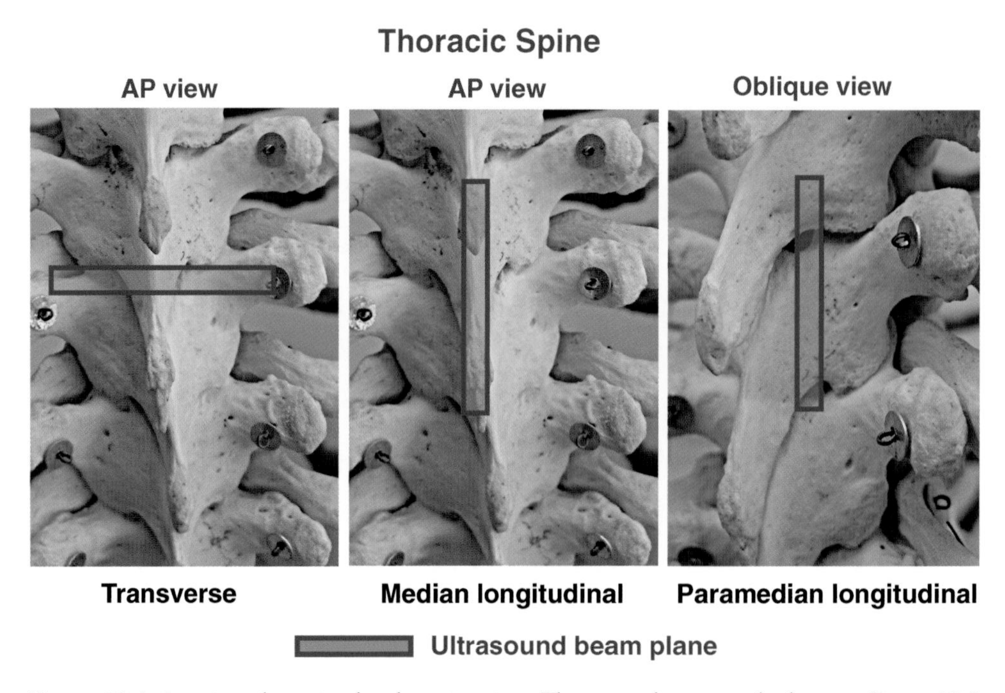

Figure 18.6. Imaging planes in the thoracic spine. The scan planes match those in Figure 18.8 ultrasound images. The longitudinal paramedian plane allows the greatest view of the dura, although it is clear that the ultrasound windows between the bony structures are very small in the thoracic spine.

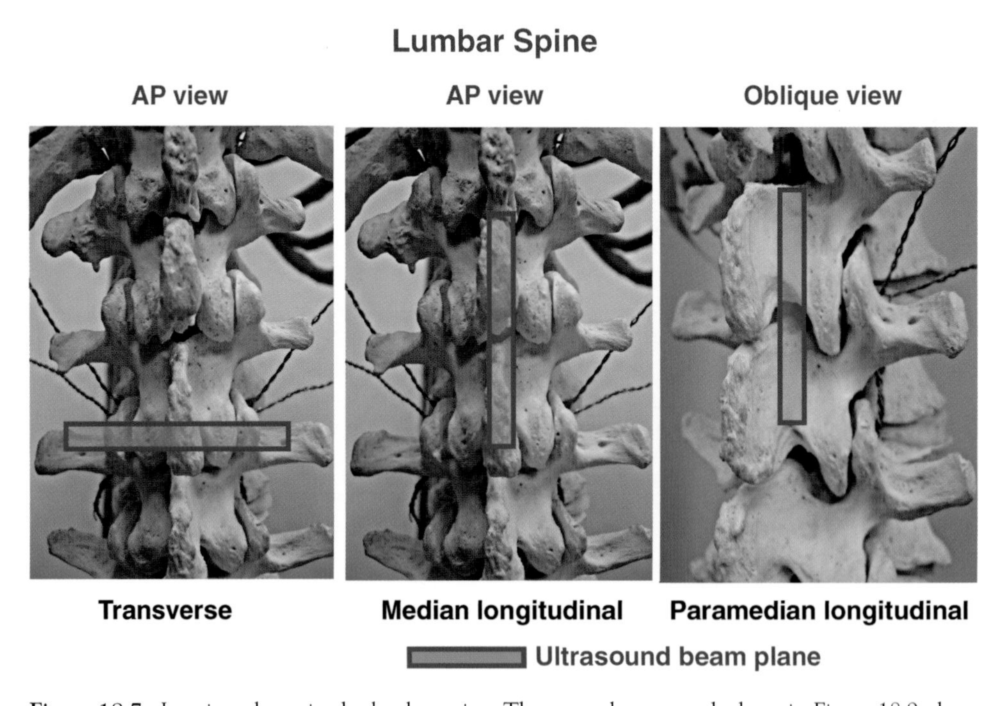

Figure 18.7. Imaging planes in the lumbar spine. The scan planes match those in Figure 18.9 ultrasound images. The longitudinal paramedian plane allows the greatest view of the dura and the ultrasound windows in the lumbar spine are significantly larger than in the thoracic spine.

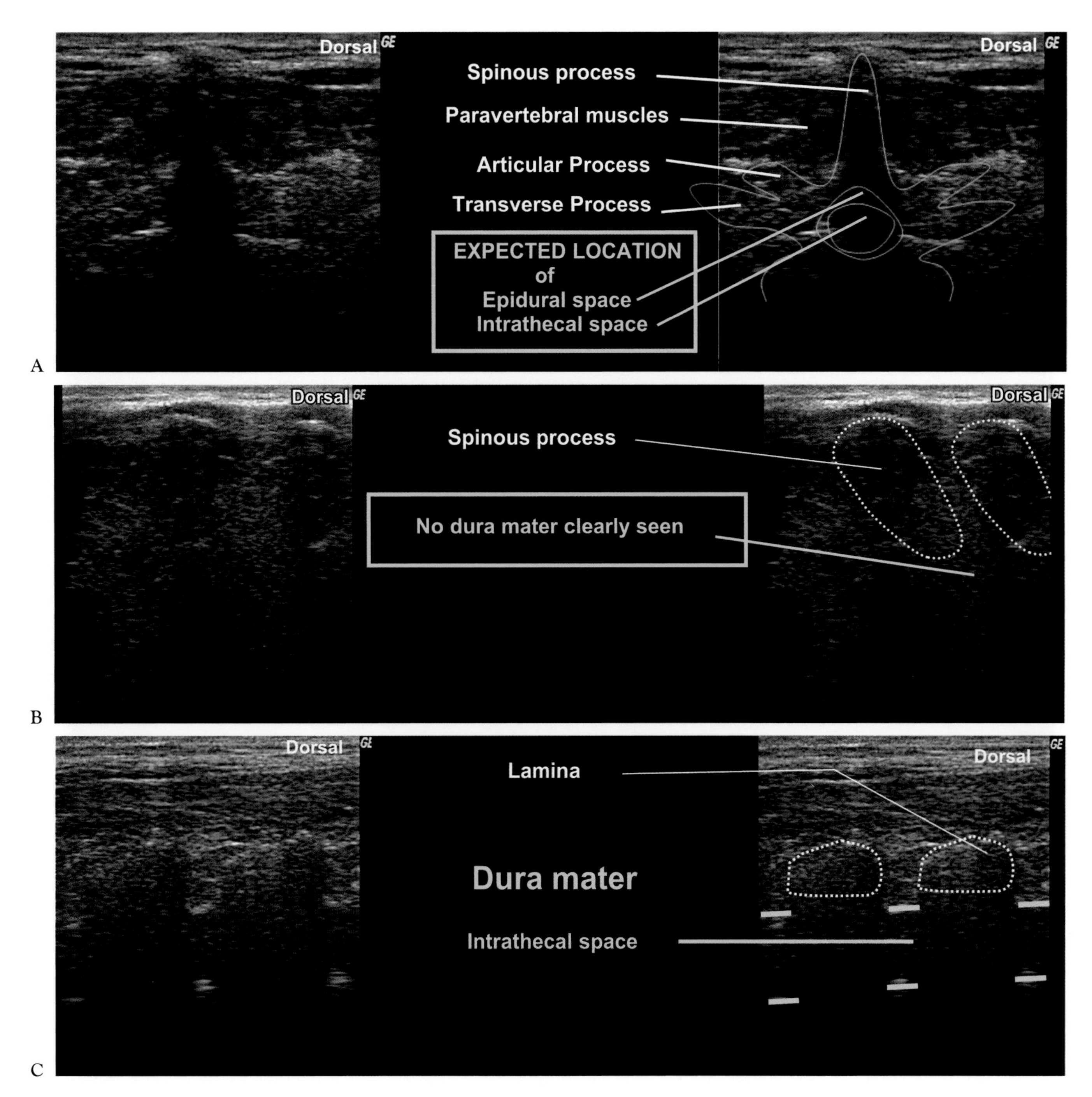

Figure 18.8. Ultrasound images at the thoracic spine in an adult in the (A) transverse, (B) longitudinal median, and (C) longitudinal paramedian planes. The paramedian longitudinal plane has a superior ultrasound window than the median longitudinal plane and illustrates the dura mater to a greater extent. (Reprinted with permission from Drs Hans Juergen Rapp (Children's Hospital, Cologne) and Thomas Grau.)

- Transverse imaging shows the spinous processes with shadowing in the midline, the facet joints laterally, and the vertebral bodies deepest, with the potential for intrathecal viewing [Figures 18.8(A) and 18.9(A)].
  - The positioning of each vertebrae is the main advantage. This may be deviant, especially in conditions such as scoliosis.
  - Needle trajectory imaging is limited except for indication of lateralization of the needle trajectory.

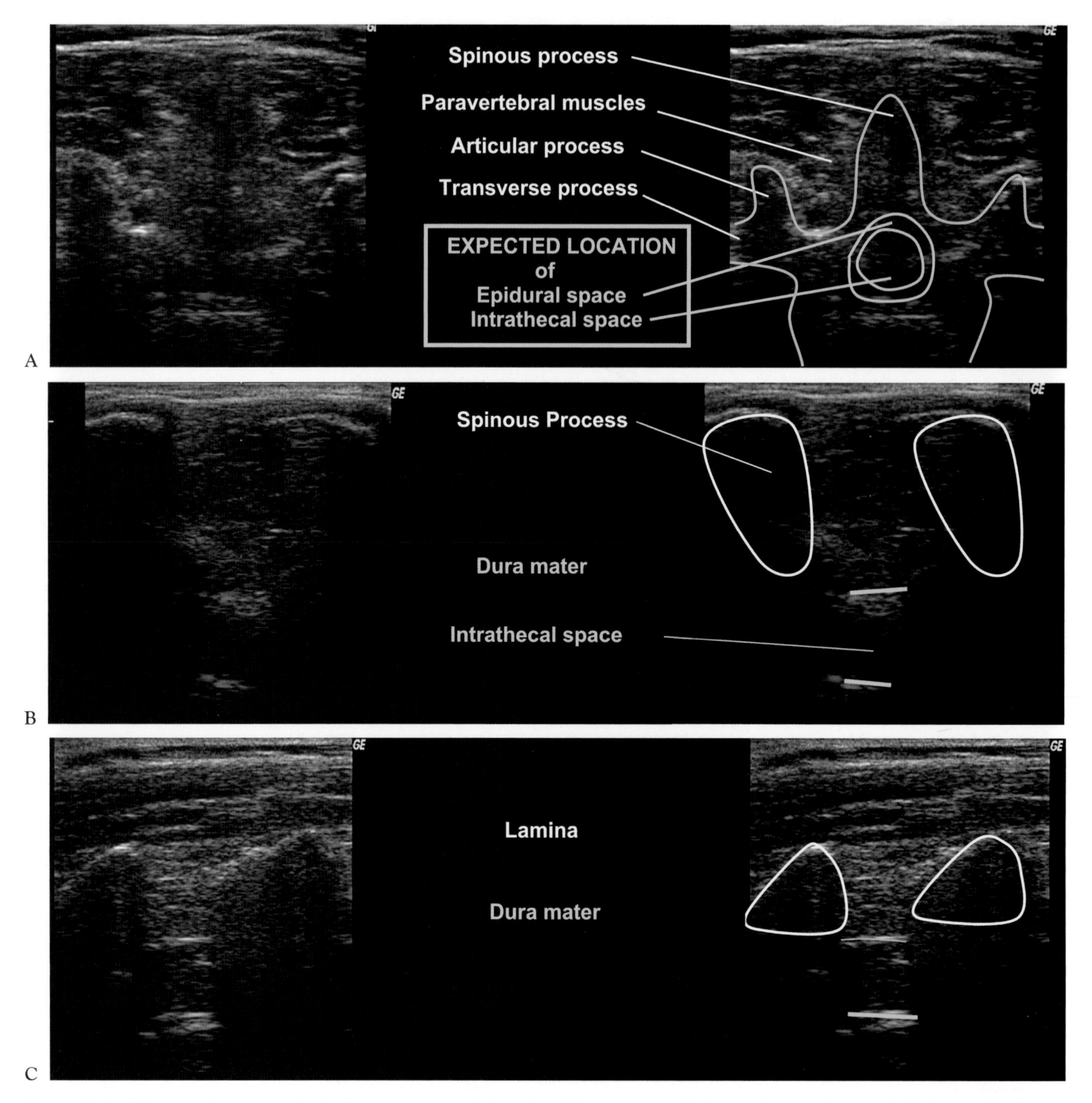

Figure 18.9. Ultrasound images at the lumbar spine in an adult in the (A) transverse, (B) longitudinal median, and (C) longitudinal paramedian planes. A greater proportion of the dura mater is seen and it is more distinct using the paramedian plane. The interspinous spaces are larger in the lumbar over the thoracic spine (seen in Figure 18.8). (Reprinted with permission from Drs Hans Juergen Rapp (Children's Hospital, Cologne) and Thomas Grau.)

- Median longitudinal/sagittal imaging depicts the spinous processes and interspinous space quite clearly and needle trajectory can be controlled through this approach [Figures 18.8(B) and 18.9(B)].
  - In young patients there is a good soft tissue window and the usually bilayered dura mater is clearly visualized, while the ligamentum flavum, intrathecal space, spinal cord, nerve roots, and fibers (including cauda equina) all have intermediate but identifiable echogenicity.

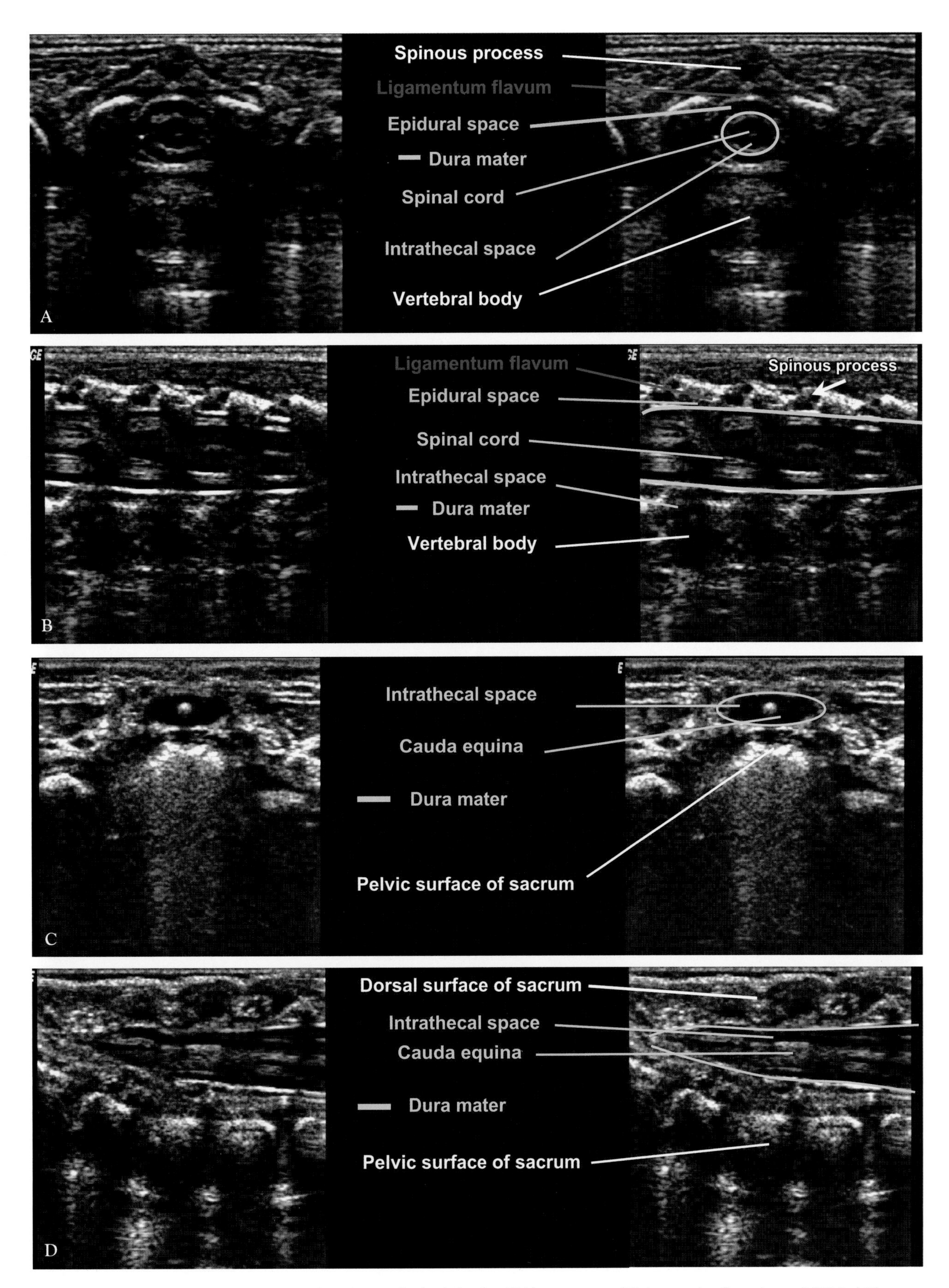

Figure 18.10. High-resolution ultrasound images at the high lumbar [(A) transverse, (B) longitudinal], and sacral [S2,3; (C) transverse, (D) longitudinal], levels in a 12-month-old infant. It is clear that there is more visibility in the infant spine due to the lack of calcification and fusion of the posterior elements of the canal. (Reprinted with permission from Drs Hans Juergen Rapp (Children's Hospital, Cologne) and Thomas Grau.)

- The advanced ossification occurring with age causes ultrasound beam reflection (i.e., increased shadowing). This problem reduces the window substantially and is most prominent in the compact thoracic spine.
  - Reasonable depiction of the dura mater and ligamentum flavum is possible in adults.
- Paramedian longitudinal imaging is an addition to the usual bidirectional ultrasound scanning plane approach, which allows greatest visibility of the dura mater [Figures 18.8(C) and 18.9(C)].
  - There is less interference from bony structures with this approach and therefore it allows enhanced depiction quality and greater interspace visualization.
  - The lamina and facet joints are visible rather than the spinous processes as in median longitudinal viewing.
  - The epidural space can be depicted in 40% to 50% of adults with this approach.
  - A remaining challenge with this technique is the tangential (out-of-plane; short-axis) relation of the needle (midline) and probe (paramedian), which only enables clear needle tip visibility and limits accurate angular positioning of the shaft.

> - Detailed anatomical descriptions of the thoracic and lumbar structures are discussed in Chapter 17.
> - The ultrasound images in this chapter clearly confirm that a paramedian longitudinal approach results in improved visibility in the adult patient.

18.3.1.2. *Indirect Visiblity*

- Continuous visualization of needle tip penetration and catheter advancement is sometimes difficult due to the ultrasound beam reflection resulting from extensive ossification.
- Needle punctures are often made visible by movements of the needle tip and displacement of the surrounding tissue (i.e., indirect means).
- Occasionally, LOR to saline can be seen as widening of the epidural space and ventral movement of the dura mater upon saline injection.
- Indeed, precise catheter tip identity is possible in children below 3 to 6 years of age (see Figure 20.15).
- Catheter advancement is generally visualized indirectly by the spread of injectate and movement of the dura in the vicinity of its tip.
  - This surrogacy limits the ability to re-assess the catheter position postprocedurally.
  - The use of metal-coiled catheters, which appear bright with striated features, may circumvent this deficiency, but other experience shows that this effect is limited.

> The ratio of visible to nonvisible structures in the sacral spine in children is higher (2:1) than in the lumbar (1:1) or thoracic spine (1:2).

18.3.2. Summary of the Ultrasound Appearance of Neuraxial Structures

The images in Figures 18.8, 18.9, and 18.10 are taken with a high-resolution, cart-based ultrasound system (see Chapter 3) and the images are often superior to those attainable with portable machines, as used in Chapter 20. In addition, images will differ with respect to patient age; because the images in Figure 18.10 are taken from a 12-month-old infant (for best illustration), they will be superior to those from an adult (Figures 18.8 and 18.9).

The images at the sacral level [Figure 18.10(C,D)] will differ from those at the high lumbar level [Figure 18.10(A,B)]

- Short-axis view at S2 to S3 (Figure 18.10C):
  - The center of the screen contains the circular/oval space, with the anechoic cerebrospinal fluid internally, the hypoechoic cauda equina, and the surrounding thin circular, hyperechoic dura.
  - Superficially (on the dorsal surface of the vertebral body), it is possible to view the linear hyperechoic subcutaneous tissue and an inverted V shape depicting the neural arches (laminae and spinous processes in older patients) as hyperechoic with dorsal shadowing.
  - Laterally and reaching dorsally, the intervertebral foramina may be seen as hyperechoic air spaces.
- Long-axis median view at S2 to S3 (Figure 18.10D):
  - The hypoechoic cerebrospinal fluid and the moderately hyperechoic fibers (with hypoechoic myelin covering) of the cauda equina form a sideways oriented broad V shape between the highly hyperechoic layers of dura mater.
  - The pulsatile character of the cauda equina is obvious in a high-resolution image.
  - The caudal entrance to the epidural space can be seen on the far inferior edge of the image, and the vertebral bodies appear dark, with hyperechoic spacing between them forming a good ultrasound window for viewing of the epidural and subdural spaces.

Chapter 3 includes a detailed description of the appearance of various tissues and substances (Table 3.2). Below is a brief comparison of the varying degrees of echogenicity of the different tissues/substances.

18.3.2.1. Hyperechogenic Tissues (Bright)

- *Dura mater*
  Appears thin, highly linear, and bright, usually with a double-layered appearance in longitudinal view; it is best viewed in a longitudinal paramedian plane.
- *Bony structures*
  Are highly reflective and bright on the surface, although they cast a dark shadow underneath.
- *Conus medullaris and cauda equina*
  Appear almost fibrillar with a nearly hyperechoic appearance.
- *Catheter*
  Appears as a double linear structure in longitudinal view and a single hyperechoic dot on short-axis view (see Figure 20.15).

18.3.2.2. Iso/Hypoechoic Structures (Identical Density; Appear Gray)

Epidural space is located beyond the relatively hyperechoic dura mater.

Spinal cord has low echogenicity, with a double line at the thoracic level.

18.3.2.3. Anechoic Structures/Substances (Black)

Upon injection of *local anesthetic*, a hypoechogenic expansion is visible at the injection location and often separates the neural and vascular structures.

Subarachnoid space is filled with cerebrospinal fluid.

18.3.2.4. Probe Characteristics

- Linear probes (5–10 MHz) have been shown to provide superior imaging to phased array probes (4–7 MHz).
- The deeper location of many epidural structures in adults, relative to some peripheral nerves, necessitates lower frequency probes.
- The lower frequencies often result in less clarity (i.e., resolution), which is a reason that ultrasound is easiest to perform in children who have more superficial spinal structures allowing higher frequency probes (5–10 MHz) with superior resolution.

18.3.3. Clinical Applications

18.3.3.1. *Preprocedural Ultrasound for Supported Needle Puncture*

- Puncture depth for use with a LOR technique of the epidural space can be measured prior to puncture as the shortest distance between the skin and epidural space (i.e., skin to ventral surface of ligamentum flavum).
  - In young children, the high-resolution capability allows very accurate width measurement of the epidural space (ligamentum flavum to dura mater).
  - There is a good correlation ($r = 0.88$) of ultrasound measured depth of the epidural space with that from LOR.
- Epidural space measurement, with the expected puncture angle, helps determine an ideal puncture point and determine the needle trajectory.
- Particularly in obese patients, ultrasound assessment of the sacral hiatus landmarks used for needle placement in the caudal epidural space may be helpful.

18.3.3.2. *Online Imaging During Processing*

18.3.3.2.1. *Caudal Needle Placement*

Caudal epidural anesthesia is commonly used to reduce the greater risk of dural puncture at higher spinal regions and to ease the technical difficulties with higher punctures in previous spinal surgical patients. This is particularly true for infants/children, in whom the procedures are performed under general anesthesia and the warnings due to paresthesia are not possible. Despite this, there is a fairly high (up to 25%) failure rate when attempting to localize the caudal epidural space and more objective tests than the "give" or "pop" have been recommended. The epidural stimulation test has shown 100% sensitivity and specificity when predicting the clinical outcomes of this block, but ultrasound can also be useful to identify landmarks during needle puncture and advancement towards the epidural space.

- Transversal (short-axis) probe orientation above the sacral hiatus in children (>1–2 years old) and adults allows visualization of the sacral cornua (bilateral horns), dorsal surface of the sacrum, posterior sacrococcygeal membrane, and sacral hiatus (Figures 20.8 and 20.9).
- Longitudinal (long-axis) viewing, in adults, between the two cornua may allow depiction of the needle trajectory to the point of sacrococcygeal membrane entrance; beyond which the characteristic "pop" can be used to confirm needle placement within the caudal epidural space.
- After epidural entrance, the short axis can be used again to confirm that the caudal needle is located in the epidural space.
- In young infants, the ultrasound probe can be placed at the midpoint of the sacrum (S2–S3) [Figure 18.10(d)], which may allow good longitudinal viewing of the needle during epidural entrance. This is possible during in-plane needling.
- Ultrasound has shown 100% accuracy (to radiographic confirmation) in adult patients to locate the sacral hiatus and to confirm needle entry into the caudal epidural space.
- The exact identification of the epidural space can be confirmed in infants as well as in adults.

Clinical Pearl

The main disadvantage of ultrasound is the problem of bony calcification leading to poor resolution and shadowing. Conversely, there is improved visibility in younger patients.

18.3.3.2.2. *Epidural Catheter Insertion*

- Compared to LOR, ultrasound (through visualizing local anesthetic spread and neuraxial structures) speeded execution and reduced bone contacts during lumbar and thoracic epidural catheter placement in 64 children. (Willschke et al., 2006)
- This study still showed a 17% bone contact rate, therefore, the bone may have been misinterpreted as soft tissue, which highlights the fact that visualization of needle tips and tissue under ultrasound guidance is subject to significant operator interpretation.
- The authors did not include ultrasound start-up and preparation time in their calculations and the catheters were only threaded 2 to 3 cm.
- There is reporting of direct visibility of lumbar LOR in pediatric patients, although visibility of thoracic puncture and LOR in young children is reduced because of increased calcification and shadowing.
- Catheter advancement from the caudal to lumbar or thoracic epidural spaces can not always be visualized in real time due to the bony sacrum, but catheter advancement and local anesthetic application can be monitored in young patients once the catheters have reached the lumbar spine.
- Without clearly visible catheters, ultrasound imaging can be difficult to perform in a dynamic manner during advancement.
- An experienced assistant is usually needed to perform the ultrasound imaging during the introduction of the catheter.

> Some clinicians find that coiled catheters are no more visible with ultrasound than conventional catheters.

18.3.3.2.3. *Direct Epidural Needle Placement*

- The needle trajectory can be predicted or followed to some extent using ultrasound.
- The paramedian longitudinal scanning plane [Figures 18.8(c) and 18.9(c)], which allows superior imaging of the neuraxial structures, only allows for a tangential approach of the needle (midline) to ultrasound plane; this out-of-plane needling technique enables clear visibility of the needle tip as a bright dot but limited needle shaft visibility for trajectory control.
- By visualizing the spread of local anesthetic and anterior movement of the posterior dural membrane, ultrasound helps determine needle and catheter placement in the epidural space.

18.4. Conclusion

Ultrasound guidance during central block procedures is very advantageous in cases where clear visibility is possible. Numerous structures can be well depicted either for measurement/assessment purposes or during dynamic processing of the needle and local anesthetic application. The needle trajectory can be predicted and the catheter advancement assessed. The main problem with this technology is the poor depiction of some anatomical structures due to significant shadowing from calcified bone as well as the limited catheter visibility after placement. Electrical stimulation in the epidural space may be greatly beneficial for the latter as it effectively determines catheter placement either during or after advancement. Both techniques can be used to provide additional safety measures during neuraxial blockade as they can help determine faulty needle or catheter placement. Integrating both into our practice could improve the success and safety of epidural anesthesia.

Suggested Reading and References

Reviews

Dalens B. Some controversies in paediatric regional anaesthesia. Curr Opin Anaesthesiol 2006;19:301–308.

Grau T. Ultrasonography in the current practice of regional anaesthesia. Best Pract Res Clin Anaesthesiol 2005;19:175–200.

Tsui BC. Innovative approaches to neuraxial blockade in children: the introduction of epidural nerve root stimulation and ultrasound guidance for epidural catheter placement. Pain Res Manag 2006;11:173–180.

Epidural Issues and Caudal Catheter Placement

Blanco D, Llamazares J, Rincon R, Ortiz M, Vidal F. Thoracic epidural anesthesia via the lumbar approach in infants and children. Anesthesiology 1996;84:1312–1316.

Bosenburg AT, Bland BAR, Schulte-Steinberg O, Downing JW. Thoracic epidural anesthesia via caudal route in infants. Anesthesiology 1988;69:256–259.

Desparmet JF. Epidural anesthesia in infants. Can J Anaesth 1999;46:1105–1109.

Fischer HB. Performing epidural insertion under general anaesthesia. Anaesthesia 2000;55:288–289.

Fischer HB. Regional anaesthesia—before or after general anaesthesia? Anaesthesia 1998;53:727–729.

Gunter JB, Eng C. Thoracic epidural anesthesia via the caudal approach in children. Anesthesiology 1992;76:935–938.

Krane EJ, Dalens BJ, Murat I, Murrell D. The safety of epidurals placed during general anesthesia. Reg Anesth Pain Med 1998;23:433–438.

Rasch DK, Webster DE, Pollard TG, Gurkowski MA. Lumbar and thoracic epidural analgesia via the caudal approach for postoperative pain relief in infants and children. Can J Anaesth 1990;37:359–362.

Tsui BC, Berde CB. Caudal analgesia and anesthesia techniques in children. Curr Opin Anaesthesiol 2005;18:283–288.

Epidural Stimulation

de Medicis E, Tetrault JP, Martin R, Robichaud R, Laroche L. A prospective comparison study of two indirect methods for confirming the localization of an epidural catheter for postoperative analgesia. Anesth Analg 2005;101:1830–1833.

Lena P, Martin R. Subdural placement of an epidural catheter detected by nerve stimulation. Can J Anesth 2005;52:618–621.

Tamai H, Sawamura S, Kanamori Y, Takeda K, Chinzei M, Hanaoka K. Thoracic epidural catheter insertion using the caudal approach assisted with an electrical nerve stimulator in young children. Reg Anesth Pain Med 2005;29:92–95.

Tsui BC, Gupta S, Finucane B. Confirmation of epidural catheter placement using nerve stimulation. Can J Anesth 1998;45:640–644.

Tsui BC, Seal R, Koller J, Entwistle L, Haugen R, Kearney R. Thoracic epidural analgesia via the caudal approach in pediatric patients undergoing fundoplication using nerve stimulation guidance. Anesth Analg 2001;93:1152–1155.

Tsui BC, Wagner A, Cave D, Kearney R. Thoracic and lumbar epidurals via the caudal approach using electrical stimulation guidance in pediatric patients: a review of 289 patients. Anesthesiology 2004;100:683–689.

Tsui BC, Wagner A, Cave D, Seal R. Threshold current for an insulated epidural needle in pediatric patients. Paediatr Anaesth 2004;99:694–696.

Tsui BCH, Gupta S, Finucane B. Detection of subarachnoid and intravascular epidural catheter placement. Can J Anesth 1999;46:675–678.

Tsui BCH, Tarkkila P, Gupta S, Kearney R. Confirmation of caudal needle placement using nerve stimulation. Anesthesiology 1999;91:374–378.

Tsui BCH, Wagner AM, Cunningham K, et al. Threshold current of an insulated needle in the intrathecal space in pediatric patients. Anesth Analg 2005;100:662–665.

Ultrasound Guidance

Bell GT, Bolton P. Caudal catheters and ultrasound [correspondence]. Pediatr Anesth 2006; 16:98–99.
Chawathe MS, Jones RM, Gildersleve CD, et al. Detection of epidural catheters with ultrasound in children. Paediatr Anaesth 2003;13:681–684.
Chen CPC, Tang SFT, Hsu T, et al. Ultrasound guidance in caudal epidural needle placement. Anesthesiology 2004;101:181–184.
Edward R. Ultrasound-guided caudal epidural injection [correspondence]. Anesthesiology 2005; 102:693.
Grau T, Leipold RW, Delorme S, Martin E, Motsch J. Ultrasound imaging of the thoracic space. Reg Anesth Pain Med 2002;27:200–206.
Huang J. Disadvantages of ultrasound guidance in caudal epidural needle placement [correspondence]. Anesthesiology 2005;102:693.
Marhofer P, Bosenberg A, Sitzwohl C, et al. Pilot study of neuraxial imaging by ultrasound in infants and children. Pediatr Anesth 2005;15:671–676.
Marhofer P, Willschke H, Kettner S. Imaging techniques for regional nerve blockade and vascular cannulation in children. Curr Opin Anaesthesiol 2006;19:293–300.
Rapp H, Folger A, Grau T. Ultrasound-guided epidural catheter insertion in children. Anesth Analg 2005;101:333–339.
Roberts SA, Galvez I. Ultrasound assessment of caudal catheter position in infants. Pediatr Anesth 2005;15:429–432.
Willschke H, Marhofer P, Bosenberg A, et al. Epidural catheter placement in children: comparing a novel approach using ultrasound guidance and a standard loss-of-resistance technique. Br J Anaesth 2006;97:200–207.

Other Epidural Placement Techniques

Ghia JN, Arora SK, Castillo M, Mukherju SK. Confirmation of location of epidural catheters by epidural pressure waveform and computed tomography catheteregram. Reg Anesth Pain Med 2001;26:337–341.
Tsui BCH, Seal R, Koller J. Thoracic epidural catheter placement via the caudal approach in infants by using electrocardiographic guidance. Anesth Analg 2002;95:326–330.

19

Paravertebral and Intercostal Blockade

Ban C.H. Tsui

19.1. Introduction

Anesthesia of thoracic and lumbar spinal nerves can be achieved by performing paravertebral blocks. These blocks are considered unilateral epidurals because they selectively block spinal nerves on the side of anesthetic application, although they also have the potential for epidural spread (i.e., they can be performed bilaterally if desired). The anesthesia includes both somatic and sympathetic effects, with a reduced hemodynamic response (to a certain extent) as compared to epidural anesthesia. There is generally less motor blockade of the extremities than with epidurals, unless lumbar spinal levels are incorporated (L2 and below). The thoracic paravertebral block is often used for breast surgery and perioperatively for thoracic surgery. Thoracolumbar paravertebral anesthesia is commonly used for inguinal herniorrhaphy and postoperative analgesia following hip surgery. This chapter will focus on ultrasound guidance during thoracic paravertebral blocks, with some discussion of intercostal nerve blockade. Lumbar paravertebral blocks are similar to those in the thoracic region with the noted absence of the ribs; they are also very similar in approach to lumbar plexus blockade (see Chapter 12).

Clinical Pearl

The dermatomal distribution of paravertebral blocks will depend on the block location and the volume of local anesthetic injected.

19.2. Clinical Anatomy

19.2.1. Skeletal Anatomy of the Trunk (Figure 19.1)

A general overview of the thoracic and lumbar spine, and their related articulations and peripheral nerves (intercostal nerves) is provided as ultrasound will enable visualization of some of these structures. The reader is referred to Chapter 17 for more detail regarding the spinal nerves and the dermatomes of the trunk.

19.2.1.1. Clinical Anatomy of the Thoracic and Lumbar Spine

- There are 12 thoracic vertebrae with several common distinguishing characteristics, including:
  - Vertebral bodies are of medium size and heart shaped (see Figure 17.1).
  - Vertebral (spinal) canals are small and circular in shape.

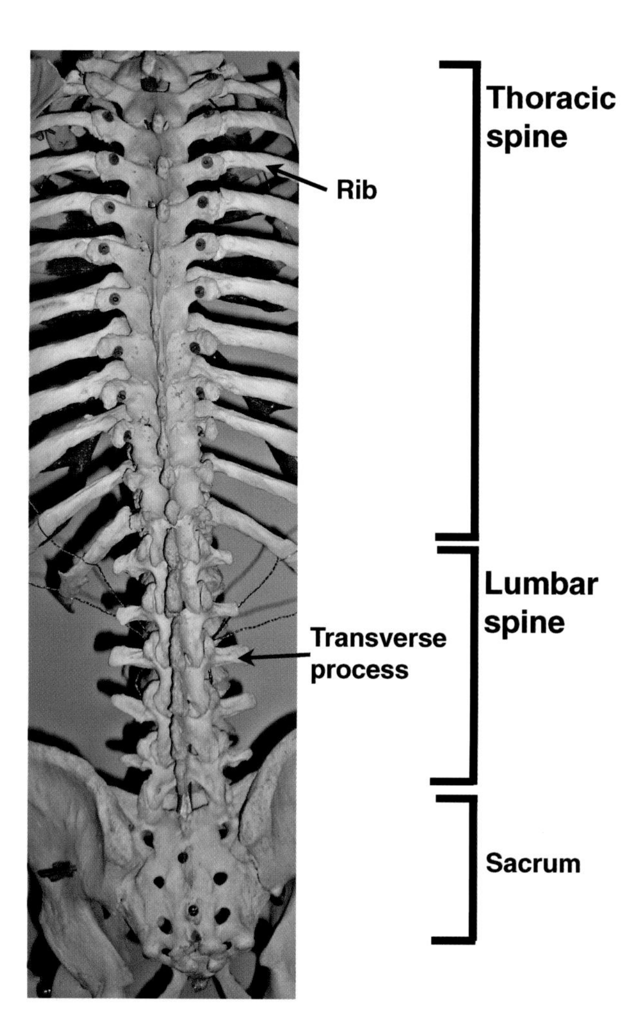

Figure 19.1. Skeletal anatomy of the trunk.

  - Laminae are relatively small.
  - Spinous processes are long and oriented inferiorly in an oblique direction.
  - Transverse processes are relatively broad and robust for articulation with the ribs and generally face posterolaterally.
- The five lumbar vertebrae are characterized by their:
  - Large and kidney-shaped vertebral bodies.
  - Triangularly shaped vertebral (spinal) canals.
  - Thick laminae.
  - Short and stout spinous processes, oriented horizontally.
  - Thick intervertebral discs (they are largest and thickest here compared to the rest of the spine).
  - Long, slender, and laterally directed transverse processes.
- In infants, the vertebral bodies and neural arches are generally completely fused by the end of the fifth year to form a complete vertebra.
- Development of the vertebral column is essentially complete at the thoracic and lumbar spine by early adulthood (20s), with the exception being inconsistent fusion between S1 and S2.

19.2.1.2. *Costovertebral Articulations*

The ribs articulate through two synovial joints with the vertebral column (see Figure 17.5).

- Costovertebral joint: Head of rib articulates through synovial joints with demifacets on adjacent thoracic vertebral bodies and the corresponding intervertebral disc of the upper vertebral joint.
- Costotransverse joint: Articular facets on the tubercles of the ribs articulate through synovial joints with the transverse processes of the thoracic vertebrae.

19.2.2. Anatomy of the Paravertebral Space and Intercostal Nerves

Thoracic spinal nerves T2 through T12 and lumbar spinal nerve L1 can be blocked for surgical anesthesia. On either side of the vertebral column, there is a wedge-shaped space through which the spinal nerves course after exiting from the intervertebral foramina on leaving the spinal cord. This paravertebral space is the main site for blockade of the spinal nerves at a point lateral to the epidural space. Just lateral to this space at the thoracic spine, the intercostal neurovascular bundle extends laterally to supply the intercostal musculature. See Figures 17.1 and 17.7 for illustration of the paravertebral space and intercostal nerves.

19.2.2.1. *Paravertebral Space*

- In the thoracic region, the boundaries of the paravertebral space are as follows (Figure 17.1):
  - Medially: Vertebral body, intervertebral disc and foramen.
  - Anterolaterally: Parietal pleura.
  - Posteriorly: Costotransverse process; approximately 2.5 cm from the tip of the spinous process, often in a slightly caudal orientation.
- Figure 19.2 shows a dissection at the thoracic spine to illustrate the paravertebral space.

19.2.2.2. *Intercostal Nerves*

- The thoracic spinal nerves, on leaving the intervertebral foramen, divide to supply the paraspinal muscles and skin of the back (dorsal ramus or branch) and the intercostal spaces (ventral ramus or branch).

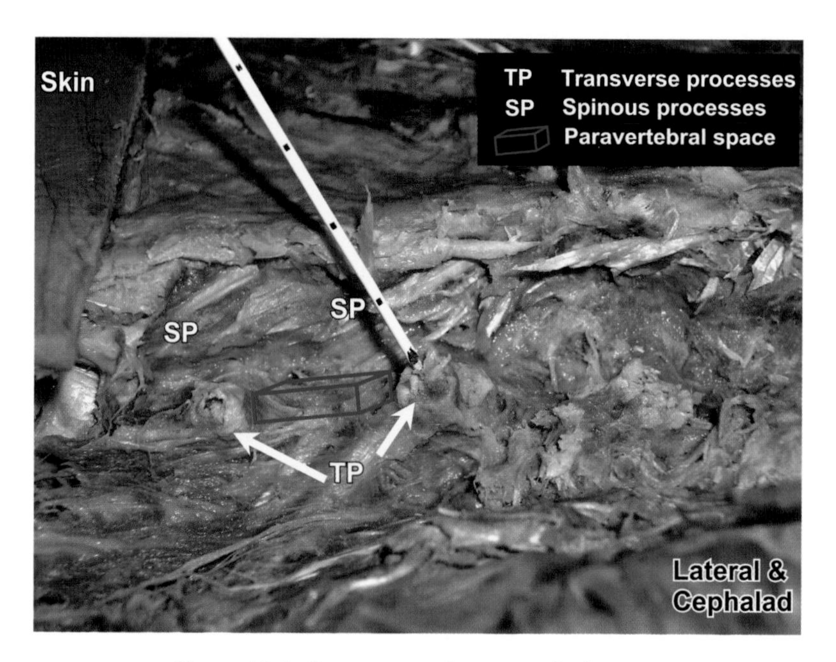

Figure 19.2. Dissection at the paravertbral space.

- The ventral rami of the thoracic spinal nerves form the 11 pairs of intercostal nerves (T1–T11) for the 11 intercostal spaces, and the subcostal nerve (T12), which courses below the 12th rib.
- The intercostal nerves give off cutaneous branches at the anterior and lateral aspects of the thoracic wall.

19.3. Patient Positioning and Surface Anatomy

19.3.1. Patient Positioning

The patient is positioned either sitting or in the lateral decubitus position. The lateral position is often used when performing the block intra- or postoperatively. Rounding out the back (increasing the thoracic kyphotic curve) in the sitting position will increase the distance between the transverse processes and facilitate injection.

19.3.2. Surface Anatomy (Figures 19.3 and 19.4)

- Spinous processes
  - Midline, with T7 at the tips of the scapulae, L4 at the level of the iliac crests, and S2 through a vertical line drawn between posterior inferior iliac spines.
  - Look for scoliosis, which may require further study of the anatomy of the spinal column (ultrasound may be good for determining the most precise needle placement site in this case).
- Transverse processes
  - Approximately 2.5 cm lateral to the spinous processes.
  - At T1, the transverse process is directly lateral to its corresponding spinous process; subsequent transverse processes are extended to increasingly cephalad locations (i.e., T7 transverse process is lateral to T6 spinous process).

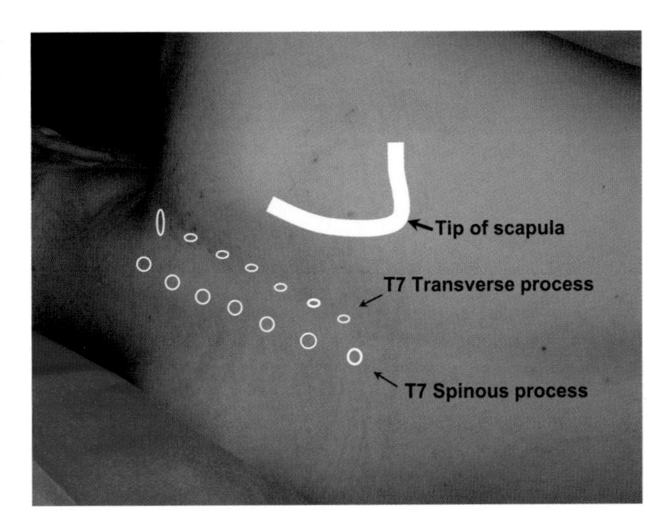

Figure 19.3. Surface anatomy for the thoracic paravertebral block.

19.4. Sonographic Imaging and Needle Insertion Technique

Figures 19.5(A,B) through 19.10(A–C) include magnetic resonance imaging (MRI) and ultrasound images depicting the anatomical landmarks used during the thoracic paravertebral block.

Prepare the needle insertion site and skin surface with an antiseptic solution. Prepare the ultrasound probe surface by applying a sterile adhesive dressing to it prior to needling as discussed earlier (see Chapters 3 and 4).

19.4.1. Scanning Technique

As was the case for the lumbar plexus/psoas compartment, extensive information on ultrasound-guided vertebral and intercostal nerve blockade is lacking. Imaging for these blocks is often used before block performance (a.k.a., preprocedural, supported, or offline imaging) rather than during (a.k.a., real-time or online imaging) to identify the deep bony structure landmarks, including the articular and transverse processes (refer to Chapters 12 and 18 for more detail regarding preprocedural scanning). Little benefit may be added from using real-time guidance and the probe may be somewhat of a nuisance. For intercostal nerve blockade, ultrasound can also be used to easily identify the ribs as landmarks.

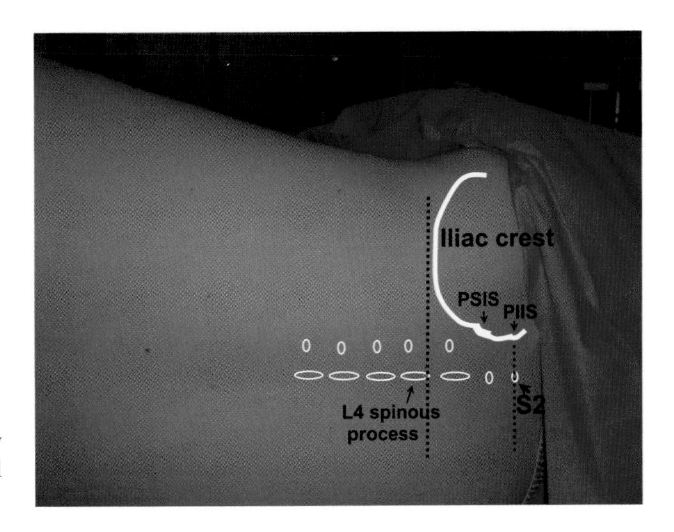

Figure 19.4. Surface anatomy for the lumbar paravertebral block.

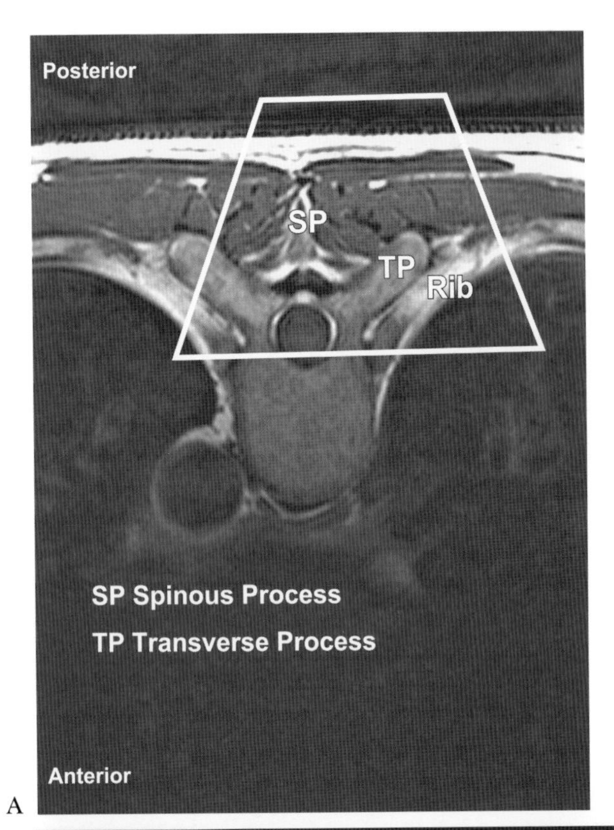

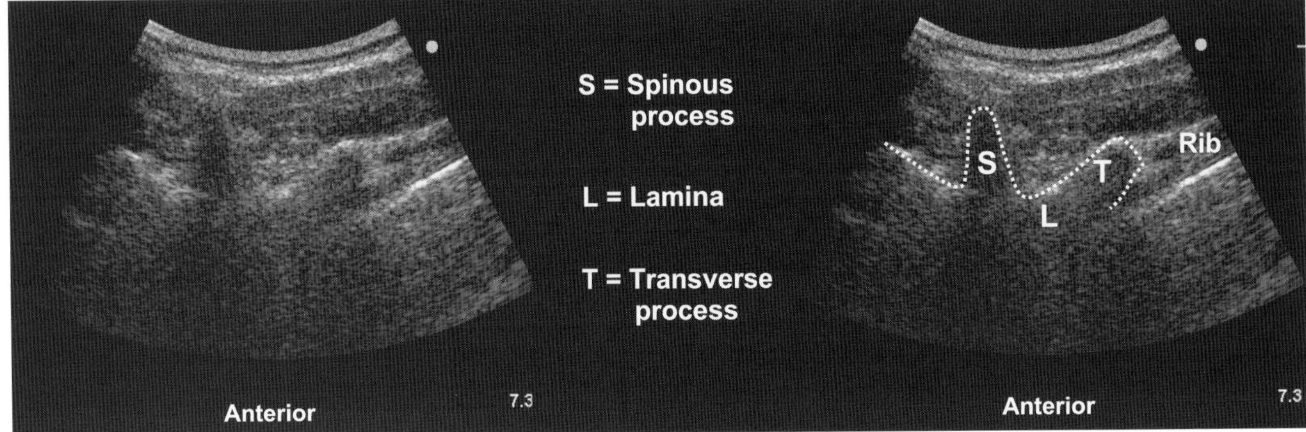

Figure 19.5. (A) MRI and (B) ultrasound images in transverse axis using a curved probe at the thoracic spine to illustrate the paravertebral space and relationship between the bony landmarks.

- Lateral scan for marking the location and depth of important landmarks:
  - Position a 5- to 7-MHz curved array ultrasound probe (lower frequency for obese patients and higher frequency linear probes for thin adult or pediatric patients) in the sagittal plane adjacent to the spinous processes of the target thoracic or lumbar region. A linear probe may be used in thin patients (Figure 19.11).
  - Scanning in a longitudinal plane at the midline will provide a view (although poorly delineated) of the spinous processes (Figure 19.6).
  - Scanning in a lateral direction will show a long-axis view of the the lamina, articular and transverse processes, and (in the thoracic spine) the ribs (Figures 19.7, 19.8, 19.9, and 19.10, respectively).
  - If intercostal blockade is required, the probe can be scanned continuously laterally to identify the costovertebral articulation and ribs.

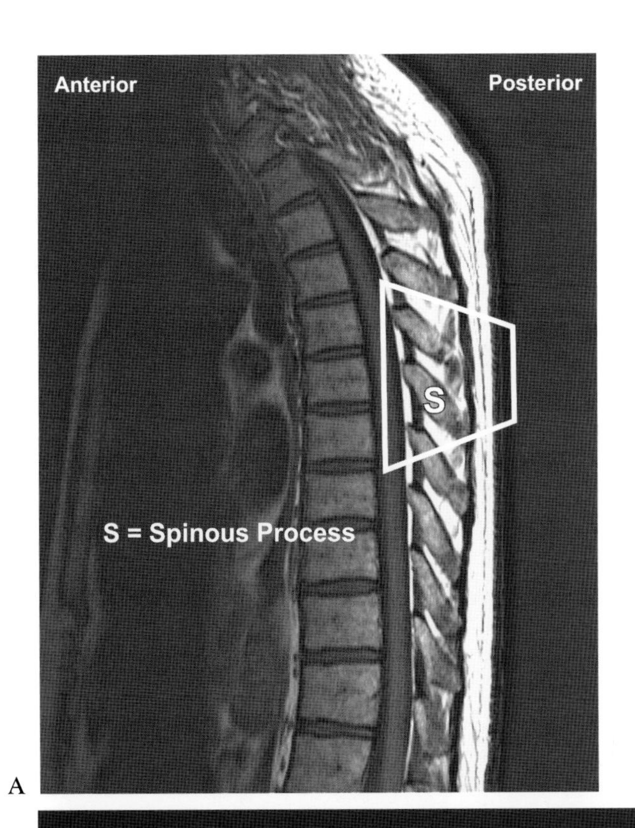

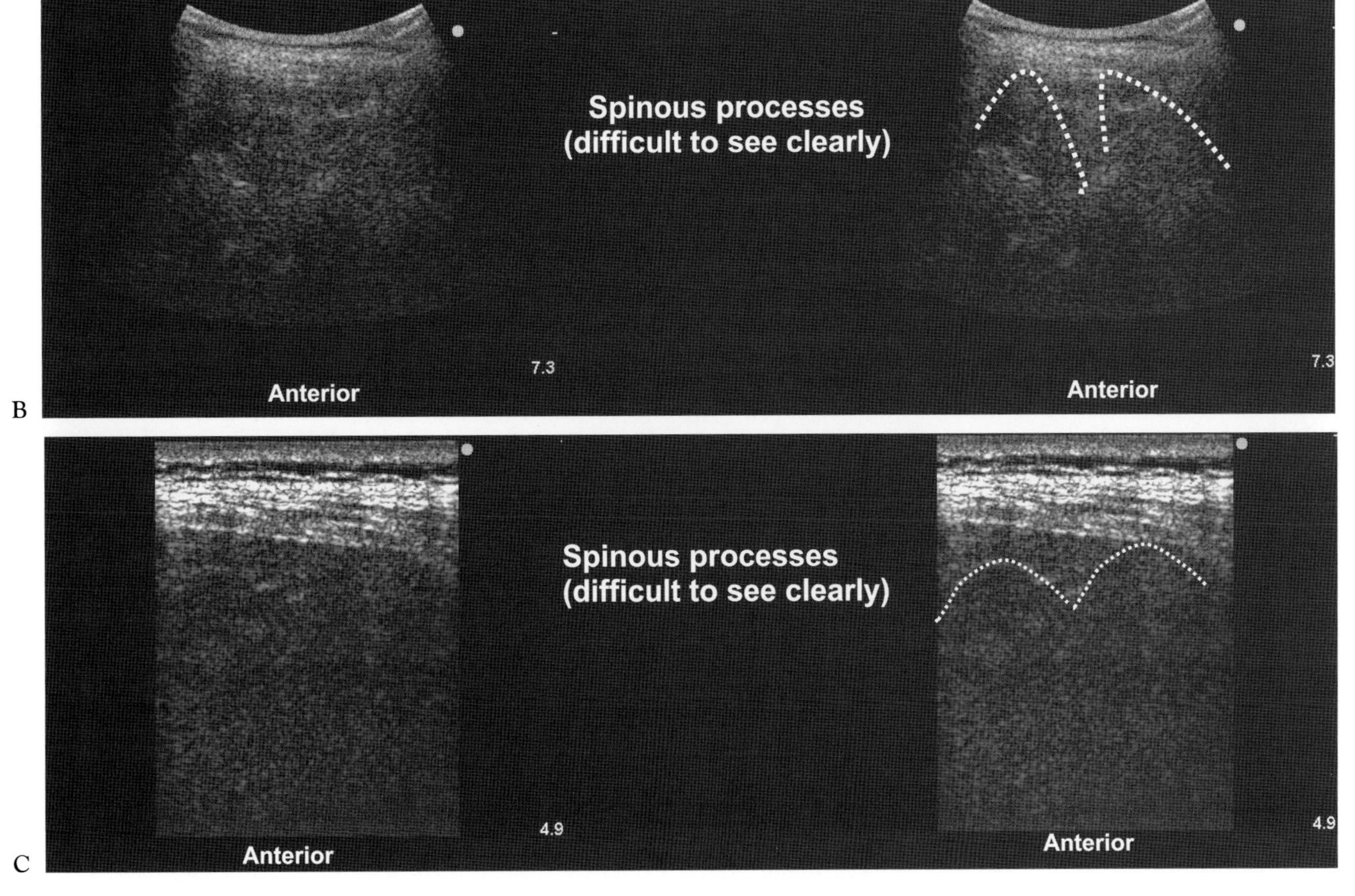

Figure 19.6. (A) MRI and (B) ultrasound images in longitudinal axis using a curved and (C) a linear probe at the thoracic spine showing the spinous processes.

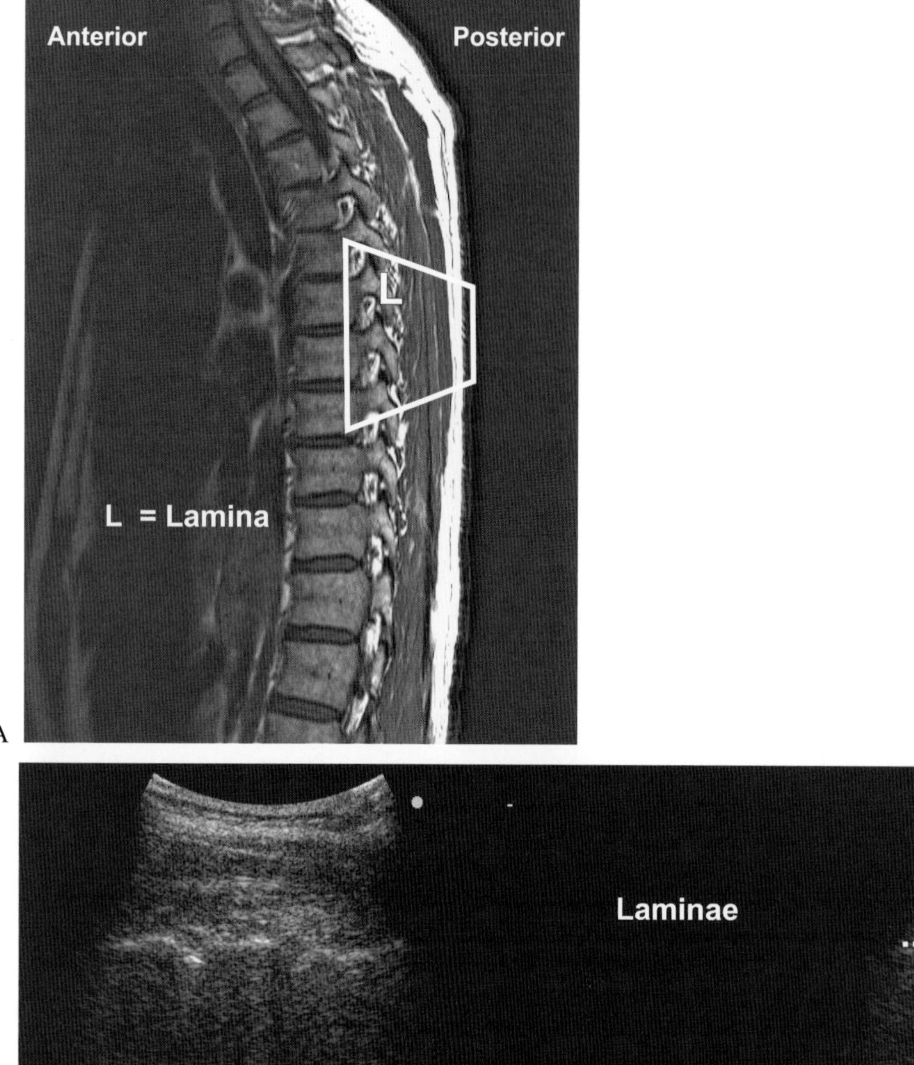

A

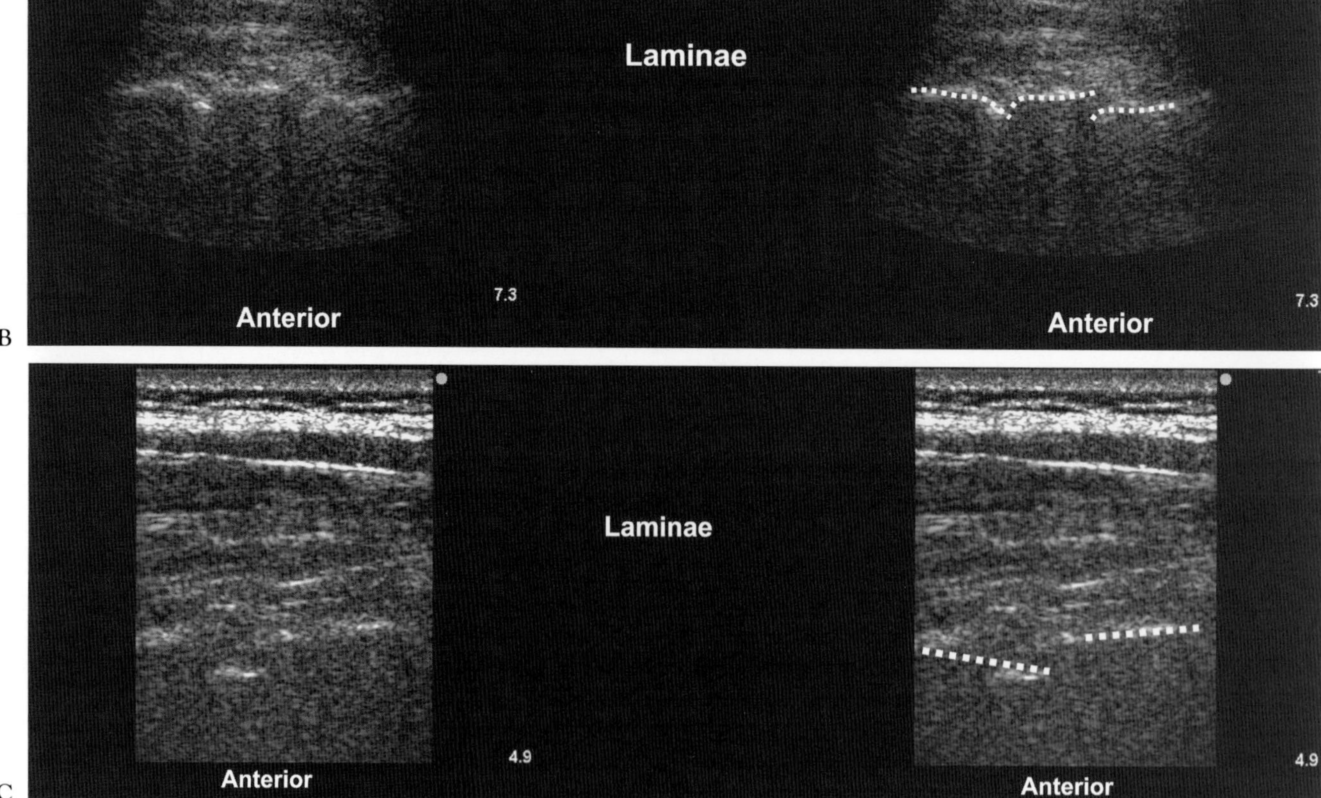

B

C

Figure 19.7. (A) MRI and (B) ultrasound images in longitudinal axis using a curved and (C) a linear probe at the thoracic spine showing the lamina.

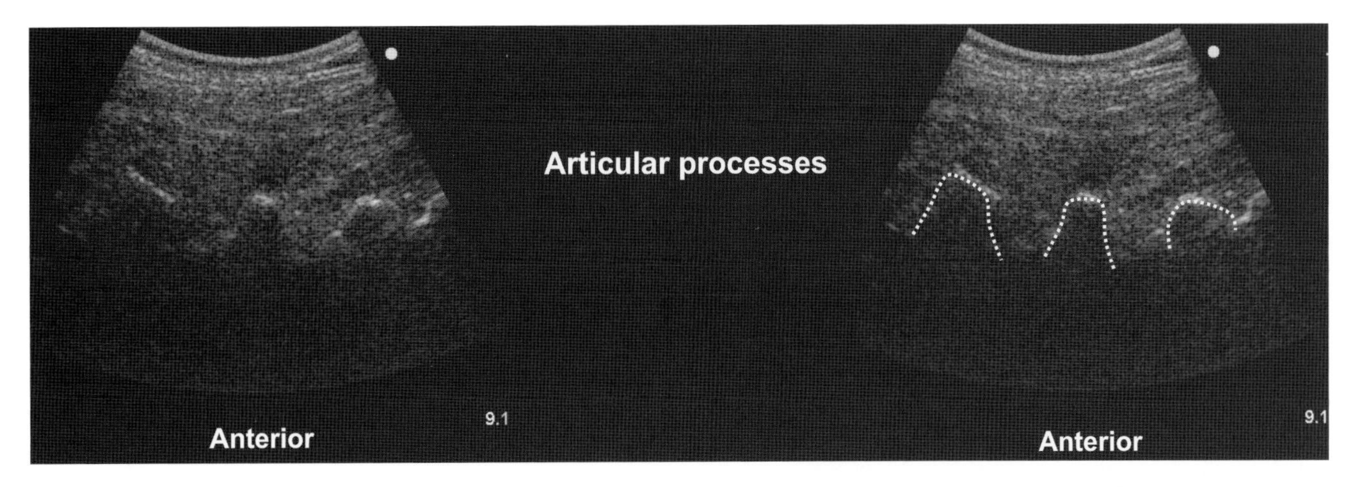

Figure 19.8. Ultrasound image in a longitudinal axis using a curved probe at the articular processes in the thoracic spine.

19.4.2. Sonographic Appearance

- The articular processes (Figure 19.8) in long axis appear as multiple lumps just lateral to the spinous processes and are short rectangular structures with hyperechoic lines with underlying hypoechoic bony shadowing.
- Moving more laterally, the transverse processes (Figure 19.9) appear and look similar to the articular processes; they will disappear when scanning beyond their tips, which can help identify them from the articular processes and mark the lateral block location.
- Beyond the transverse processes, the heads of the ribs (Figure 19.10) appear as long shadows within hyperechoic borders, deep to the linear hyperechoic muscle fibers of the paravertebral muscles.
- Pleura can often be seen lateral and deep to the transverse process as well as deep to the ribs.

19.4.3. Needle Insertion Technique

- Theoretically, both in-plane (IP) and out-of-plane (OOP) techniques can be used for paravertebral or intercostal blocks (Figures 19.12 and 19.13; see Chapter 4).
- Because multiple injection levels are generally needed to completely cover all the dermatomes of the surgical area in clinical practice, the author uses ultrasound imaging for a preblock assessment (supported ultrasound) to visualize and measure the depth of needle penetration required to contact the transverse processes. This eliminates the potential risks associated with real-time guidance (see sidebar on Needling below), while improving the accuracy of the blind procedure (see Chapter 12 and 18 for more discussion on preprocedural and real-time ultrasound imaging). This is particularly true for intercostal nerve blockade.
- In this chapter, we focus on identifying important landmarks instead of using real-time imaging during needling.

19.4.3.1. *Paravertebral Nerve Block (Needle Insertion after Landmark Identification)*

- Insert the needle perpendicular to the skin, at the level of the transverse processes, as previously marked by ultrasound imaging (usually 2.5 cm lateral from the spinous processes), and note the depth of the transverse process.
- As with the conventional blind procedure, the needle is inserted until bone (transverse process) is contacted (usually at a depth of 2–4 cm in the thoracic region and 6–8 cm in the lumbar region); however, ultrasound may be used in some cases to measure the depth of the plexus, which would reduce the need for needle contact with bone.

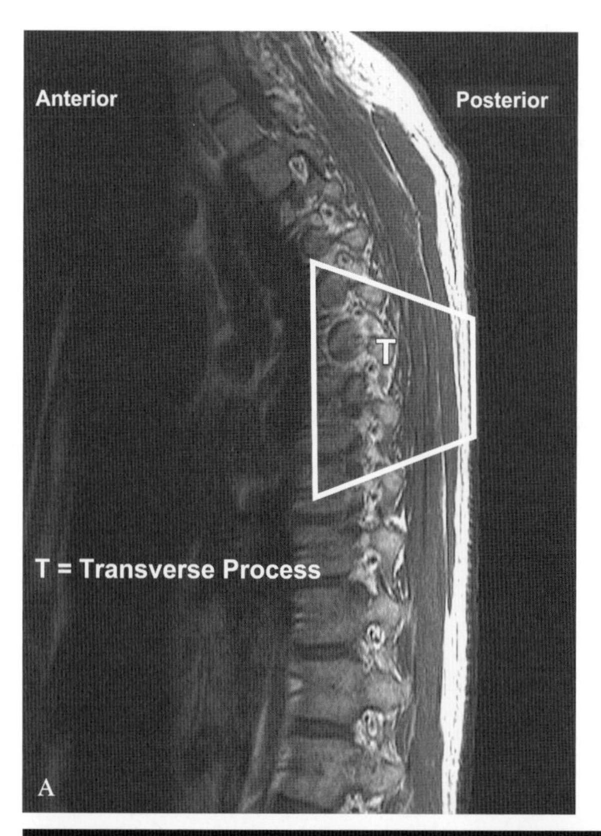

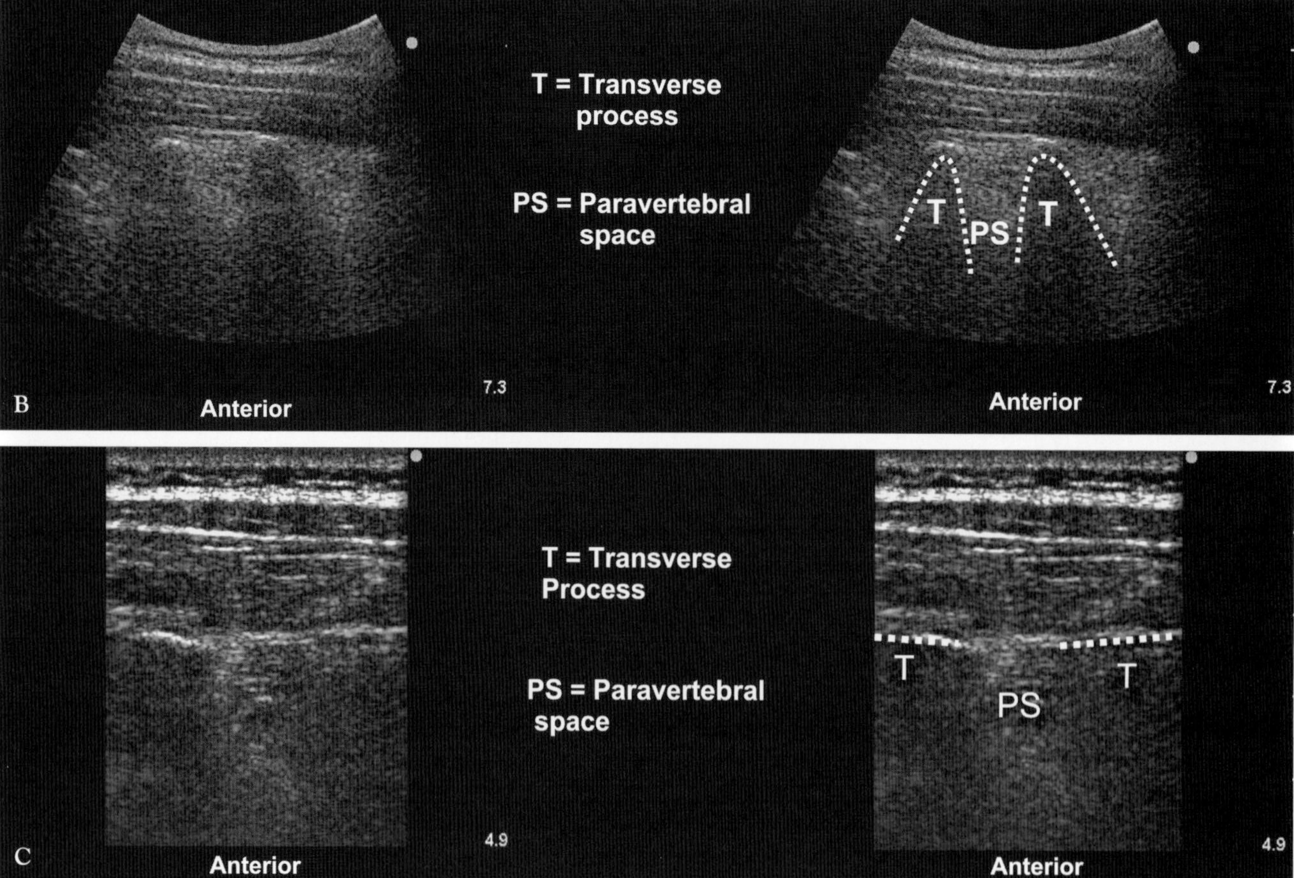

Figure 19.9. (A) MRI and (B) ultrasound images in longitudinal axis using a curved and (C) a linear probe at the thoracic spine showing the transverse processes. Curved lower frequency probes can provide superior penetration to view the transverse processes.

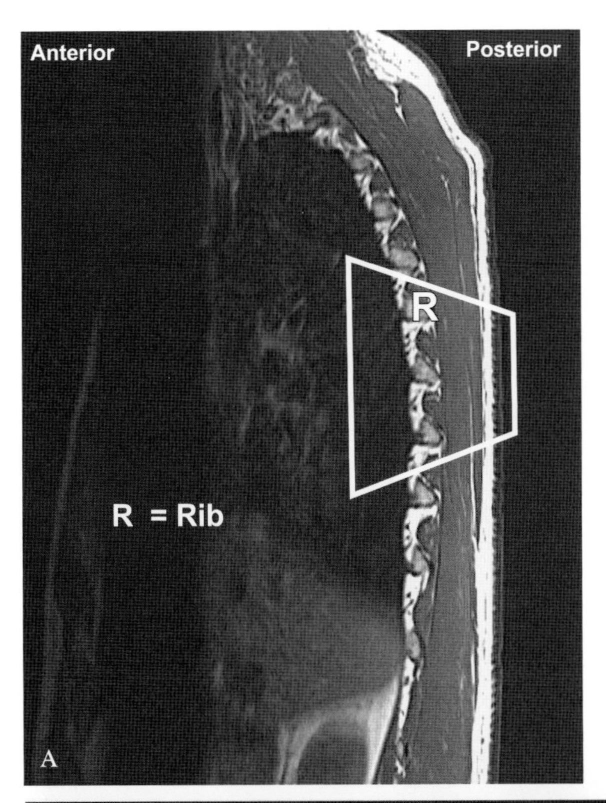

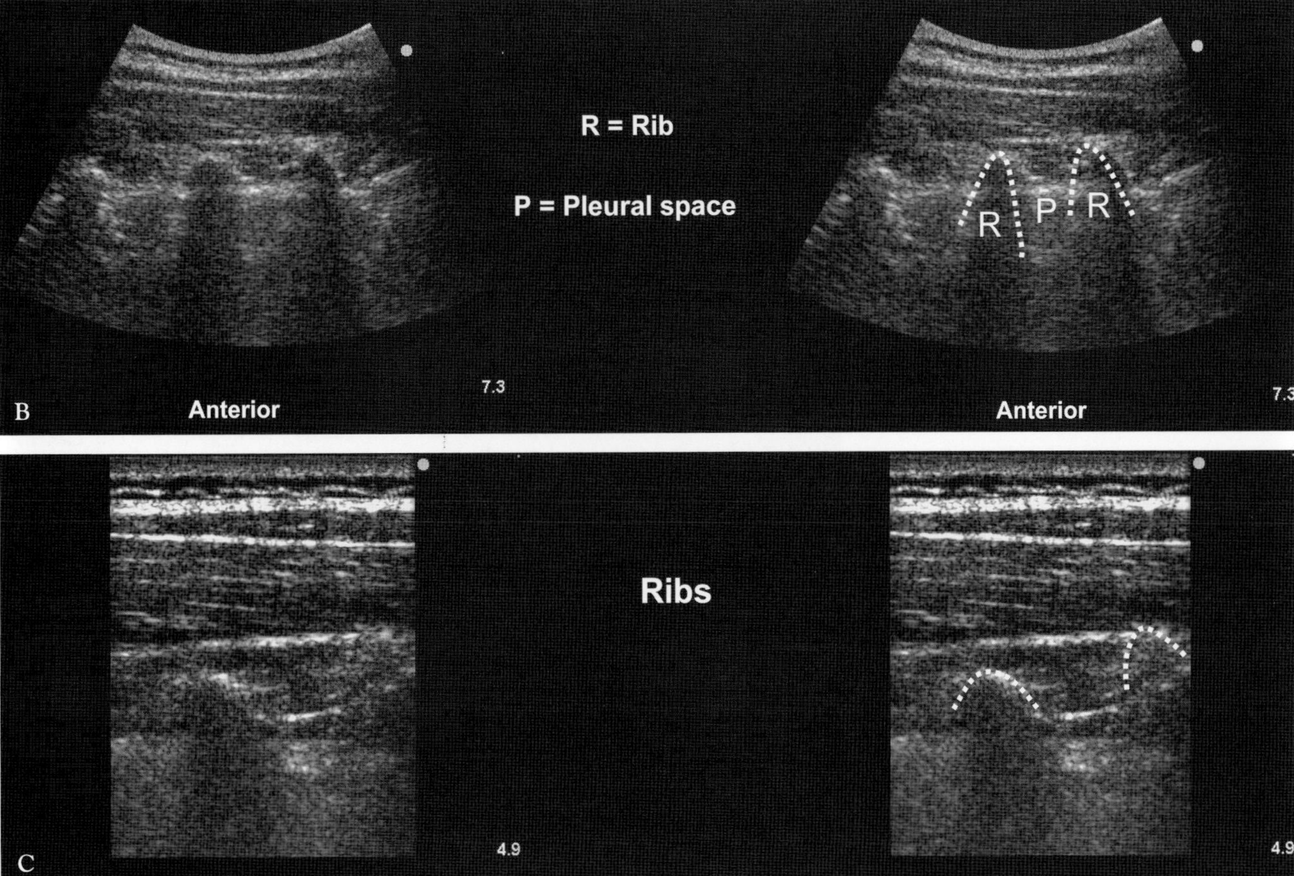

Figure 19.10. (A) MRI and (B) ultrasound images in longitudinal axis using a curved and (C) a linear probe at the rib necks. The pleural cavity is located deep to the ribs.

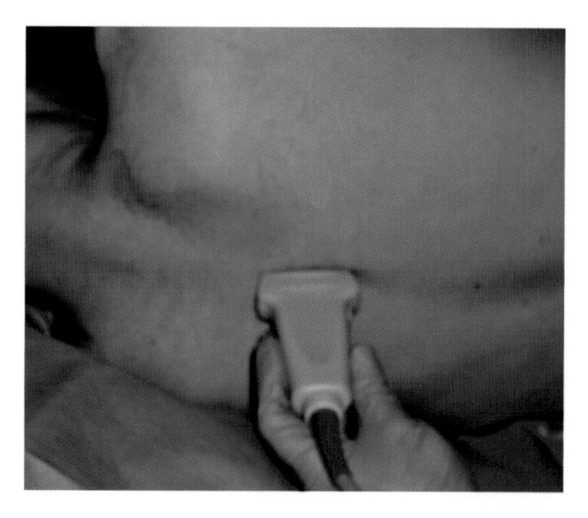

Figure 19.11. Scanning in a lateral direction in longitudinal axis with a linear probe. A curved probe may be advantageous for increased depth of penetration.

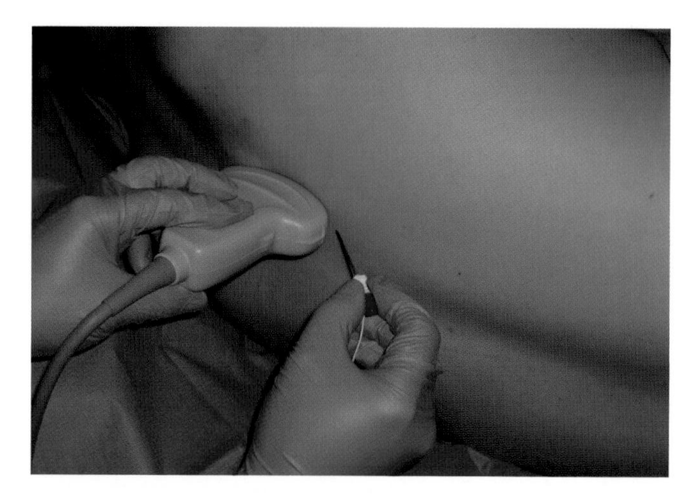

Figure 19.12. Needling technique using a curved probe in longitudinal axis and an in-plane (IP) needle alignment.

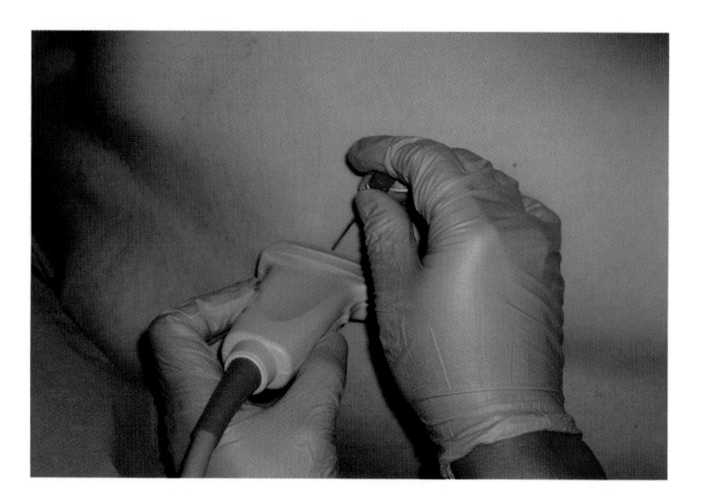

Figure 19.13. Needling technique using a linear probe in longitudinal axis and an out-of-plane (OOP) needle alignment. This needling technique may be risky, with either medial or lateral needle insertion, as discussed in the sidebar on needling.

- Withdraw the needle to skin level and reinsert it 10° superiorly (to target the spinal nerve corresponding to the spinous process) or inferiorly (corresponding to the vertebral level below the spinous process) and 1 cm deeper than the point of bone contact.
- There will be a subtle give at the midpoint between these landmarks (spinous and transverse processes) indicating entrance into the paravertebral space; however, it may be difficult to see any nerve structures with ultrasound.
- A lumbar paravertebral block at L3 to L5 is essentially the same as the lumbar plexus block.

19.4.3.2. *Intercostal Nerve Block*

- Once the probe locates the rib in the sagittal/longitudinal plane, note the depth and mark the location of the rib.
- Insert the needle as with the traditional blind procedure.

Needling

The needle should not be inserted with a significant medial direction as there is a risk of spinal cord injury from intraforaminal injection. Likewise, a lateral direction bears the risk of pneumothorax. If choosing to use real-time ultrasound guidance during block procedure please note:

- With the probe placed in the sagittal/longitudinal plane, OOP needling may be more risky as it often requires the medial or lateral angulations described above (Figure 19.13).
- Similarly, an IP needling approach can be more risky when the probe is placed in the coronal/transverse plane.

19.5. Nerve Stimulation

19.5.1. Paravertebral Block

- Using nerve stimulation during needle insertion from the level of the transverse process through entry into the paravertebral space has been described.
- However, this block is commonly performed blindly and based on surface landmarks and the feeling of a tactile "pop" without nerve stimulation. Thus, the available information on using nerve stimulation for this block is very limited.

19.6. Local Anesthetic Application

Local anesthetic application is difficult to view with this block.

Suggested Reading and References

Awad IT, Duggan EM. Posterior lumbar plexus block: anatomy, approaches, and techniques. Reg Anesth Pain Med 2005;30:143–149.

Ganapathy S, Nielsen K, Steele S. Outcomes after paravertebral blocks. Int Anesth Clin 2005; 43:185–193.

Grau T, Leipold RW, Delorme S, Martin E, Motsch J. Ultrasound imaging of the thoracic space. Reg Anesth Pain Med 2002;27:200–206.

Jamieson BD, Mariano ER. Thoracic and lumbar paravertbral blocks for outpatient lithotripsy. J Clin Anesth 2007;19:149–151.
Kirchmair L, Tanja E, Jorg W, Bernhard M, Kapral S, Mitterschiffthaler G. A study of the paravertebral anatomy for ultrasound-guided posterior lumbar plexus block. Anesth Analg 2001; 93:477–481.
Naja MZ, Gustafsson AC, Ziade MF, et al. Distance between the skin and the thoracic paravertebral. Anaesth 2005;60:680–684.
Pusch F, Wilding E, Klimscha W, Weinstabl C. Sonographic measurement of needle insertion depth in paravertebral blocks in women. Br J Anaesth 2000;85:841–843.

20

Caudal and Epidural Blockade

Ban C.H. Tsui

20.1. Introduction

20.1.1. Caudal Blocks: Single-Shot Blocks and Advancement of Catheters Cephalad from the Caudal Spine

Single-shot caudal epidural anesthesia is suitable for blockade of the lumbar and sacral dermatomes. Although needle puncture may be considerably safer at the sacral hiatus than at other regions in the spinal canal because it is below the spinal cord, there is still a high failure rate (up to 25%) of placing needles into the caudal canal and inadvertent vascular puncture occurs with some frequency (5%–9% of patients). Usually, a "pop" or "whoosh" is detected as the needle enters the sacral canal through the sacral hiatus and posterior sacrococcygeal membrane, and this sign (together with ease of advancement of the intravenous catheter and local anesthetic injection) is classically used to determine correct needle placement (Figure 20.1).

The development of the epidural electrical stimulation test has added to the current repertoire of methods that assess correct needle placement in the caudal canal and is a more objective method than those currently available. Ultrasound may be useful to determine the best puncture site for caudal needle placement. Although direct visibility of the needle puncture of the sacrococcygeal membrane can be difficult in adults, due to bony shadowing of the sacrum, it is possible to view the needle entrance to the sacral hiatus (in longitudinal view) and the needle tip may be appreciated in transverse view after epidural space entrance. As with other spinal levels, ultrasound imaging at the sacral spine may be most beneficial in young infants as there is less ossification and therefore a good ultrasound window in this region. The main disadvantage with both ultrasound and nerve stimulation is that they do not provide immediate warning in cases of intravascular puncture.

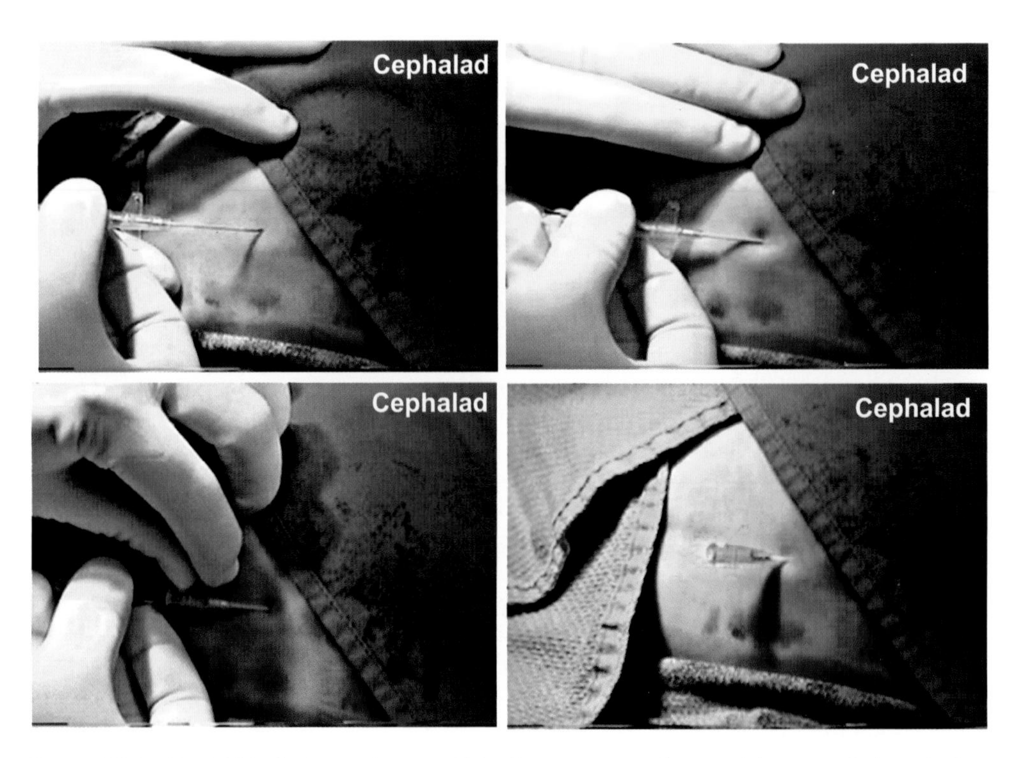

Figure 20.1. Caudal blockade involves needle/catheter entry at the sacral hiatus and through the posterior sacrococcygeal ligament (upper left). As the needle enters the sacral canal and epidural space there is traditionally a "pop" (upper right). The ease of intravenous cannula advancement and local anesthetic injection is also used to confirm caudal epidural space localization.

Epidural anesthesia may also be administered effectively using epidural catheters. Advancing catheters from the sacral (or low lumbar) epidural space to lumbar or thoracic levels has the advantage of reducing the risk of direct spinal cord trauma (especially when there are no sensory warnings, as in anesthetized pediatric patients) and may be technically easier in patients with prior spinal surgery at higher levels. Confirmation of both proper catheter placement in the epidural space as well as monitoring the catheter's cephalad advancement are both important, and ultrasound and electrical epidural stimulation may both be beneficial because of the dynamic nature of these techniques. The epidural stimulation test can provide warning of intrathecal, and possibly intravascular, needle or catheter placement (intrathecal from motor responses to currents <1 mA and intravascular from motor response despite repeated local anesthetic administration; see Chapter 18).

A procedure using epidural electrocardiographic (ECG) monitoring to guide catheters to target locations has also been developed for use when neuromuscular blockade or prior local anesthetic injection limits the use of the epidural stimulation test. The placement of the epidural catheter is determined by comparing the ECG signal from the tip of the catheter to a signal from a surface electrode positioned at the target segmental level.

20.1.2. Lumbar and Thoracic Epidurals

Epidural needle placement may fail for several reasons, including anatomical pecularities (e.g., limited interlaminar space, ossified or calcified ligamentum flavum, enlarged facet joints, or rotated vertebrae), faulty identification of the midline (e.g., obesity, scoliosis), and poor patient compliance or cooperation. In children, however, these issues may not be significant, but because they are anesthetized, the absence of any sensory warning of intrathecal placement adds inherent risks to the procedure. When catheters are advanced within the thoracic epidural space, less resistance is encountered than that within lumbar levels, possibly because of the reduced length of the catheter in the space and the significant resistance at the lumbar spine where significant curvature develops.

Both epidural stimulation and ultrasound may be useful for identifying epidural needle entry, as adjuncts to other tests such as loss-of-resistance (LOR) to saline. The epidural stimulation test may be especially beneficial for providing a warning of misplacement of the needle, especially if it is in the subdural or subarachnoid spaces or abutting up against a nerve root. The main benefit of ultrasound imaging is the ability to gauge depth and space (e.g., diameter of epidural space) measurements prior to the procedure, which can help refine the point of needle puncture and angle of needle insertion. One may visualize the disruption caused by the injection of fluid into the epidural space when using the LOR technique in the lumbar region in pediatric patients, but this observation is limited in the more compact thoracic spine (Figure 20.2; also see Figures 17.3, 18.6 and 18.7).

The distance of catheter threading will determine which technique to use with continuous blocks. The epidural stimulation test is optimal when threading catheters lengthy distances into the epidural space, but has only moderate application during direct placement of the catheter. In these cases, the LOR to saline will accurately determine epidural placement and ultrasound-guidance can be helpful. The epidural stimulation test is useful in both situations, however, in warning against unintentional intrathecal or intravascular local anesthetic injection.

20.2. Clinical Anatomy

Knowledge of the anatomy of the spinal column will provide an understanding and appreciation of the limitations with using ultrasound and nerve stimulation for neuraxial anesthesia. The limited bony calcification in young patients allows adequate visualization through ultrasound and justifies the use of ultrasound guidance in this population. Epidural stimulation can be used successfully for needle placement in adults at the thoracic and lumbar spinal levels, although the caudal route as utilized for catheter advancement is most

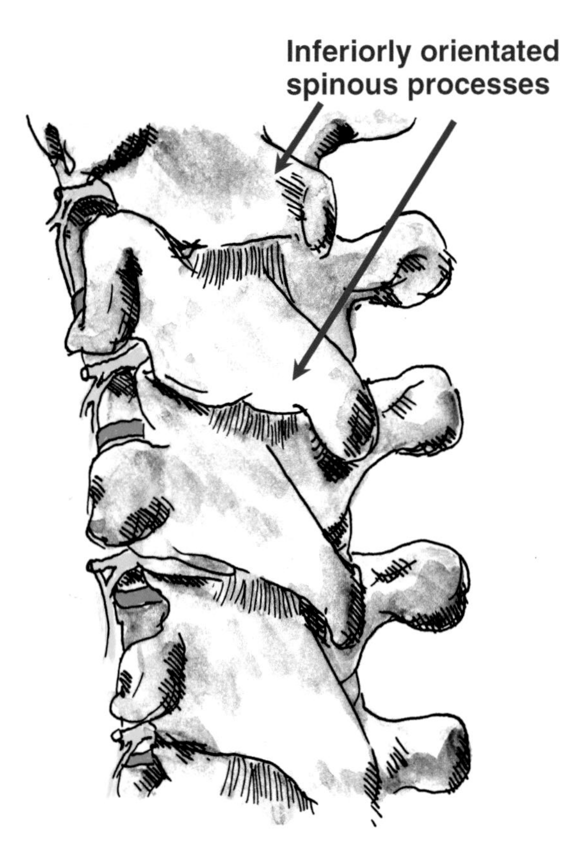

Figure 20.2. The thoracic spine in a paramedian view. The spinous processes are overlapping and the area is very compact with little space for ultrasound beam entry (i.e., limited ultrasound window) to visualize local anesthetic injection (spread) or dural movement to confirm epidural placement.

successful in pediatric patients. This is because the pediatric (particularly those <2 years of age) spinal column has yet to incorporate a significant lumbar curvature that hinders catheter advancement from caudal to cephalad positions.

Anatomy of the spinal column, its costovertebral articulations, spinal nerve meninges, and peripheral distribution are discussed in detail in Chapter 17. Most relevant for epidural anesthesia are the caudal epidural space, developmental and mature anatomy of the sacrum, lumbar and thoracic vertebrae, and the spinal nerve meninges. Figures 17.4 and 17.8 are definitely worth reviewing and Figures 20.3 and 20.4 are provided here for an overview of critical anatomy and appreciation of the sacral hiatus route for epidural needle/catheter entry to avoid the spinal cord.

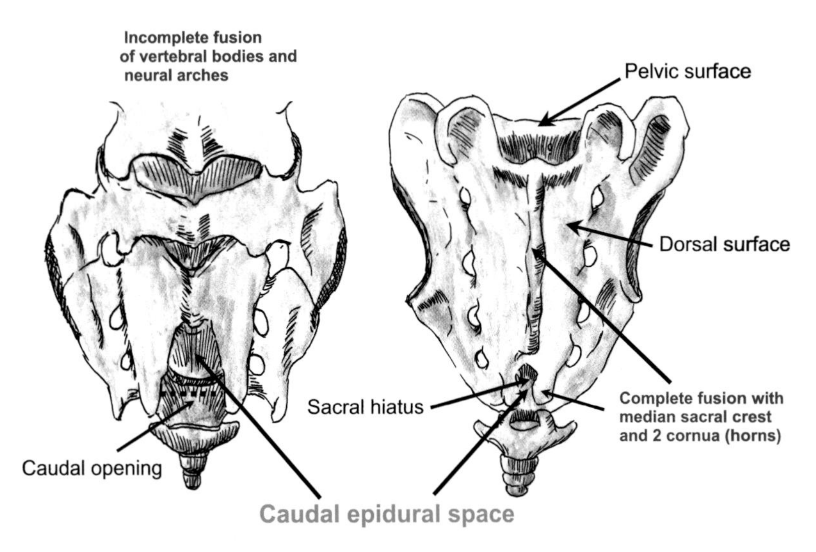

Figure 20.3. Posterior views of the developing and mature sacrum. The caudal opening in infants is much larger than in adults (sacral hiatus) and there is significant space for beam penetration into the caudal epidural space. The lack of fusion throughout the pediatric sacrum (S1 and S2 body fusion can take years) also helps with ultrasound visibility of the needle trajectory and local anesthetic application in the sacral canal.

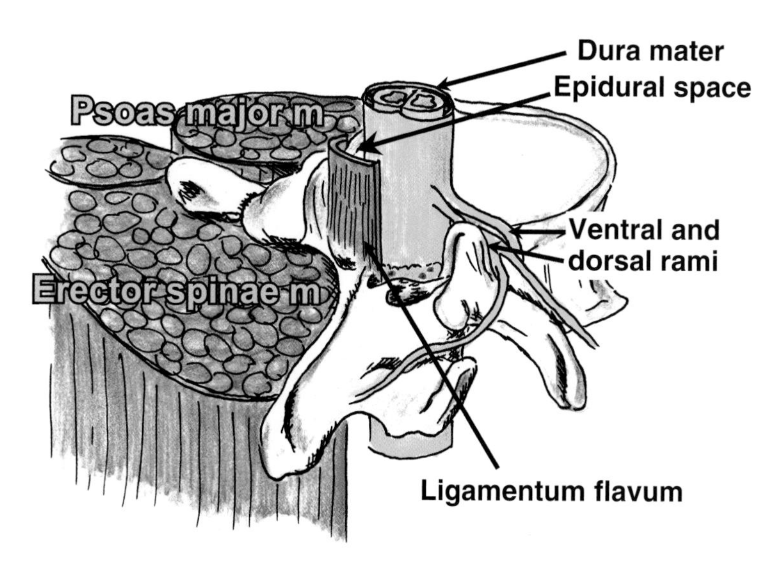

Figure 20.4. Lumbar vertebra with spinal cord and meninges and its relation to the paraspinal muscles.

20.3. Patient Positioning and Surface Landmarks

20.3.1. Patient Positioning

Position the patient in the lateral position. In some patients, there may be excessive subcutaneous tissue that will make identification and palpation of surface landmarks difficult. Under these circumstances, ultrasound imaging may be especially helpful in viewing and localizing the landmarks.

20.3.2. Surface Anatomy

20.3.2.1. *Caudal Epidural Space* (Figure 20.5)

- Iliac crests
  - Approximately at the level of the L4 spinous process
- Posterior superior iliac spines (PSIS)
  - Approximately 4 to 5 cm lateral to S1
- Median sacral crest*
  - Fused spinous processes of sacrum (on dorsal surface)
  - May be difficult to palpate in patients with excessive subcutaneous tissue
- Sacral hiatus*
  - Sacral cornua (horns) can be palpated approximately 5 cm above the tip of the coccyx
  - The sacral hiatus lies at the midpoint between these cornua

*These landmarks are suitable as reference points in older children and adults only. Refer to Figure 20.3 for more illustration.

20.3.2.2. *Lumbar and Thoracic Spine* (Figures 20.6 and 20.7)

- Spinous processes*
  - Midline, with T1 most prominent, T7 at tips (inferior angles) of scapulae, L4 at level of iliac crests, and S1 on horizontal line drawn between the two posterior superior iliac spines
  - Look for scoliosis

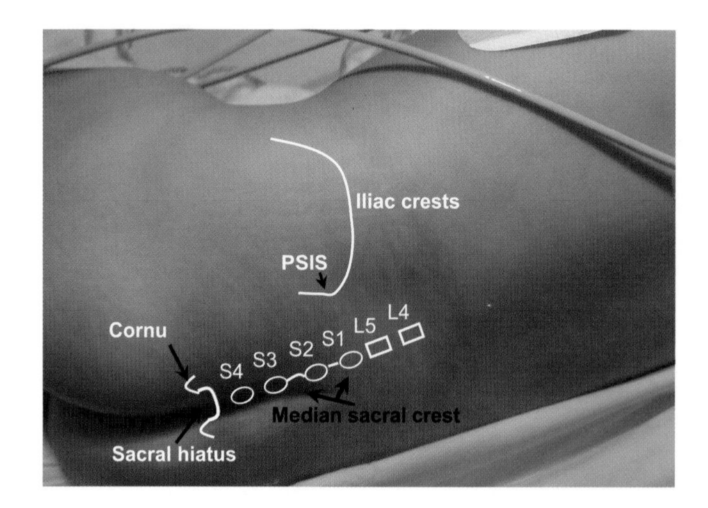

Figure 20.5. Patient positioning and surface landmarks for caudal block.

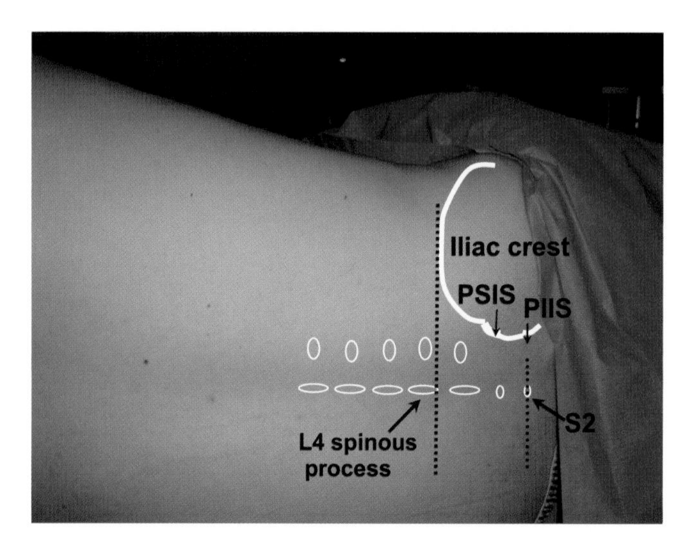

Figure 20.6. Patient positioning and surface landmarks for lumbar epidural anesthesia.

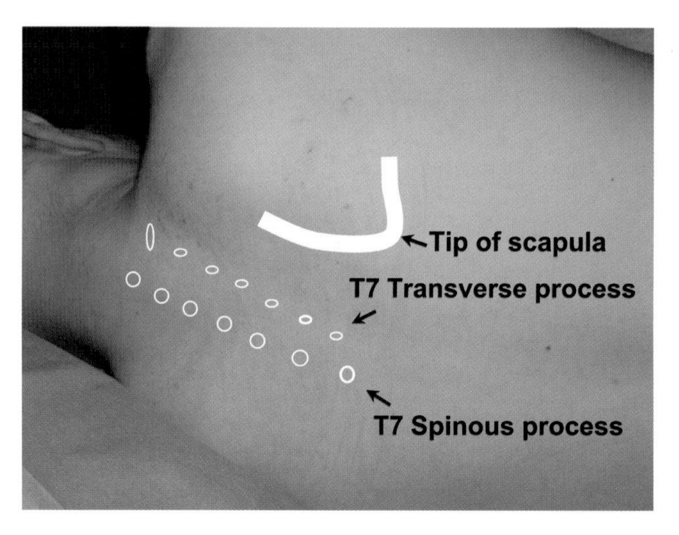

Figure 20.7. Patient positioning and surface landmarks for thoracic epidural anesthesia.

- Transverse processes
  - Approximately 2 cm (thoracic) and 2.5 cm (lumbar) lateral to spinous processes; this distance will be reduced in young infants

*The neural arches, forming the spinous processes, are not completely fused until the end of the first year (except for at L5, in which they fuse significantly later), so it is common to palpate two separate bony landmarks in infants. In adults, the spinous processes of the cervical and lumbar vertebrae are fairly horizontal, while those at the thoracic spine are orientated along a steep inferior inclination, with significant overlapping so that each of the spinous processes palpated will be below the level of its respective vertebral body.

20.4. Single-Shot Caudal Anesthesia

20.4.1. Sonographic Imaging and Ultrasound-Guided Block Procedure

20.4.1.1. Scanning Technique

- Begin with a short-axis (transversal) probe (5–12 MHz linear) orientation at the level of the fifth sacral vertebra to identify landmarks by visualizing the sacral cornua (bilateral horns of sacrum), dorsal surface of the sacrum (see Figure 20.3), posterior sacrococcygeal ligament, and sacral hiatus (Figure 20.8).
- Upon skin puncture, rotate the probe 90° for long-axis (longitudinal) viewing between the two cornua (Figure 20.9), which may allow in-plane (IP) imaging of the needle trajectory to the point of entrance to the sacrococcygeal ligament; beyond this barrier the characteristic "pop" can be used to confirm needle placement within the caudal epidural space.
- Linear probes are advantageous in most patients; curvilinear array transducers with lower frequencies may be beneficial with older and/or obese patients.
- Footprint will depend on the patient's size; in very thin patients small footprints will be most appropriate.
- After entry into the caudal epidural space, the probe can be rotated from a longitudinal to a transverse orientation to locate the needle in short axis (as a dot) between the sacrococcygeal ligament and the pelvic (ventral) surface of the sacrum (i.e., caudal epidural space).

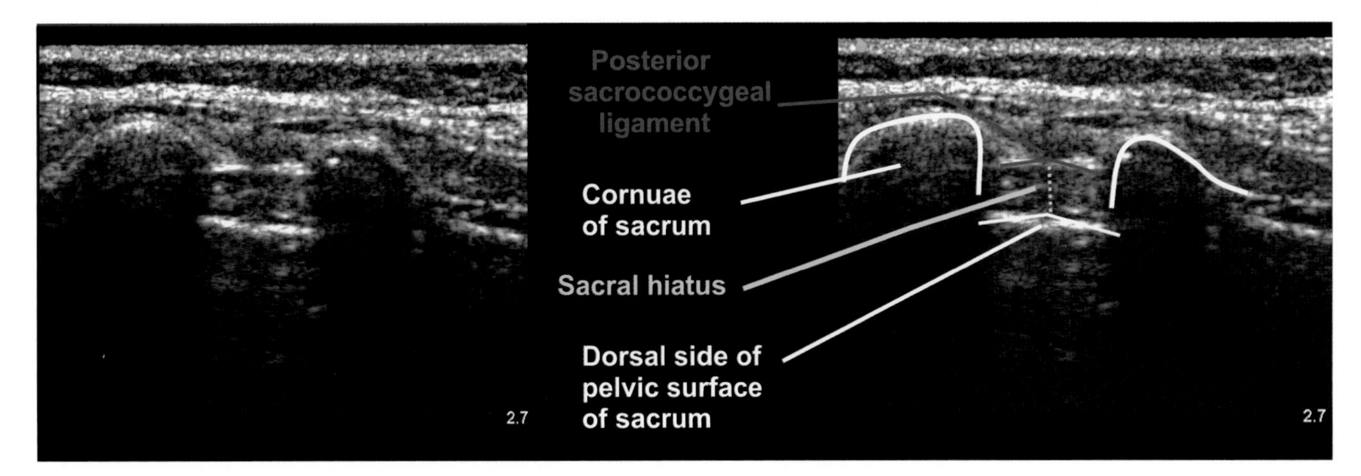

Figure 20.8. Transverse/short-axis image captured by a linear probe at the level of the sacral hiatus and capturing the sacral hiatus space in a 10-year-old patient.

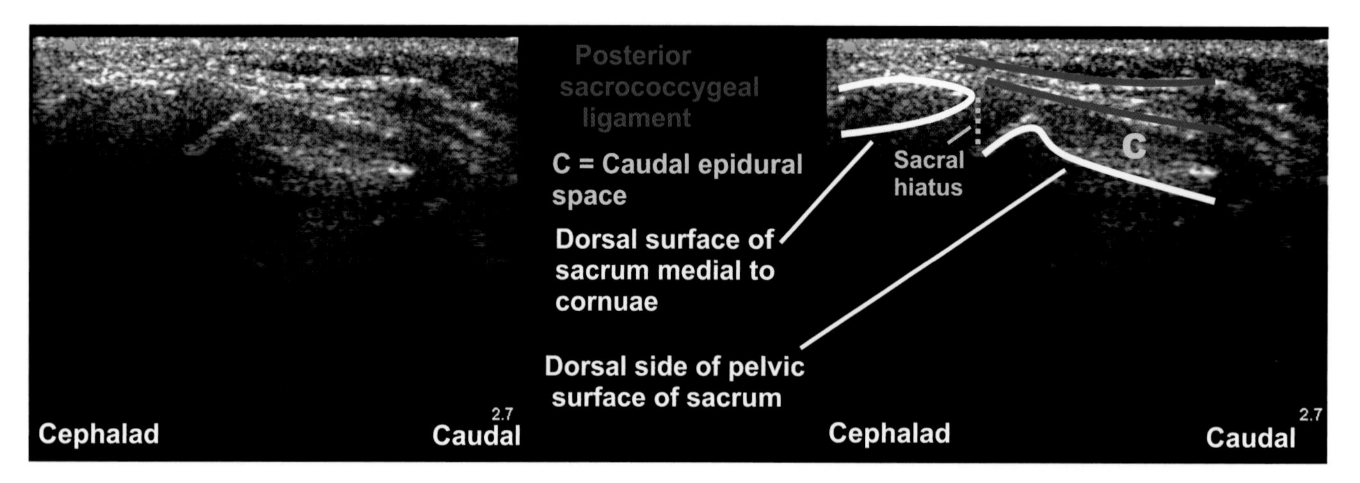

Figure 20.9. Longitudinal/long-axis image captured by a linear probe placed between sacral cornua of a 10-year-old patient.

- For young infants, the probe (7–12 MHz linear) can be placed over the midsacral level (S2–S3) due to the limited ossification of the sacral vertebrae (see Figure 18.10). The long-axis view will allow clear visibility of the needle trajectory through the caudal entrance into the epidural space.

20.4.1.2. *Sonographic Appearance*

Chapter 18 describes and illustrates the appearance of the sacral epidural space and related structures in an infant (12 months old) using a high-resolution ultrasound machine. The images here are captured from using a portable machine (MicroMaxx, SonoSite, Inc., Bothell, WA, USA) with lower resolution, although they may represent a more practical and perhaps realistic approach for regional anesthesia practitioners.

In children (e.g., 10 years old):

- Short-axis view at sacral hiatus (Figures 20.8):
  - Superficially, the two sacral cornua are seen as hyperechoic inverted U-shaped structures beneath the variably echogenic linear subcutaneous tissue.
  - Deep and between the cornua are two hyperechoic bands resembling the posterior sacrococcygeal ligament and the dorsal side of the pelvic surface of the sacrum (see Figure 20.3); the hypoechoic space between these is the sacral hiatus.
  - Deep to the cornua and bands, the image may show lateral darkening and a medial hypoechogenic epidural space; this will be variable.
  - The needle can be seen as a highly hyperechoic dot within the sacral hiatus following sacrococcygeal membrane puncture (not shown).
- Long-axis view at sacral hiatus (Figure 20.9):
  - The sacrococcygeal ligament appears broad, hyperechoic, and linear, slanted at a caudal angle.
  - The dorsal surface of the sacrum appears hyperechoic deep and cephalad to the membrane.
  - The dorsal side of the ventral (pelvic) surface of the sacrum appears dark at the bottom of the image, with a moderately hypoechogenic space between the ligament and bone resembling the sacral hiatus (with the caudal epidural space cephalad and beneath the dorsal surface of the sacrum).
  - The caudal epidural needle may appear as a hyperechoic and highly linear structure outside the epidural space; it is not visible within the epidural space due to the beam reflection from the dorsum of the sacrum (not shown).

20.4.2. Needle Insertion and Local Anesthetic Application

In pediatric patients, the procedure for instituting caudal anesthesia is performed following general anesthesia in most cases, whereas in adults, for the most part, caudal anesthesia is performed while the patient is fully awake.

Position the probe at the sacral hiatus for patients older than 1 year, and place it at S2 to S3 in infants.

- Insert a 21- to 22-ga needle perpendicular to the skin and in the midline at the sacral hiatus.
- With the probe placed longitudinally, the needle can be seen in long axis as it advances to and penetrates the sacrococcygeal ligament.
- Advance the needle until a "pop" is felt, signifying caudal epidural space entrance.
- In infants, because of reduced fusion and calcification of the dorsal sacrum, this longitudinal plane may allow visibility of the needle tip beyond the ligament and within the epidural space.
- In adults, once the needle reaches the ligament, the shadowing from the overlying bone tissue will obstruct the view of the needle and neural structures.
- Rotate the probe to short axis to confirm the needle as a bright dot in the epidural space and inject the local anesthetic.
- Local anesthetic may be seen as an expansion of hypoechogenicity and indirectly through dural movement.
- Using a color Doppler mode with the probe placed transversely at the low lumbar (adults) or midsacral (infants) region, observe the Doppler signal indicating the flow of local anesthetic in the epidural space. [Figure 20.10(A,B) illustrates (a) pre-injection and (b) postinjection of the local anesthetic at L4 in an adult.] The epidural space will expand slightly as the local anesthetic is injected.

20.4.3. Epidural Stimulation Guidance and Block Technique

20.4.3.1. Procedure

- An insulated, sheathed 22-ga needle is required for the epidural stimulation test.
- After sterile preparation, connect a nerve stimulator to the needle.
- Attach the cathode lead of the nerve stimulator to the insulated needle and the grounding anode lead to an electrode on the patient's body surface.
- Set the nerve stimulator to low frequency and pulse width (1 or 2 Hz; 0.1 or 0.2 ms).
- Perform skin puncture in a direction perpendicular to the skin at the level of the sacral cornuae (located by palpation).
- Advance the needle until the characteristic give or "pop" is felt, indicating entrance into the caudal epidural space.
- Carefully and slowly increase the current intensity until motor activity begins.
- The correct motor response is contraction of the anal sphincter (S2–S4) at current threshold generally between 1 to 15 mA.
- Localized muscular twitches of the gluteal or back muscles is an incorrect response and indicates that the needle is likely in the subcutaneous space outside the sacrococcygeal ligament.
- Refer to Table 18.1 for characterizing the response, particularly with respect to subarachnoid placement.
- Once aspiration is negative for cerebrospinal fluid, an epinephrine test dose (0.5 μg/kg) should still be administered to identify inadvertent intravascular placement indicated by specific ECG changes (i.e., >25% increase in T wave or ST segment changes irrespective of chosen lead).
- The presence of any physical signs of subcutaneous bulging or tissue resistance upon the injection of local anesthetic indicates improper needle placement and an unsuccessful caudal block.

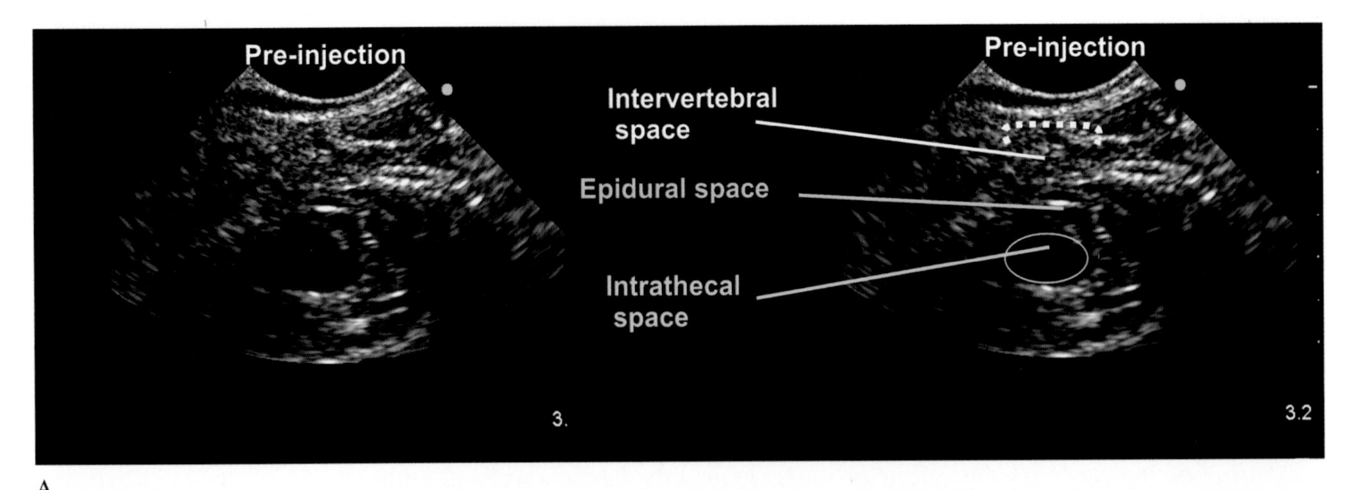

A

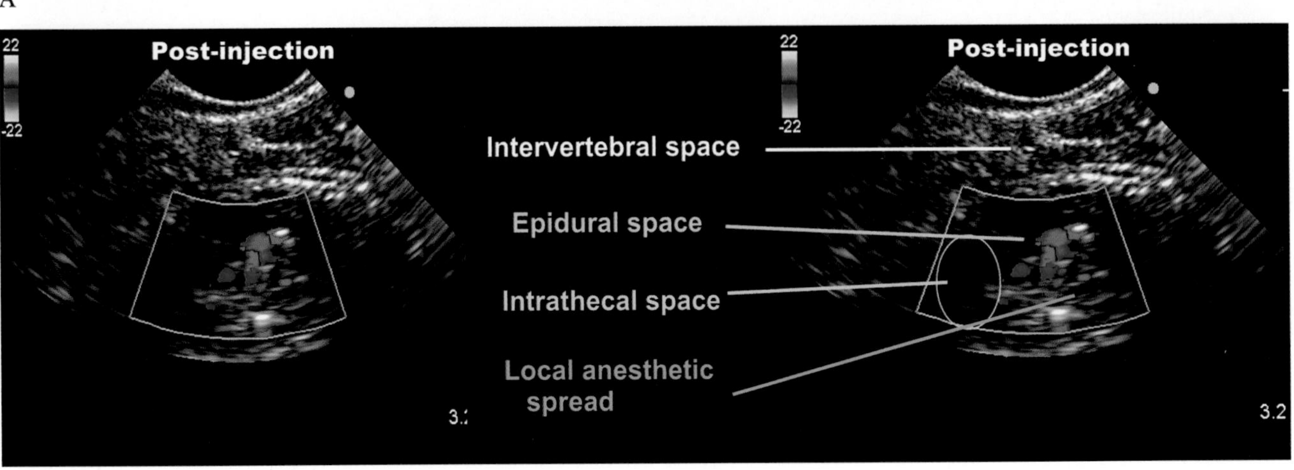

B

Figure 20.10. Color Doppler for confirming local anesthetic spread into the lumbar (L4) epidural space. Pre-injection (A) there is no illumination and a central circular intrathecal space; postinjection (B) the local anesthetic appears as a medley of colors and slightly expands the epidural space.

20.5. Catheter Advancement from the Caudal Epidural Space

20.5.1. Sonographic Imaging and Ultrasound-Guided Block Procedure

This technique is most suitable for young infants (0–6 months) because, due to incomplete ossification of the vertebrae, the catheter tip and a greater number of anatomical structures are more easily visualized. The thoracic spine provides less of an ultrasound window due to its smaller size and overlapping spinous processes.

20.5.1.1. Scanning Technique (e.g., 5–10 MHz "Hockey Stick" Probe)

- An assistant must perform the ultrasound imaging during catheter placement.
- During caudal cannula placement and epidural catheter advancement, follow the scanning technique described earlier (Section 20.4) for caudal needle placement in young infants.

- For viewing the lumbar and thoracic regions of the spine, position the probe in a longitudinal median or paramedian plane (probe lateral to the spinous processes).
- Either alignment may be suitable for the lumbar spine, although the paramedian may be superior as it allows clear visibility of the dura, and dural movement upon catheter entrance has been shown to be more useful than ligamentum flavum penetration (as seen best through median alignment).
- The paramedian position (whether transverse or longitudinal axis) is the best choice for the thoracic spine as there is more ossification here and the long, obliquely oriented spinous processes overlap each other significantly.

20.5.1.2. *Sonographic Appearance*

- The appearance of the caudal epidural space will match that seen with single-shot anesthesia (see Figure 18.10 and Figures 20.8 and 20.9).
- In the lumbar spine in a 10-year-old patient:
  - Transverse axis (Figures 20.11 and 18.9), similar to the sacral region in this age group (Figure 20.8):
    - The center of the screen contains the circular intrathecal space within the vertebral (spinal) canal, with the internal anechoic cerebrospinal fluid and hypoechoic intrathecal nerve roots (not viewed in Figure 20.11) surrounded by a thin circular layer of hyperechoic dura.
    - Superficially, it is possible to view the linear layer of hyperechoic subcutaneous tissue and an inverted ∀ shape of the pedicles and spinous processes.
  - Paramedian longitudinal axis (Figure 20.12):
    - The image contains an alternating dark (dorsal shadowing from bone) and bright (ultrasound window) pattern (mainly intervertebral spaces).
    - If seen, the conus medullaris and cauda equina have a hyperechoic and almost fibrillar appearance.
    - Hypoechoic cerebrospinal fluid lies adjacent to the spinal nerve roots and within the linear hyperechoic dura mater.
    - The ligamentum flavum may be seen on the dorsal aspect of the dura, and would also indicate the epidural space.
- In the thoracic spine of a 10-year-old patient:
  - Transverse viewing (Figure 20.13):
    - The "starry night" appearance of the paravertebral muscles is evident on either side of the hypoechoic matter (shadowing) from the long and thin spinous process.
    - The articular and transverse processes may be depicted through shadowing if the image is clear and field of view large enough.

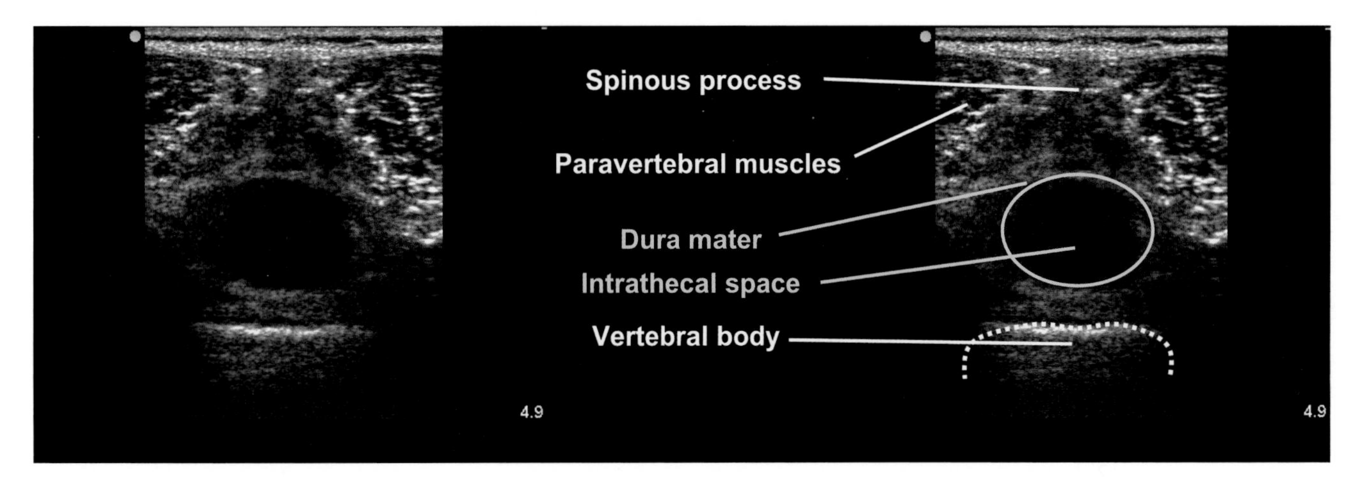

Figure 20.11. Image from a transverse scan in the lower lumbar spine of a 10-year-old patient.

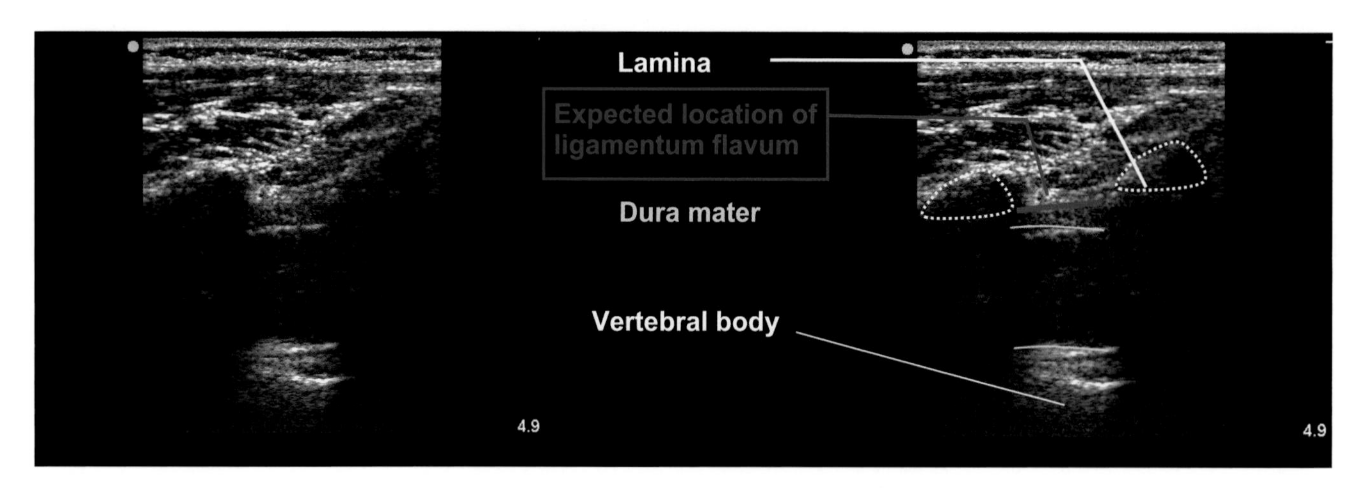

Figure 20.12. Image form a longitudinal paramedian scan in the lower lumbar spine of a 10-year-old patient.

  - The central window of the spinal canal viewed in the lumbar and sacral spine is not nearly as well depicted in the thoracic region (in patients older than a few months) due to the compact nature of the bony elements.
  - Generally, the hyperechoic meninges are not delineated and the dura position is estimated at best.
- Paramedian longitudinal viewing (Figure 20.14):
  - Appears similar to that seen at the lumbar spine except the spinal cord appears hypoechoic with the surrounding dura appearing as a shorter thin hyperechoic line between shadows from the overlaying spinous processes.
  - The ligamentum flavum may be seen and the epidural space determined to some extent.

- Catheter visibility (14-month-old patient):
  - The tip of the catheter may be seen upon entry and during advancement at the lumbar spine [Figure 20.15(A,B)], although more than one imaging plane may be required; in children older than 3 to 6 years of age, the catheter tip may not be clearly identified following insertion.
  - Generally, the catheter is viewed indirectly through observing movement of the dura upon fluid injection; the very hypoechoic local anesthetic will appear to expand the epidural space and cause ventral movement of the dura.
- Local anesthetic injection:

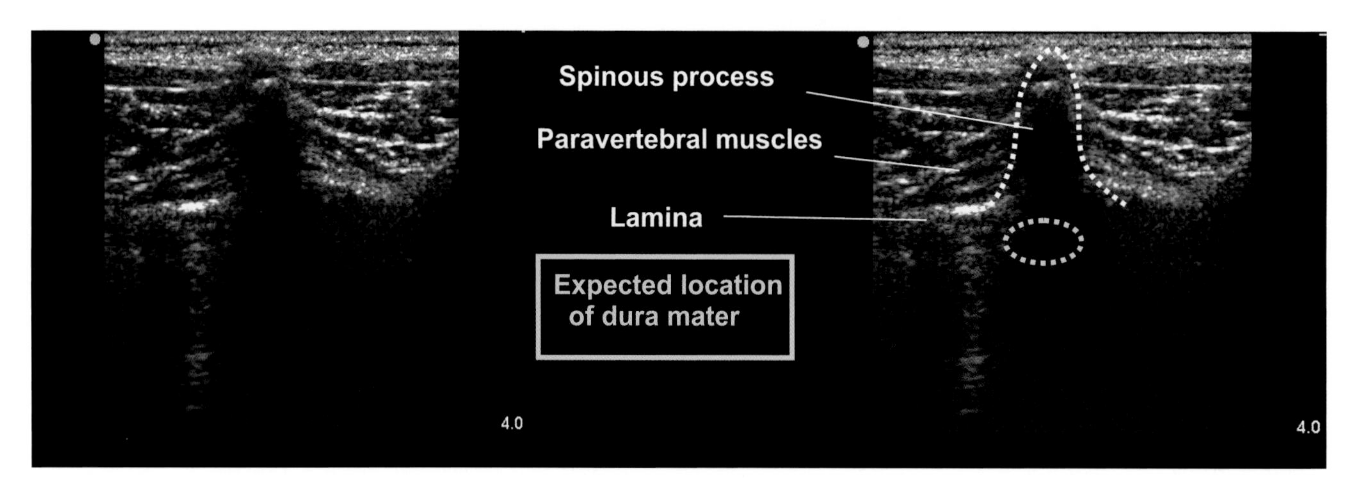

Figure 20.13. Image from a transverse scan in the thoracic spine of a 10-year-old patient.

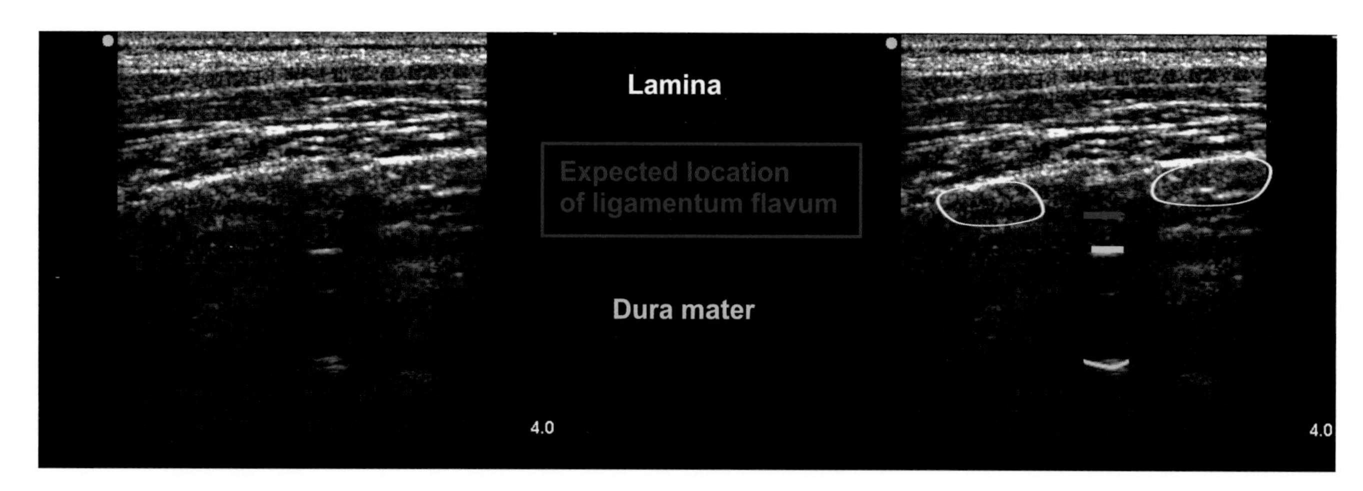

Figure 20.14. Image from a longitudinal paramedian scan in the thoracic spine of a 10-year-old patient.

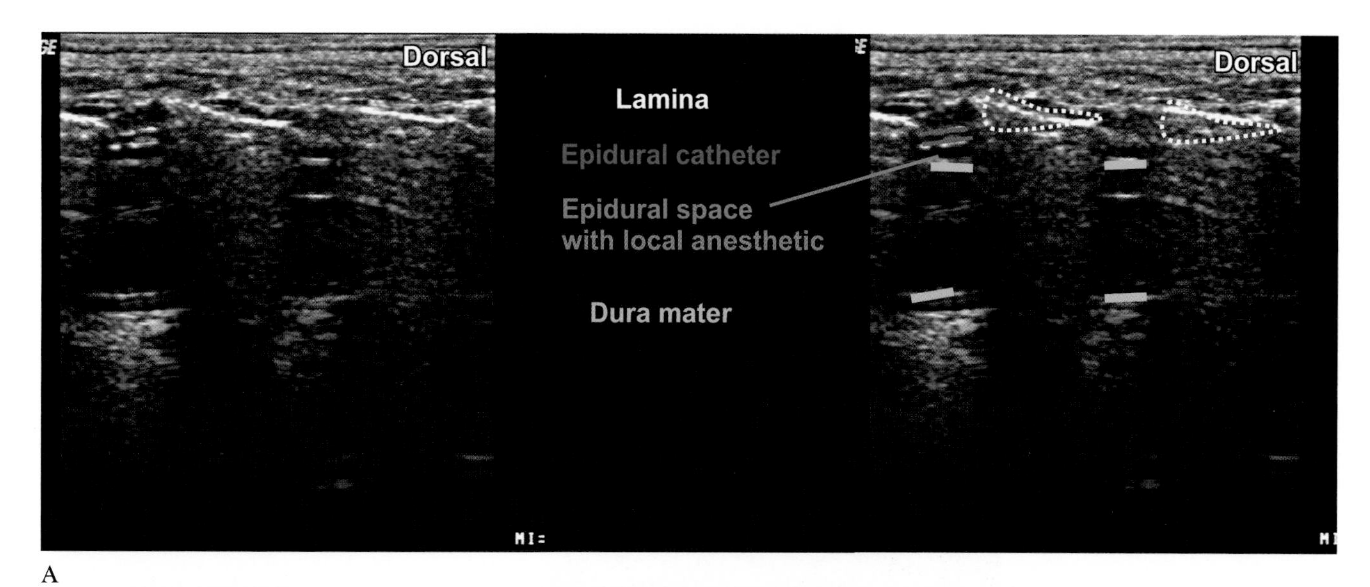

A

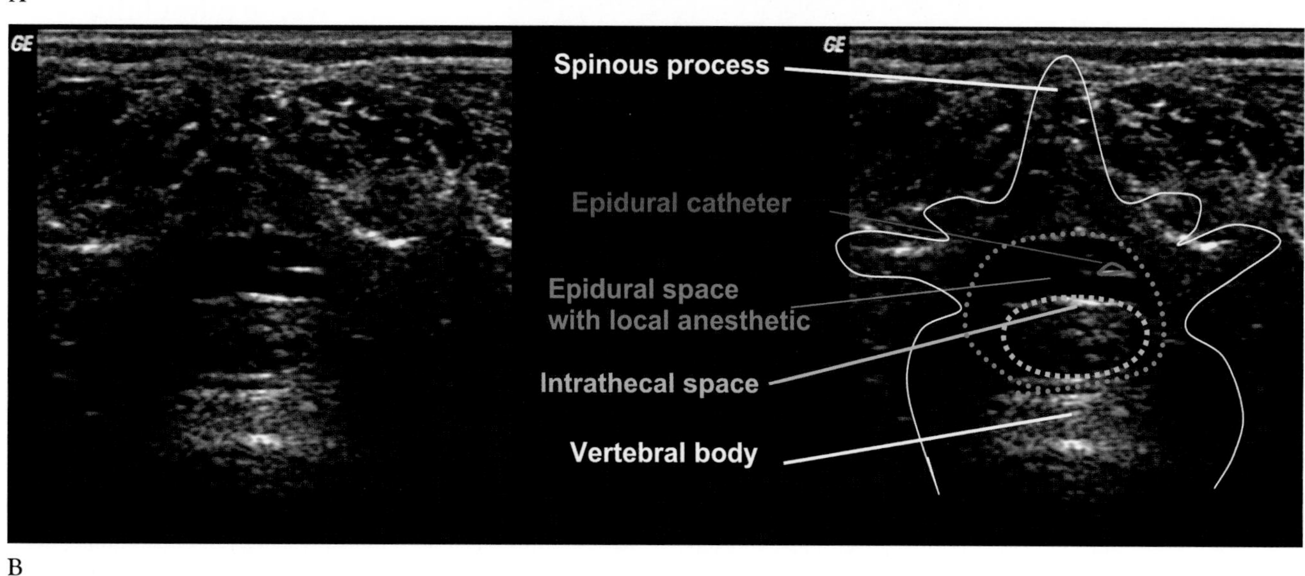

B

Figure 20.15. Epidural catheter visibility during advancement. Longitudinal (A) and transverse (B) views of an epidural catheter at the lumbar spine are shown in a 14-month-old patient. (Reprinted with permission by Drs Hans Juergen Rapp (Children's Hospital, Cologne) and Thomas Grau.)

- In general, local anesthetic can not be seen directly but occasionally, caudad and cephalad spread can be appreciated indirectly from displacement of the dura on the ultrasound screen.

20.5.2. Catheter Insertion and Local Anesthetic Application

- Measure the length of catheter required on the exterior of the patient's body.
- Perform the block using an 18-ga IV cannula and a 20-ga epidural catheter (standard or stimulating if using electrical epidural stimulation).
- If using epidural stimulation, follow the procedure in the next section while viewing the catheter using ultrasound.
- If using ultrasound alone with the classical "pop" at the caudal epidural space, visualize catheter advancement either directly (in young infants) or with the aid of local anesthetic injection causing movement of the dura.
- If using the epidural stimulation test, once catheter tip placement is deemed correct, rule out inadvertent intrathecal placement (Table 18.1) and inject local anesthetic to check for inadvertent intravascular injection (see Section 18.2.6 for clinical applications of the epidural stimulation test). Ultrasound may also be of use in this regard if the movement of dura is clear and the catheter tip is highly visible in the epidural space.

20.5.3. Epidural Stimulation Guidance Technique (Figure 20.16)

20.5.3.1. *Procedure (Refer to Chapter 18)*

- Estimate the length of a 20-ga styletted epidural stimulating catheter or metal-containing epidural catheter necessary to thread to the required distance.

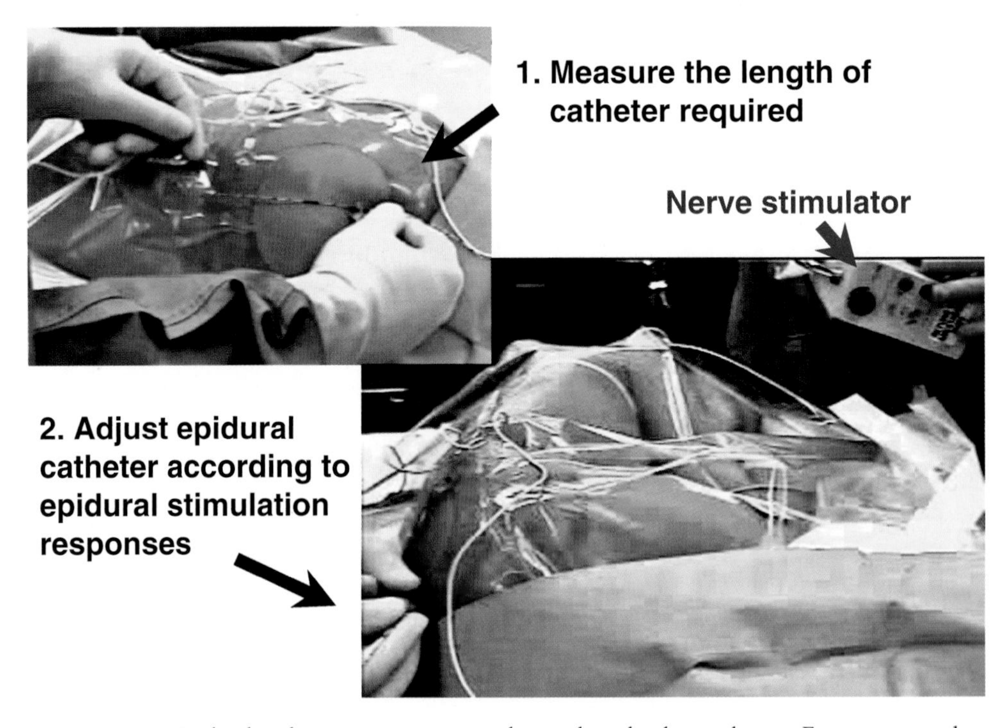

Figure 20.16. Epidural catheter insertion using electrical epidural stimulation. First, estimate the length of a styletted metal-containing catheter required for advancement; then insert the catheter into the caudal epidural space using traditional methods (i.e., "pop") and advance the catheter. Observe the responses to nerve stimulation to confirm epidural placement and the segmental level of catheter tip location.

- Adjust the stylet to a point within the distal end of the epidural catheter where there is the desired stiffness.
- After sterile preparation, insert an 18-ga IV catheter, using similar technique to that of the single-shot approach into the caudal epidural space; correct placement will be characterized by the typical give or "pop" upon penetration of the sacrococcygeal ligament (Figure 20.1).
- Connect a nerve stimulator to the stimulating epidural catheter by the electrode adapter.
- Prime the stimulating catheter and adapter with sterile normal saline (1–2 mL).
- Attach the cathode lead of the nerve stimulator to the metal hub of the adapter and the grounding anode lead to an electrode on the patient's body surface.
- Set the nerve stimulator to low frequency and pulse width (1 Hz; 0.2 ms).
- For caudal continuous anesthesia:
  - Advance the catheter a few millimeters and gradually apply current to the catheter until motor activity or twitch response in the anal sphincter (S2–S4) is visible.
- For threading to lumbar or thoracic spine:
  - Advance catheter while gradually applying current.
  - Follow progressive motor responses through cranial advancement until desired level is reached [from lower limbs and lumbar (back) to intercostals to thoracic and upper limbs].
  - Minor resistance to the passage of the catheter can be overcome by injecting normal saline through the advancing epidural catheter and/or simple flexion or extension of the patient's vertebral column.
- Inject a test dose of local anesthetic to rule out intravascular placement (see below).
- Compare the total characteristics of the response to Table 18.1 to determine catheter placement and make any required adjustments.
- If the catheter does not reach the desired level, it can be pulled back and re-inserted.
- Once optimally positioned, withdraw the 18-ga IV catheter and the stylet.
- Affix the catheter immediately cephalad to the site of insertion with several layers of occlusive dressing.

20.5.3.2. Local Anesthetic Application (Test) to Confirm Avoidance of Intravascular Placement

- After aspirating to rule out intrathecal placement, inject a test dose of local anesthetic (e.g., 0.05mL/kg (up to 3 mL) lidocaine 1.5% with 1 : 200,000 epinephrine) to confirm catheter placement and to ensure it is not placed in the intravascular space.
- If catheter placement is correct, with local anesthetic injection, the current threshold should increase and the motor response cease.
- If the catheter tip is within the intravascular space, the local anesthetic will disperse systemically and the motor response will remain the same with repeated doses of local anesthetic.
- Once intravascular placement is ruled out, the catheter can be fixed to the skin as described above.

> **Clinical Pearl**
>
> Clinicians must remain extremely vigilant throughout these procedures because all techniques of epidural catheter placement are associated with the potential risk for neurological injury. Therefore, under no circumstances should any force be used to advance the catheter.

20.5.4. Electrocardiograph Monitoring Technique (Figure 20.17)

One downfall of the epidural stimulation technique is that it cannot be performed reliably if any significant clinical neuromuscular blockade is present or local anesthetics have been administered in the epidural space. To overcome this limitation, an alternative technique using ECG monitoring was developed by the author. Using epidural ECG, the anatomical position of the epidural catheter is determined by comparing the ECG signal from the tip of the catheter to a signal from a surface electrode positioned at the target segmental level. Thus, the advancement of an epidural catheter from the lumbar or sacral region into the thoracic region can easily be monitored and placed within two vertebral spaces of the targeted level under ECG guidance.

20.5.4.1. *Procedure*

- Place left-leg (red in figure) and left-arm (black in figure) electrodes at their standard positions.
- Record a standard reference ECG (lead II) by connecting the right-arm electrode (white in figure) to a skin electrode on the patient's back at the target spinal level.
- Subsequently, connect the right-arm electrode to the metal hub of an electrode adapter to record a tracing from the epidural catheter.

20.5.4.2. *Interpreting the Electrocardiographic Method*

- When the epidural catheter tip is positioned in the lumbar and sacral regions, the amplitude of the QRS complex is relatively small as the recording electrode (epidural tip) is

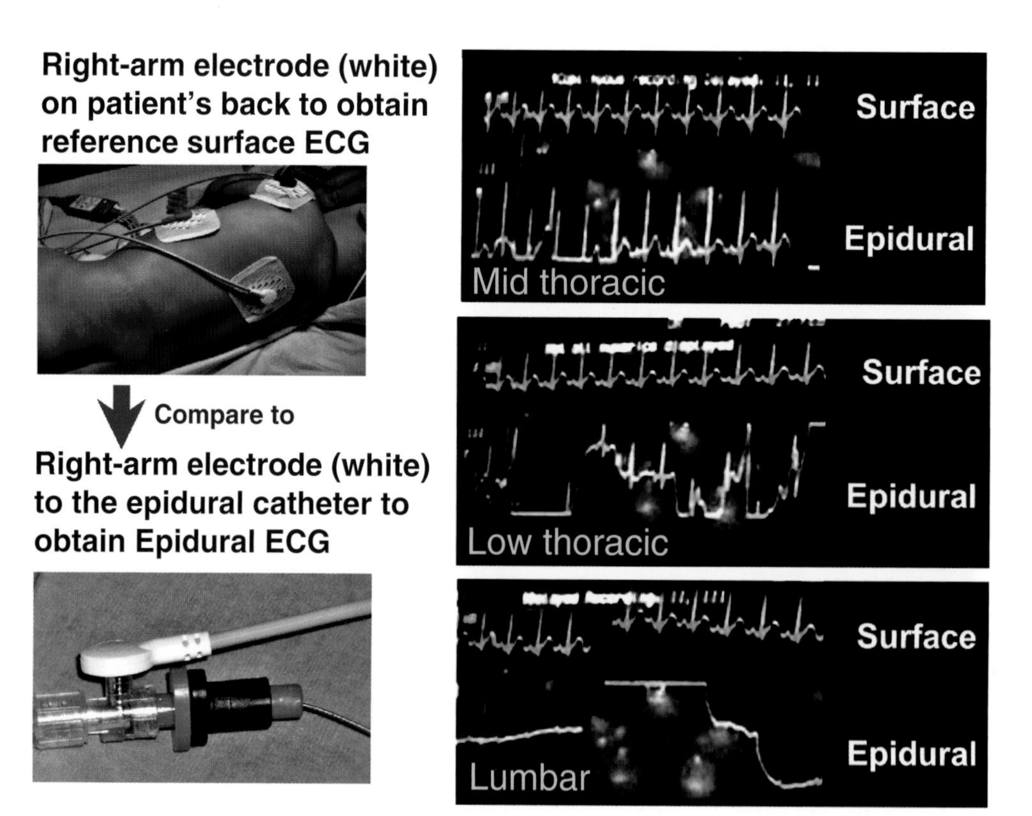

Figure 20.17. ECG monitoring technique. This test can be used when the epidural stimulation test is precluded by neuromuscular blocking drugs or previous local anesthetic injection. The ECG signal from the tip of the catheter is compared to a signal from a surface electrode positioned at the target segmental level; the catheter can be placed reliably within two segmental levels.

at a considerable distance from the heart and the vector of the cardiac electrical impulse is at approximately a 90° angle.

- As the epidural tip advances toward the thoracic region, the amplitude of the QRS complex increases as the recording electrode comes closer to the heart and becomes more parallel to the cardiac electrical impulse.
- As the catheter tip passes the target level, the amplitude of QRS should match the amplitude of the reference surface electrode.

20.5.4.3. *Limitations*

- The ECG technique cannot warn of a catheter placed in the subarachnoid or intravascular space.
- In addition, this technique may not be suitable when threading catheters a short distance because the ECG changes may be too subtle to observe.

20.6. Direct Lumbar and Thoracic Epidurals

20.6.1. Sonographic Imaging and Ultrasound-Guided Block Procedure

Figures 20.18 to 20.20 describe the scanning and appearance of the lumbar spine of an adult, while those in Figures 20.21 to 20.23 describe the thoracic spine. The magnetic resonance imaging (MRI) scans in Figures 20.18 and 20.21 can be used for reference with the corresponding ultrasound images. The ultrasound images are captured using a portable machine and will be of inferior quality, yet more practical, than those from a cart-based high-resolution system.

20.6.1.1. *Scanning Technique*

- Use a low-frequency probe to scan the lumbar and thoracic spine in transverse and longitudinal planes.
- Figures 20.19(A,B) and 20.22(A,B) show the scanning and ultrasound appearance in a transverse median plane at the lumbar spine and thoracic spine, respectively. Using a flexed spine will be advantageous for viewing in this plane as it will provide more of an ultrasound window between the vertebrae. The spinous processes will be evident and the expected position of the dura can be estimated, although longitudinal viewing will be superior in this respect in most cases. Longitudinal imaging in a paramedian [see Figure 20.20(A,B)] position may provide somewhat superior viewing.
- Figures 20.20(A,B) and 20.23(A,B) show the scanning and ultrasound appearance in a paramedian longitudinal plane at the lumbar and thoracic spine, respectively. As described in Chapter 18, the longitudinal paramedian plane will provide the best ultrasound window with reasonably good visibility of the dura mater for surrogate marking of the puncture site and LOR depth.
- Ultrasound imaging in young children would result in a superior image quality.
- Preprocedural scanning can be beneficial to assess the vertebral column (transverse and longitudinal views) and measure the epidural space and LOR depths (longitudinal only with the machine and probes used for the images in this book; see Chapter 18).
    - Depth of the epidural space = skin-to-epidural distance, which can be estimated by measuring the depth of what appears to be the ventral surface of the ligamentum flavum.
- For ultrasound guidance during epidural anesthesia techniques, an assistant must perform the imaging to allow the anesthesiologist to use both hands.

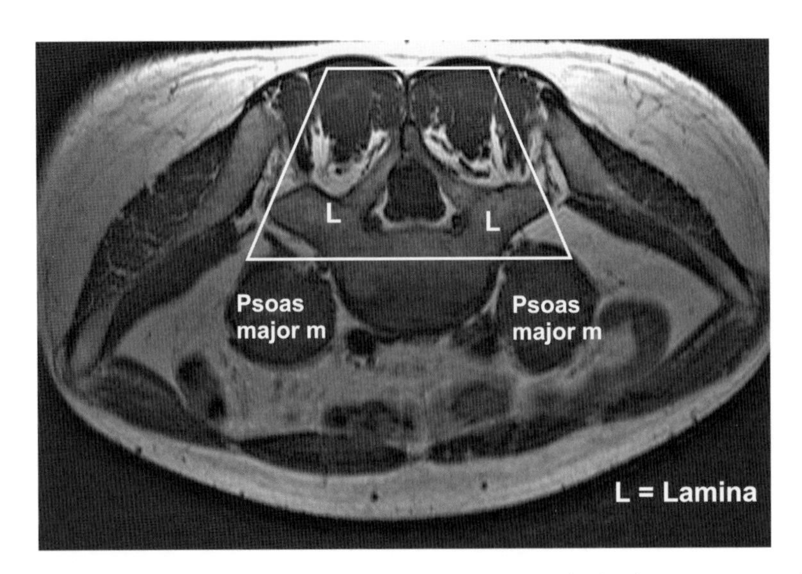

Figure 20.18. Transverse image captured by MRI at the lumbar spine in an adult.

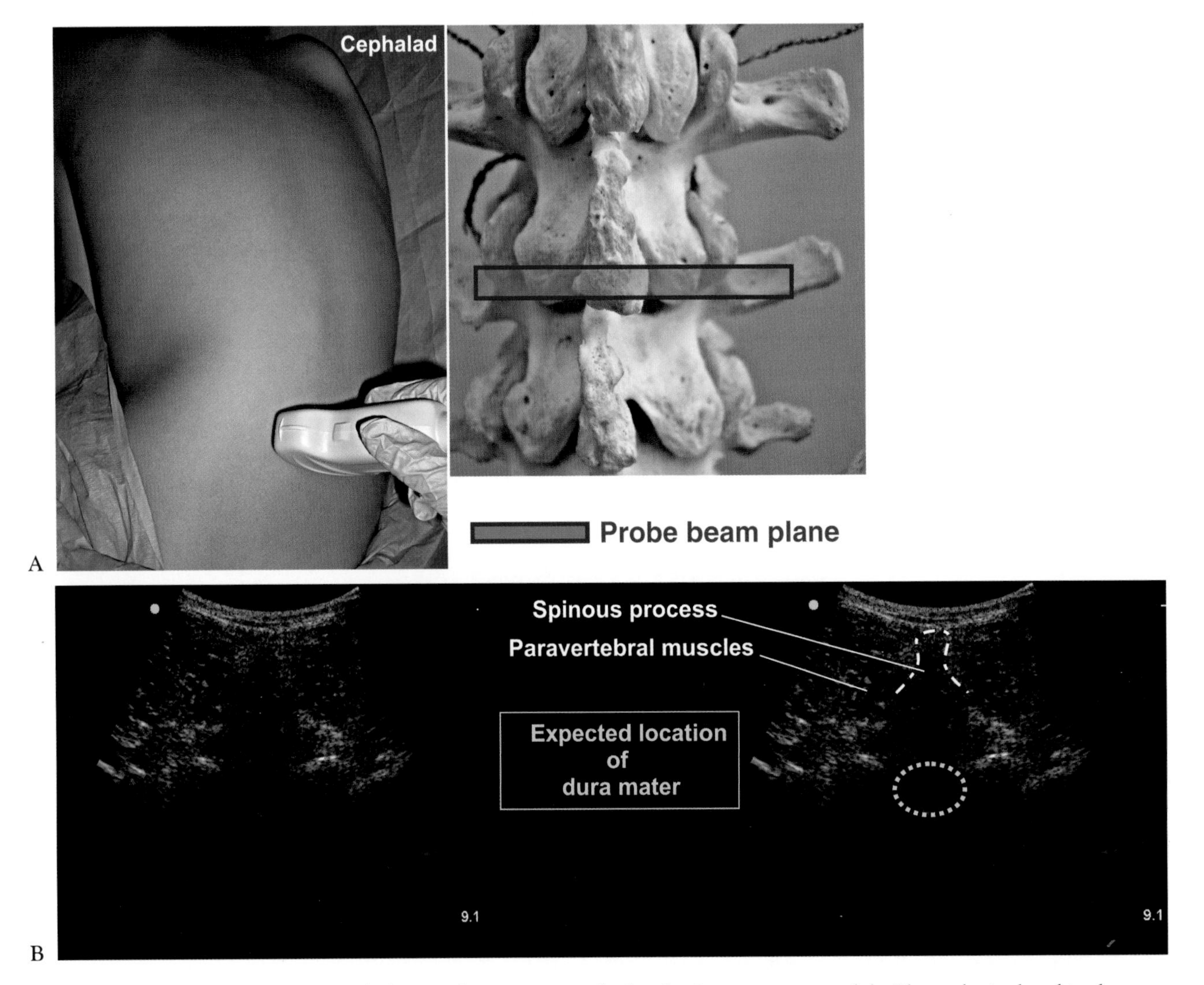

Figure 20.19. Transverse scanning and ultrasound appearance in the low-lumbar region in an adult. The probe is placed in the transverse plane in a median position. (A) The probe position and beam plane used during this scanning method are illustrated in a volunteer and a skeleton model. (B) The corresponding ultrasound image.

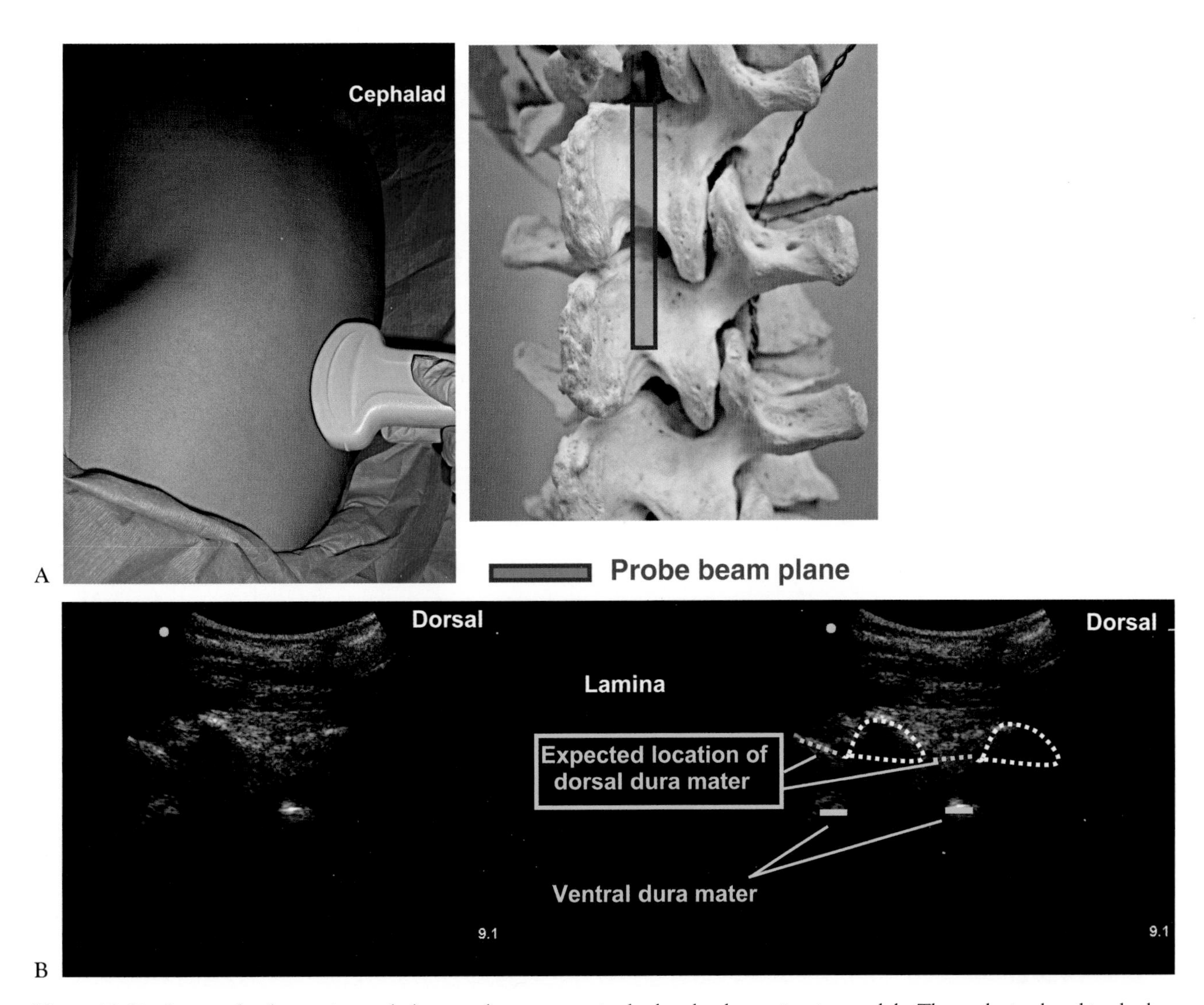

Figure 20.20. Longitudinal scanning and ultrasound appearance in the low-lumbar region in an adult. The probe is placed in the longitudinal plane in a paramedian position. (A) The probe position and beam plane used during this scanning method are illustrated in a volunteer and a skeleton model. (B) The corresponding ultrasound image.

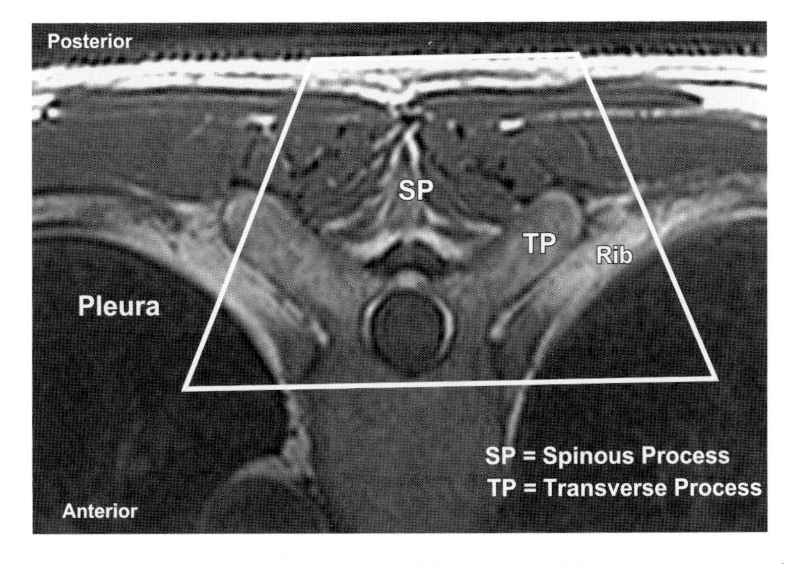

Figure 20.21. Transverse image captured by MRI at the midthoracic spine in an adult.

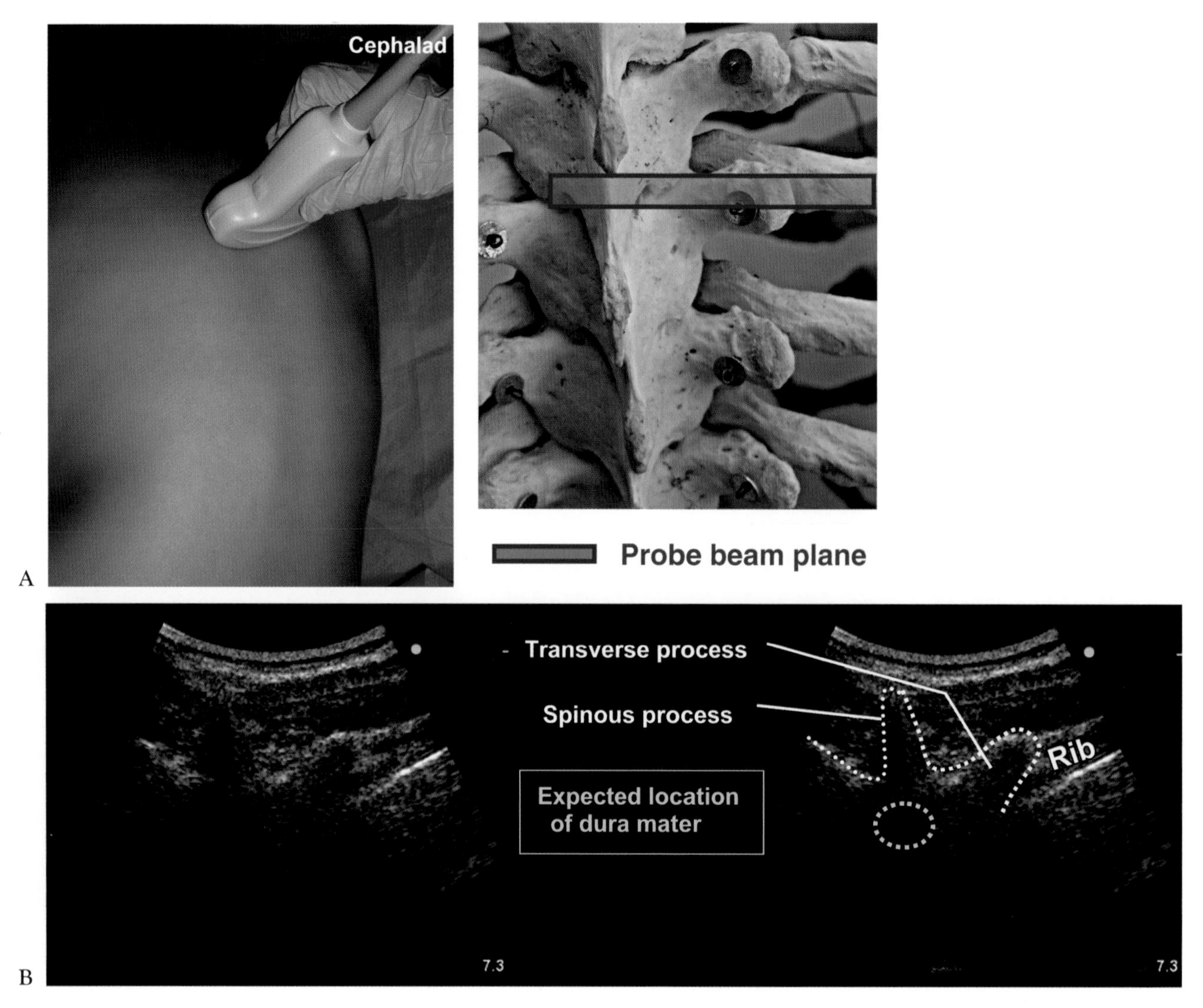

Figure 20.22. Transverse scanning and ultrasound appearance in the midthoracic region in an adult. The probe is placed in the transverse plane in a median position. (A) The probe positioning and beam plane used during this scanning method are illustrated in a volunteer and a skeleton model. (B) The corresponding ultrasound image.

- During both epidural needle and catheter insertion, the probe will be tangential (out-of-plane) to the midline placement of the needle and catheter (if using paramedian longitudinal scanning) and only the needle/catheter tip will be viewed adequately, if at all.

20.6.1.2. *Sonographic Appearance*

See Section 20.5 for description and illustration of the lumbar and thoracic spine, and catheter and local anesthetic visibility. Similarly, the appearance of the spinal canal elements will be superior with young infants, as will be the identification of the catheter and local anesthetic. The compact structure of the thoracic spine will limit the visibility of all structures/substances significantly.

20.6.1.3. *Needle Insertion Technique*

- Preprocedural measurements (i.e., ultrasound supported technique):
  - Use short- and long-axis scanning with a paramedian probe alignment.
  - Ultrasound can be used for assessing neuraxial anatomy and measuring various distances in the vertebral (spinal) canal, depending on visibility, including those from skin and bone to dural, epidural, and intrathecal structures (see Section 18.3.3).

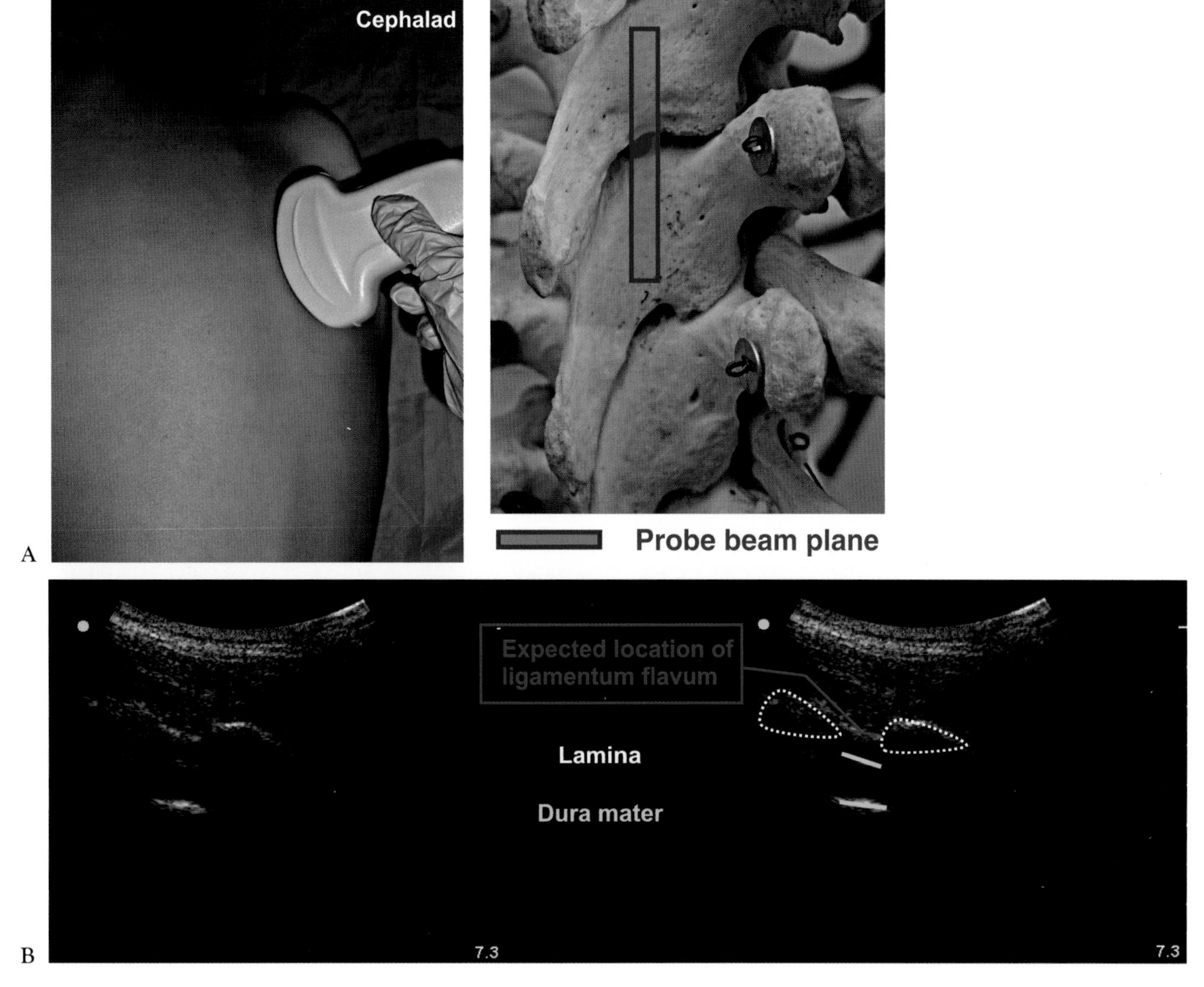

Figure 20.23. Longitudinal scanning and ultrasound appearance in the midthoracic region in an adult. The probe is placed in the longitudinal plane in a paramedian position. (A) The probe positioning and beam plane used during this scanning method are illustrated in a volunteer and a skeleton model. (B) The corresponding ultrasound image.

- Ultrasound-guided determination of epidural space depth may be beneficial (see Section 18.3.3).
- Determination of ideal puncture location and trajectory can be performed.
- Preprocedural assessments can be performed prior to real-time ultrasound guidance or in isolation before proceeding with standard LOR technique.

- Real-time (i.e., online) guidance:
  - Dynamic ultrasound guidance may be of limited value in the thoracic region in patients older than a few months of age.
  - The puncture needs to be made with a midline approach at the required segment since the probe is best aligned along the paramedian plane and longitudinally (Figure 20.24).
    - The needle shaft and probe beam are out-of-plane (OOP) and only the needle tip may possibly be seen.
  - An assistant is required during ultrasound-guided neuraxial technique.
  - It is very important to secure sterility of the probe, for example, with long sleeve covers (see Chapters 3 and 4).

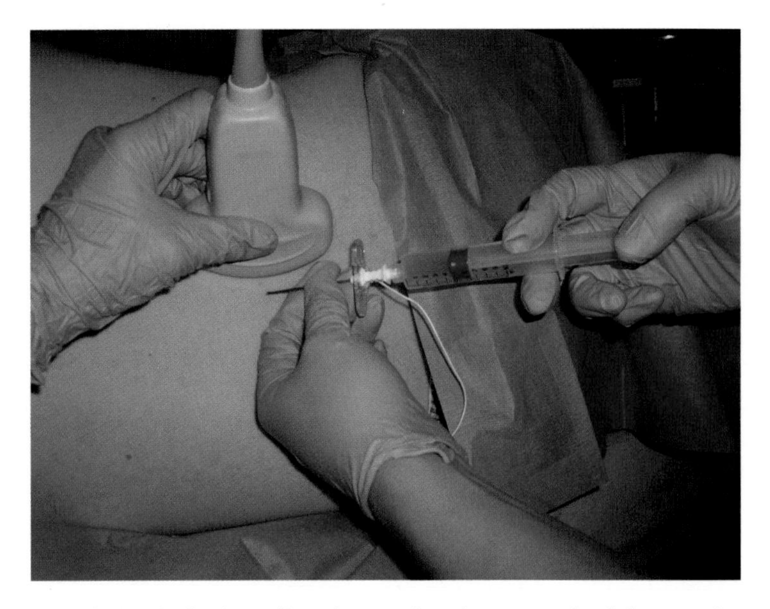

Figure 20.24. Real-time (online) needling during a low-thoracic epidural showing the out-of-plane alignment of the needle (median) and probe (paramedian). An assistant must perform the ultrasound imaging.

  - LOR technique is still required since there is no guarantee of visualizing the needle penetrating the ligamentum flavum. Confirmation of epidural space localization will generally occur in a similar way as for single caudal injections, thereby, through the visibility of a test dose of local anesthetic and the resulting movement of the dura.
- When performing ultrasound-guided epidural placements in small babies, a short needle should be used.
- After epidural space confirmation, the injection of the local anesthetic solution will be seen with its caudad and cephalad spread.

20.6.1.4. *Catheter Insertion and Confirmation*

- To confirm correct needle insertion, we recommended using LOR to saline technique despite the availability of ultrasound guidance or epidural stimulation testing.
- Once the needle is positioned in the epidural space, as confirmed by direct visualization of penetration and, in particular, the dural movement upon entrance of a test dose of local anesthetic, the catheter is introduced.
- Visibility of the catheter tip may be possible upon entry and during advancement with local anesthetic injection.
- If using epidural stimulation, follow the procedure as described in the next section while viewing the catheter using ultrasound. The epidural stimulation test may be best used for confirming correct epidural needle entrance (i.e., preventing intrathecal or intravascular placement), while its use in short-distance (2–5 cm) catheter advancement may be limited.
- Once catheter tip placement is confirmed to be correct, rule out intrathecal placement and inject local anesthetic (if the movement of the dura is obvious and catheter tip highly visible, this may help confirm epidural placement; Figure 20.15).

20.6.2. Epidural Stimulation Test for Direct Lumbar and Thoracic Continuous Epidurals

During direct lumbar and thoracic epidural placement, the epidural stimulation test can, in theory, be of value in confirming epidural needle entrance, particularly if patients are deeply sedated or under general anesthesia (e.g., pediatric patients). This is because the electrical stimulation test can provide an additional safety measure to alert the clinician of needle proximity to the intrathecal space, spinal cord, or nerve roots. However, there is no clinical evidence to support this contention at the moment.

20.6.2.1. *Procedure*

Catheter insertion and confirmation have been discussed in Section 20.5. In general, a stylet will usually not be required for the shorter distances of catheter advancement and estimating the length of catheter required is not of significant importance. Local anesthetic test doses should be used to rule out intravascular placement.

Suggested Reading And References

Chen CPC, Tang SFT, Hsu T, et al. Ultrasound guidance in caudal epidural needle placement. Anesthesiology 2004;101:181–184.

Grau T. Ultrasonography in the current practice of regional anaesthesia. Best Pract Res Clin Anaesthesiol 2005;19:175–200.

Rapp H, Folger A, Grau T. Ultrasound-guided epidrual catheter insertion in children. Anesth Analg 2005;101:333–339.

Tsui BC, Berde CB. Caudal analgesia and anesthesia techniques in children. Curr Opin Anaesthesiol 2005;18:283–288.

Tsui BC, Gupta S, Finucane B. Confirmation of epidural catheter placement using nerve stimulation. Can J Anesth 1998;45:640–644.

Tsui BC, Wagner A, Cave D, Kearney R. Thoracic and lumbar epidurals via the caudal approach using electrical stimulation guidance in pediatric patients: a review of 289 patients. Anesthesiology 2004;100:683–689.

Tsui BCH, Seal R, Koller J. Thoracic epidural catheter placement via the caudal approach in infants by using electrocardiographic guidance. Anesth Analg 2002;95:326–330.

Tsui BCH, Tarkkila P, Gupta S, Kearney R. Confirmation of caudal needle placement using nerve stimulation. Anesthesiology 1999;91:374–378.

Index